The Prostate Cancer Dilemma

Nelson N. Stone • E. David Crawford

Editors

The Prostate Cancer Dilemma

Selecting Patients for Active Surveillance, Focal Ablation and Definitive Therapy

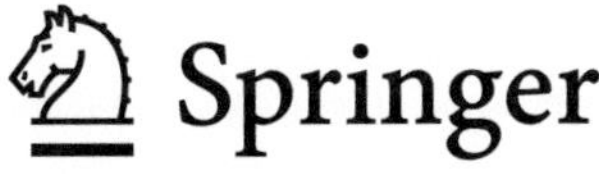

Editors
Nelson N. Stone
Professor of Urology and Radiation
 Oncology
Department of Urology
The Icahn School of Medicine
 at Mount Sinai
New York, NY, USA

E. David Crawford
Professor of Urology/Surgery,
 Radiation Oncology
University of Colorado
Denver, Aurora, CO, USA

Videos can also be accessed at http://link.springer.com/book/10.1007/978-3-319-21485-6

ISBN 978-3-319-36443-8   ISBN 978-3-319-21485-6   (eBook)
DOI 10.1007/978-3-319-21485-6

Springer Cham Heidelberg New York Dordrecht London

Springer International Publishing AG Switzerland is part of Springer Science+Business Media
(www.springer.com)

Preface

The Prostate Cancer Dilemma: Selecting Patients for Active Surveillance, Focal Ablation and Definitive Therapy is the first textbook to provide a complete description of the newest technologies to diagnose and manage the most common prostate cancer diagnosed today: low risk disease. Over 50 % of men diagnosed with prostate cancer by transrectal biopsy appear to have this type of cancer. But do they really? And if they do, is it safe to observe them or should they have more aggressive therapy? Follow a typical patient and see how these issues are addressed by reading the valuable contributions of all of the coauthors of this textbook. In addition to the many state-of-the-art photographs accompanying this book, several procedure videos are also available online.

A 52-year-old man visits his primary care physician for his annual checkup. He asks her about being tested for prostate cancer. She tells him about the controversy surrounding PSA testing and that the USPTF has given PSA a grade D recommendation. In Chap. 1, Drs. Andriole and Manley summarize the history of the discovery of PSA and how it became such an integral part of prostate cancer management. Basic biology and physiology of PSA is discussed to provide insights about its current and future applications. Salient points in the arguments for and against PSA screening are presented. A thorough review of the randomized trials (both US and European) that led to the "D" recommendation is undertaken. Lastly, new PSA markers that may help distinguish between benign, low grade, and aggressive cancer are evaluated.

The patient asks about prostate cancer pathology. He wants to know if he has a biopsy and it is positive what type of cancer and how dangerous might it be. In Chap. 2, Dr. Lucia discusses how prostate cancer pathology has changed over the last 30 years. In 1966, Donald Gleason described the varied architectural appearances of a large number of prostatic adenocarcinomas and demonstrated that the degree of glandular differentiation and infiltration of the surrounding stroma by tumor cells reflected the biology of the tumor. Those tumors that displayed well-formed acinar structures had favorable outcomes compared with those that had progressively more poorly formed acini. Those tumors that formed only sheets, cords, or single cell arrangements behaved aggressively and were often lethal.

Over the ensuing years modifications of Dr. Gleason's original system arose from outcomes experience with prostate cancer grading on biopsy and prostatectomy specimens evolved. In 2005, 80 genitourinary pathologists from around the world (members of the International Society of Urologic Pathologists) participated in a survey of practice patterns and a consensus conference to document and assess cancer grading trends and refined the guidelines for Gleason grading. Most notable among the items addressed were (1) restrictions on assigning very low-grade patterns (grades 1 and 2) on biopsy specimens, (2) refining the separation between patterns 3 and 4, (3) assigning grade to cribriform patterns of cancer, and (4) scoring biopsies that contain minor amounts of high-grade patterns or tertiary-grade patterns. By the mid-1990s, it was recognized that prostate cancer often has multiple foci of discrete tumors in surgical prostatectomy specimens in more than 50 % of the cases. These findings increased the risk that standard transrectal biopsies, where limited tissue is removed, might mislead the clinician as to the type and extent of cancer present. Dr. Lucia also discusses the new role of molecular pathology and how what appears to the eye of the pathologist as low-grade cancer might have a more ominous clinical course.

The primary care physician examines the patient and finds a sizable lesion occupying the entire left lobe of the prostate. She tells him that her suspicion for prostate cancer is increased. He asks what the implications of these findings are. In Chap. 3, Drs. Leapman and Cooperberg discuss the American Joint Commission on Cancer Tumor, Lymph Node, Metastasis (TNM) clinical staging systems and compare it to the newer Cancer of the Prostate Risk Assessment (CAPRA) method. CAPRA is based on a 10-point system, designed to provide an approximate doubling of risk with every 2-point increase in the total score. Tissue-based assays and how their addition to the CAPRA score improves outcome predictability are also discussed. The patient's physician now orders a PSA and refers the patient to a urologist for further evaluation.

In Chap. 4, Drs. Leapman and Shinohara discuss the "gold standard" for diagnosing prostate cancer, the transrectal ultrasound-guided prostate biopsy. The urologist tells the patient that a 12-core biopsy procedure incorporating the apical and lateral peripheral zone improves cancer detection rates over a 6-core procedure. Despite taking an increased number of samples, limitations of systematic TRUS prostate biopsy include both over- and under-sampling of disease, misrepresentation of the removed tissue, and an increased rate of biopsy-related complications. The urologist explains that additional ultrasonographic parameters including contrast-enhancement, power Doppler imaging, and elastography may improve the discrimination of suspicious lesions during biopsy. He also tells the patient new technology allows him to refine the selection for biopsy candidates by utilizing novel serum biomarkers which offer specificity beyond PSA and clinical parameters alone. The patient's PSA is 8.5 ng/ml and he agrees to have a 12-core TRUS biopsy. On the left 2 of 6 cores are positive for Gleason 6 prostate cancer with 33 % of both cores positive; all 6 cores are negative on right.

The urologist tells the patient he may qualify for active surveillance but he is not sure if the transrectal biopsy may have missed more significant disease. He tells him about transperineal mapping biopsy (TPMB) and mpMRI-targeted biopsy. In Chaps. 5 and 6 TPMB is discussed. The TPMB technique uses a grid placed against the perineum and in a sterile fashion directs biopsy specimens be taken at 5 mm intervals using a combination of transverse and sagittal imaging. In contrast to the TRUS method where 12–18 samples are typically taken, with the TPMB 50 or more biopsies can be taken. On average the TPMB finds 30 % more cancers when a TRUS biopsy is negative, upgrades low risk cancers that were initially diagnosed by TRUS, and excludes patients from focal therapy because of a high incidence of multifocality. Dr. Crawford introduces a new software program which creates a real-time 3D model of the prostate generated from intraoperative axial (transverse) images. Once the 3D representation is obtained, a biopsy plan is generated. During the biopsy phase, the image position and the virtual biopsy sites (in axial and longitudinal) can be adjusted to match the US contours of the prostate, urethra, and rectum. This "real-time" image-guided procedure also allows matching of the virtual biopsy sites to the biopsy needle in the gland. The 3D reconstruction creates a highly accurate method to biopsy the gland and to provide a roadmap for focal therapy. Dr. Skouteris reviews their experience with elastography and how it can improve the diagnosis and staging of prostate cancer in Chap. 7. He compares the biopsy results of elastography suspicious lesions to those detected by mapping technique in a number of men biopsied at is center in Athens, Greece.

While interested in the TPMB procedure, the patient already knows he has prostate cancer and is looking for a less invasive method of further assessing his gland. In Chap. 8, Dr. Taneja and associates describe the advantages of utilizing mpMRI in both the diagnosis and focal treatment of prostate cancer. This chapter provides a detailed review of the different aspects of an mpMRI, for example diffusion weighted imaging (DWI) and the apparent diffusion coefficient (ADC) and how these "parameters" improve the differentiation between benign and malignant tissue. These authors also compare mpMRI biopsy results to radical prostatectomy specimens and provide important data about tumor volume and location setting the stage for using mpMRI for focal ablation. An mpMRI is ordered and a Pi-RADS 4/5 0.5 cm^3 lesion is seen in the anterior of the gland. An mpMRI-targeted biopsy is performed on this lesion which demonstrated a Gleason 3 + 4 lesion.

Finally to help the patient decide how aggressive the cancer is the urologist tells him about a variety of new genetic markers. In Chap. 9, Drs. Shore and Ventii discuss the use of genomic and proteomic markers/assays and their ability to improve the precision of risk assessment and shared educational patient–physician review, thus enhancing decision-making for physicians and patients, especially when the traditional clinical parameters (PSA, DRE, pathology) may not provide the most accurate assessment of indication for biopsy nor indication for treatment option. A patient with low-risk, newly diagnosed prostate cancer may benefit from a more precise, personalized assessment of their individual tumor biology. Even patients with a histologic diagnosis of Gleason 3 + 4 tumors can have a more indolent course once analyzed with these new genetic markers.

The patient now has a clearer understanding of his disease characteristics and is deciding on treatment. He knows he has intermediate to low risk disease and realizes that there are advantages to active surveillance. In Chap. 10, Dr. Klotz tells us that active surveillance is an effective solution to the widely recognized problem of overtreatment of screen detected prostate cancer and that it could reduce overall mortality without an increase in prostate cancer deaths and provide substantial cost savings. However, the patient is a little reluctant to "leave" his cancer untreated and is concerned about the side effects of entire gland treatment. He inquires about a "lumpectomy" where only the lesions are treated. Dr. Barqawi (Chap. 11) summarizes the morbidity associated with conventional treatment of prostate cancer by radical prostatectomy or radiation therapy and argues for a less invasive method of treating the disease. Accurate lesions location by TPMB and resolving multifocality by treating just the index lesion are proposed. In Chap. 12, Dr. Onik discusses different energy modalities for applying focal therapy and makes a case for treating high-grade disease by inducing an immunologic system response. Finally, in Chap. 13, Dr. Pinto et al. show how mpMRI-guided therapies can potentially achieve equivalent oncologic efficacy to traditional whole gland therapies such as surgery and radiation, while avoiding the side effects of conventional treatment.

New York, NY, USA   Nelson N. Stone, M.D.
Aurora, CO, USA   E. David Crawford, M.D.

Contents

Part II   Treatment

Contributors

Gerald L. Andriole, M.D. Division of Urologic Surgery, Washington University in St. Louis, Barnes Jewish Hospital, St. Louis, MO, USA

Paul Arangua, B.S., M.P.H. Urologic Oncology, University of Colorado Denver, Aurora, CO, USA

Craig Baer, Ph.D. BCSi Inc., Colorado Springs, CO, USA

Al Barqawi, M.D., F.R.C.S. Division of Urology, Department of Surgery, University of Colorado Denver School of Medicine, Aurora, CO, USA

Marc A. Bjurlin, D.O. Division of Urologic Oncology, Department of Urology, NYU Langone Medical Center, New York, NY, USA

Matthew R. Cooperberg, M.D., M.P.H. Department of Epidemiology, University of California, San Francisco, San Francisco, CA, USA

Epidemiology & Biostatistics, University of California, San Francisco, San Francisco, CA, USA

E. David Crawford, M.D. Professor of Urology/Surgery, Radiation Oncology, University of Colorado, Aurora, CO, USA

Jesse Elliott, B.A. Software Development, BSCi Inc., Colorado Springs, CO, USA

Michele Fascelli, B.A. Urologic Oncology Branch, National Cancer Institute – National Institutes of Health, Bethesda, MD, USA

Arvin K. George, M.D. Urologic Oncology Branch, National Cancer Institute— National Institutes of Health, Bethesda, MD, USA

Amichai Kilchevsky, M.D. Urologic Oncology Branch, National Cancer Institute – National Institutes of Health, Bethesda, MD, USA

Laurence Klotz, M.D. Sunnybrook Health Sciences Centre, Toronto, ON, Canada

Kevin Krughoff, B.A. Division of Urology, Department of Surgery, University of Colorado Denver School of Medicine, Aurora, CO, USA

Michael S. Leapman, M.D. Department of Urology, University of California, San Francisco, San Francisco, CA, USA

M. Scott Lucia, M.D. Anatomic Pathology, Department of Pathology, University of Colorado School of Medicine, Aurora, CO, USA

Brandon J. Manley, M.D. Division of Urologic Surgery, Washington University in St. Louis, Barnes Jewish Hospital, St. Louis, MO, USA

Neil Mendhiratta, B.A. School of Medicine, NYU Langone Medical Center, New York, NY, USA

Gary Onik, M.D. Mechanical Engineering, Carnegie Mellon University, Ft. Lauderdale, FL, USA

Peter A. Pinto, M.D. Prostate Cancer Division, Urologic Oncology Branch, National Cancer Institute, Bethesda, MD, USA

Katsuto Shinohara, M.D. Department of Urology, University of California, San Francisco, San Francisco, CA, USA

Neal D. Shore, M.D., F.A.C.S. Carolina Urologic Research Center, Myrtle Beach, SC, USA

Vassilios M. Skouteris, M.D. Prostate Brachytherapy Department, Hygeia Hospital, Hygeia Group, Maroussi, Athens, Greece

Nelson N. Stone, M.D. Professor of Urology and Radiation Oncology, Department of Urology, The Icahn School of Medicine at Mount Sinai, New York, NY, USA

Samir S. Taneja, M.D. Division of Urologic Oncology, Department of Urology, NYU Langone Medical Center, New York, NY, USA

Karen Ventii, Ph.D. Emory University, Atlanta, GA, USA

Spyros D. Yarmenitis, M.D. Radiology Department, Hygeia Hospital, Hygeia Group, Maroussi, Athens, Greece

Georgios P. Zacharopoulos, M.D., M.Sc., Ph.D. Ultrasound Department, Hygeia Hospital, Hygeia Group, Maroussi, Athens, Greece

Editor's Biography

Nelson N. Stone, M.D. Dr. Stone, an internationally recognized entrepreneur and academician, is Professor of Urology and Radiation Oncology at the Icahn School of Medicine at Mount Sinai, NY. Professor Stone earned his medical degree from the University of Maryland in 1979. He completed a general surgical residency in 1981 at the University of Maryland, followed by residency in urology at the University of Maryland. Dr. Stone then completed a fellowship in urologic oncology at Memorial Sloan Kettering Cancer Center and a research fellowship in biochemical endocrinology at Rockefeller University in 1986. He then became chief of urology at Elmhurst City Hospital, eventually being promoted to full professor of Urology and Radiation Oncology at Mount Sinai in NYC.

From the outset, Dr. Stone recognized the need to develop innovative technologies for urologic diseases and specifically prostate cancer. He was one of the first adopters combining academic achievement with medical inventions. He recognized the need to develop an alternative to radical surgery for his patients with prostate cancer and invented the real-time 3D brachytherapy (radioactive seed) program in 1990. Now he has turned his attention to the development of a 3D imaging and biopsy system to more accurately diagnose and localize individual prostate cancer lesions.

Dr. Stone serves on the editorial board of many scientific journals and is a member of many professional societies, including the Prostate Conditions Education Council, the Society for Minimally Invasive Therapy, the New York State Urological Society, the American Association of Clinical Urologists, and the American Urologic Association. Dr. Stone has participated in approximately 25 research studies on prostate cancer and has authored over 400 articles, abstracts, and book chapters, most on prostate cancer.

E. David Crawford, M.D. With his vast experience and knowledge in the urology field, Dr. Crawford is Professor of Surgery, Professor of Radiation Oncology, and Head of the Section of Urologic Oncology at the University of Colorado Denver Health Sciences Center and School of Medicine. He serves as associate director of the University of the Colorado Comprehensive Cancer Center, also in Denver.

Dr. Crawford received his medical degree from the University of Cincinnati. His postgraduate training included an internship and residency in Urology at the Good Samaritan Hospital in Cincinnati. He was subsequently awarded a Genitourinary Cancer fellowship with Dr. Donald G. Skinner at the University of California Medical Center in Los Angeles.

Dr. Crawford is a nationally recognized expert in prostate cancer. The recipient of more than 69 research grants, he has conducted research in the treatment of advanced bladder cancer, metastatic adenocarcinoma of the prostate, hormone-refractory prostate cancer, and other areas of urological infections and malignancies. He has authored or coauthored over 400 articles, which have been published in such journals as Urology, the New England Journal of Medicine, and the Journal of the National Cancer Institute. He has published five textbooks. He is also an editorial reviewer or consultant for a large number of publications, including Urology, Journal of Urology, the New England Journal of Medicine, Cancer, and the Journal of Clinical Oncology.

Dr. Crawford is an active member of many national and international organizations, including the American Society of Clinical Oncology, American Urological Association (AUA), and the American Association for the Advancement of Science. Within the AUA, he is a member of the Committee to Study Urologic Research Funding and the Prostate Cancer Clinical Trials Subcommittee. He currently serves on the board of governors, the GU committee, and the scientific advisory board of the Southwest Oncology Groups, and chairs the Prostate Conditions Education Council.

Part I
Diagnosis

Chapter 1
History of Prostate-Specific Antigen, from Detection to Overdiagnosis

Brandon J. Manley and Gerald L. Andriole

Abbreviations

PSA	Prostate-specific antigen
PAP	Prostatic acid phosphatase
DRE	Digital rectal exam
kDa	Kilodaltons
hK2	Human kallikrein 2
FDA	Federal Drug Administration
WHO	World Health Organization
IRP	International Reference Preparation
BPH	Benign prostatic hyperplasia
AUA	American Urological Association
ACA	American Cancer Association
USA	United States of America
CPDR	Center for Prostate Disease Research
SEER	Surveillance epidemiology, and end results
PLCO	Prostate lung, colorectal and ovarian screening
ERSPC	European randomized study of screening for prostate cancer
PIVOT	Prostate cancer intervention versus observation trial
PCPT	Prostate cancer prevention trial
REDEEM	Reduction by dutasteride of clinical progression events in expectant management
TRUS	Transrectal ultrasound
CAP/ProtecT	Comparison arm for prostate testing for cancer and treatment trial
PCOS	Prostate cancer outcomes study

B.J. Manley, M.D. • G.L. Andriole, M.D. (✉)
Division of Urologic Surgery, Washington University in St. Louis, Barnes Jewish Hospital,
4960 Children's Place, Campus Box 8242, St. Louis, MO 63110, USA
e-mail: andrioleg@wudosis.wustl.edu

© Springer International Publishing Switzerland 2016
N.N. Stone, E.D. Crawford (eds.), *The Prostate Cancer Dilemma*,
DOI 10.1007/978-3-319-21485-6_1

The discovery and integration of prostate-specific antigen (PSA) has substantially changed the diagnosis, treatment, and management of prostate cancer. Only a few discoveries in the medical field over the last half century can rival the profound impact of PSA. While the current opinions of the appropriate use of PSA as a screening tool can be debated, its impact and the way it has directed the course of prostate cancer research can not.

For many younger clinicians it may be hard to imagine managing a prostate cancer patient without the use of PSA. Prior to the identification of PSA, there were many attempts to identify tumor markers for prostate cancer by several research groups around the world.

The Pursuit and Discovery of PSA

Many trace the initial pursuit for a prostate cancer marker to Gutman and Gutman in 1938 when they found elevated serum phosphatase levels in metastatic prostate cancer patients [1]. Later in 1941, Huggins and Hodges demonstrated this finding was likely related to the presence of bony metastasis in such patients [2]. While the use of serum phosphatase in prostate cancer was eventually found to be limited as a clinically useful tumor marker due to its poor sensitivity and specificity, it did pave the way for many groups to began focused research in the field.

Over the next decade, prostatic acid phosphatase (PAP) was identified as a potential tumor marker. Several different assays to measure PAP were developed to aid in the clinical management of prostate cancer patients. Early assays measured total enzyme activity of PAP, mainly calorimetric, which involved the use of reagents that change color in the presence of a specific substrate [3]. Later, newer techniques using radioimmunoassays were able to moderately improve the specificity of testing for PAP [4]. Ultimately, while PAP was found to be a more specific marker, it lacked the sensitivity for prostate cancer needed to be clinically useful, as it was noted to be elevated in several benign prostatic diseases and even after digital rectal exam (DRE) [5]. It was also found only to be elevated in 20–30 % of patients with clinically localized prostate cancer.

The work with PAP and other markers brought to light the need for a more sensitive and reliable tumor marker. There was also a shift in focus to find a marker that was present or elevated in those patients with clinically localized disease, as these patients could possibly benefit from a serum assay test that could be useful to monitor or even initiate treatment.

Many groups claimed to have conducted the research that led to the discovery of PSA. One of the earliest reports on the identification of prostate-specific antigens was by Rubin Flocks in 1960 [6]. In 1966, a Japanese forensic scientist, Mitsuwo Hara, partially characterized and reported on a protein many consider similar to PSA. He labeled the protein "gamma-seminoprotein" and proposed its use as forensic evidence in rape cases because of its presence in seminal fluid [7]. Later Li and Beling further purified this protein and reported it to have a molecular weight of

31 kilodaltons (kDa) [8]. Similar reports and characterization were done by Sensabaugh and his group confirming this protein to have specificity for human semen [9]. Years later, through the work of Wang and Papsidero the purification of this protein demonstrated that it was identical to that of PSA found in human serum [10, 11]. More definitively, in 1970 and 1972 Albin published his reports of a purified antigen isolated from prostate tissue [12, 13].

In 1979, T. Ming Chu and his research group purified and characterized PSA and demonstrated its presence in both benign and malignant prostate tissue [11, 14]. These studies confirmed that PSA was highly specific for prostate tissue and was produced by prostatic epithelial cells. This group was also credited with the first development of an immunoassay that could be used for human serum testing although it was much less sensitive than those used today detecting PSA at a minimal concentration of 500 ng/ml compared to modern assay's detecting PSA at <0.01 ng/ml [11]. In 1987, early work in the clinical applications of PSA by Chu's group and Thomas Stamey demonstrated a use for PSA in monitoring the course of patients known to have prostate cancer [15].

More precise testing using protein sequencing has determined that many of the groups from the 1960s and 1970s were most likely describing prostate-specific antigen or one of its natural analogues [16].

Shortly after its discovery much of the interest on PSA focused on determination of its physiologic role. In 1984 Chu et al. reported that PSA was a protease and later through studies by Lilja its role in the proteolytic cleavage of seminal vesicle proteins was published [17, 18]. They described the role of PSA as cleaving the gel-forming proteins from the seminal vesicles (semenogelins I, II and fibronectin) which initiates liquefaction of the ejaculate, thereby increasing the motility of sperm and aiding in fertilization. These studies and others also identified several other prostatic proteins similar to PSA, notably human kallikrein 2 (hK2). Similar to PSA, it is expressed by prostatic tissue and has a similar role in cleaving of seminal vesicle proteins, although it is much more potent enzymatically [19].

Later in the 1980s PSA was confirmed to belong to the human kallikrein family of serine proteases, and it was given formal nomenclature and labeled human kallikrein 3 (hK3) [20]. There are currently 15 other members of this family that have been described in the literature and many of them are believed to play some role in many human cancers [21]. The relationship between PSA and hK2 is worth noting. These two share many common features but also some key differences. PSA and hK2 share 80 % amino acid sequence homology but hK2 is present in 1–2 % of the amount of PSA found in typical prostate tissue [22]. In vitro studies have demonstrated that hK2 has the ability to autoactivate, while PSA does not have this characteristic and for this reason some have proposed a role for hK2 in regulating the activity of PSA [23].

Further studies into the physiologic role of PSA also uncovered two forms of PSA most commonly found in patients serum. One form was smaller than the other (36 kDa compared to 90–100 kDa) and it was found later by Lilja and Stenman that the smaller form was that of free PSA and the larger was complexed PSA (also known as bound PSA) [24]. Studies showed that PSA was most commonly complexed with alpha-1-antichymotrypsin, a protease inhibitor [25]. Only 10–30 % of PSA was present in an uncomplexed form. Free PSA represented the inactive form and was typically higher in patients with begin prostatic conditions. Other studies demonstrated that the level of free PSA was lower in prostate cancer patients and this subsequently led to the development of immunoassays to test specifically for it [26]. The ratio of free PSA to total PSA has proven useful in its clinical application and ability to increase the positive predictive value for positive prostate biopsies [27].

The Golden Years of PSA Testing

The Federal Drug Administration (FDA) approved the first commercial immunoassay for PSA testing in 1987. Around this time Stamey et al. and Oesterling reported the half-life of PSA to be 2.2 ± 0.8 and 3.2 ± 0.1 days respectively [15, 28]. Subsequently several assays were developed for PSA testing including Tandem-R PSA®, Pros-check PSA®, Tandem-E PSA®, IRMA-count PSA®, and Abbott IMX PSA®. Myrtle et al. was one of the first to attempt to give the reference range for a "normal" PSA value with the use of the Tandem R PSA® assay [29]. He studied the reported PSA values in a population of 472 men without a history of prostate cancer, most of which were below the age of 60 years. Other larger studies attempted to find the ideal value for initiating prostate biopsy looking at more clinically relevant patient populations (i.e., over 50 years of age) and varied in their suggested cutoff values between 2.8 and 4.0 ng/ml using a standard deviation of ±2 [30, 31]. Ultimately it was the screening test reported from a cohort of 6630 men aged 50–74 years of age using a cutoff value of 4.0 ng/ml that led to the FDA's approval of screening with PSA [32–35]. Consequently the value of 4.0 ng/ml became most commonly used for initiating prostate biopsy, although at the time several groups felt this value to be too aggressive and proposed a cutoff value of 10 ng/ml. Notably in 2004 the National Comprehensive Cancer Network recommended a lower cutoff of 2.5 ng/ml citing the number of cancers missed with higher cutoffs and the benefits in patient outcomes reported at that time.

Early use of these commercial assays used in the clinical setting led to inconsistent results and created the need for standardization of PSA testing. Graves et al. called for an international standardization of PSA assays in 1990, which led to the principles used in PSA testing today [36]. The issue he described centered around the fact that each assay detected different molar ratios of the various forms of PSA found in the serum (free vs. bound to proteins) and therefore different results were obtained with different assays from the same serum [37]. As many of the initial PSA screening trials were done using the Tandem R PSA® assay from Hybritech, newer assays that came on the market were initially "standardized" to the values of this assay. With time it became apparent that there was increasing variability between these assays and their reported PSA values. Naturally this raised many concerns, especially when following patients' PSA values could dictate the decision to perform a prostate biopsy. In an effort to mitigate these effects, a group of researchers and experts convened at Stanford University in 1994 and proposed a method of standardization that later was adopted by the World Health Organization (WHO) who issued the First International Reference Preparation (IRP) for PSA in 1999. Unknowingly the standardization from the WHO produced PSA values that were approximately 22 % lower than that of the traditional results from the Tandem R PSA assay®. These discrepancies had the potential to cause serious confusion among physicians and potentially resulted in some patients not being offered biopsy, especially when following patients by such metrics as PSA velocity.

In 1990, the idea for the incorporation of PSA as part of the initial work up for diagnosing prostate cancer was introduced by Cooner [38]. He described using PSA testing as part of a "three-legged stool" which included DRE and transrectal ultrasound guided prostate biopsies. This algorithm was believed to be superior for prostate cancer screening since DRE alone found that 70–80 % of patient had locally advanced or metastatic disease at diagnosis [39]. Subsequent to his initial study, Cooner and several other groups attempted to improve the specificity of PSA testing for prostate cancer by reporting on age-specific PSA values [40–42]. These studies were done in part due to the fact that patients with benign prostatic hyperplasia (BPH) had increased PSA levels making one "normal" value for all men unreliable. The introduction of PSA density (prostate volume/PSA) and PSA velocity (changes over time) was an attempt to compensate for these limitations [43].

In 1991, Catalona et al. used a PSA cutoff of 4.0 ng/mL in the initial screening of prostate cancer patients and suggested the use of PSA as a screening test for prostate cancer [32, 40]. Over the next couple of years several medical groups including the American Urological Association (AUA) and American Cancer Association (ACA) endorsed annual PSA screening for men over 50 years of age.

During this time PSA screening was hailed as dramatically improving the detection of curable prostate cancer. Gann et al. found in men diagnosed with prostate cancer an elevated PSA preceded an abnormal DRE by an average of 6.2 years [42]. Incorporation of PSA screening into clinical practice resulted in an increase of prostate cancer detection from 1987 to 1992 of 85 %. By 1997, 75 % of prostate cancers were diagnosed by elevated or abnormal PSAs in the United States of America (USA) [44, 45]. Stage migration of prostate cancer also dramatically shifted during this time with Catalona et al. publishing a report in 1993 that 70–80 % of men were being diagnosed with organ confined disease compared to historical cohorts of 20–30 % [33]. The Center for Prostate Disease Research (CPDR) reported that the percentage of patients presenting with metastatic disease decreased from 19.8 % in 1989 to 3.3 % by 1998 [46].

The Trials and Tribulations of PSA Screening

After PSA screening came into practice in the USA in the late 1980s and especially in the early 1990s, the incidence of prostate cancer diagnosis rapidly increased, with mortality rates subsequently declining [47]. Etzioni and colleagues used modeling data from Surveillance, Epidemiology, and End Results (SEER) Medicare and screening standards used in the Prostate, Lung, Colorectal and Ovarian screening trial (PLCO) to show that PSA screening alone could not account for the decrease in prostate cancer mortality seen during the 1990s [48]. Their work and others highlighted the fact that while PSA screening certainly played a role in the mortality decrease for prostate cancer patients, especially in the USA, the increase in new and more aggressive treatments also contributed to this decline. Tapering enthusiasm for PSA screening, Albertsen and colleagues published data that showed that many patients in the pre-PSA screening era, when followed without treatment, were destined to die of causes other than prostate cancer [49].

Opposition to PSA's use and specifically PSA screening became more common by the late 1990s and early 2000s. Concern grew that the results of the emerging retrospective studies showing improved diagnosis and survival of prostate cancer patients using PSA screening were confounded by lead time and length time biases. Around this time several large randomized studies testing the hypothesis that PSA screening could decrease prostate cancer-specific mortality were initiated.

The two largest and most discussed studies regarding PSA screening are the Prostate, Lung, Colorectal and Ovarian screening trial (PLCO) in the USA and the European Randomized Study of Screening for Prostate Cancer (ERSPC) [50, 51]. Several other large studies also contributed to the evaluation of the benefits and risks of PSA screening including Prostate Cancer Intervention Versus Observation Trial (PIVOT), Prostate Cancer Prevention Trial (PCPT), and Reduction by Dutasteride of Clinical Progression Events in Expectant Management (REDEEM) trial [52–54]. It is essential that all physicians who treat or manage prostate cancer patients read and understand the results of these trials.

The primary objectives of both ERSPC and PLCO were nearly identical. The main endpoint in both studies was prostate cancer mortality. One of the main differences between the two studies was the population in Europe, at least during the early years of the study, had less exposure to PSA testing and thus offered a less "contaminated" control group. Unfortunately, men enrolling in the US study had significant exposure to PSA testing compromising the PLCO control group. In this regard many consider the PLCO trial to be one of comparing systematic PSA screening to "opportunistic" screening as evidenced by the fact that the absolute difference in those who underwent PSA screening at anytime during the study between the screening and control group was only 33 %.

There was also some other differences between the trials that deserve mention. In PLCO the contamination rate was reported to be 54.8 % with patients obtaining a PSA outside the trials design [55]. The best reported rate of contamination in ERSPC published was 30.7 %, although this data is hard to come by in Europe [56]. It should be mentioned that for the power calculations used in the design of the ERSPC trial a contamination rate of 20 % was employed. There was also a large difference between the two trials with regard to performing indicated prostate biopsies. In PLCO the rate of biopsy was 41 % in patients indicated for biopsy during the first year of the study and rose to 64 % with the third year of screening. In ERSPC the rate was 85.8 % for patients indicated within its trial design [57]. This difference likely contributes to the lower rate of cancer detection seen in the PLCO screening arm and may have impacted comparison between the two arms in regard to prostate cancer mortality.

The randomization of patients in both trials also had some notable differences, along with the indications for biopsy. Patients aged 50–74 years were randomized to the two arms but later a "core age group" was defined in reporting much of the data from ERSPC, which had patients aged 55–69. Men in the screening arm were screened at 4-year interval, except in Sweden in which they were screened at 2-year intervals. Indications for biopsy varied among the constitute centers for the ERSPC trial. Initially some centers required a PSA over 4.0 ng/dl and an abnormal DRE as an indication for biopsy. After 1997, all centers, minus Finland, recommended biopsy for a PSA over 3.0 ng/dl. In Finland DRE was required to be positive for PSA in the 3–3.9 ng/dl range and later this changed to having a free/total ratio of PSA of equal to or less than 0.16. In Italy patients with a PSA of 2.5–3.9 ng/dl had DRE and transrectal ultrasound (TRUS) performed. When performing biopsies a lateral sextant method was applied in all centers but the execution of these was left to individual study groups within ERSPC. Medical contraindications were the only exception listed for not performing an indicated biopsy. After a diagnosis of prostate cancer, treatment decisions were left to the discretion of local providers.

PLCO initially randomized patients aged 60–74 years old, later they included patients aged 55–60 and also used prior PSA testing with 3 years of entry to the trial to reduce contamination between the two arms. In PLCO screening with DRE and PSA was offered yearly for the first 4 years and then with PSA alone for another 2 years. Recommended indications for prostate biopsy were "community standard" where initially a PSA value above 4.0 ng/dl and/or abnormal DRE. In later years a significant percentage of patients underwent biopsy for a PSA 2.5–4.0 ng/dl. The biopsy extent and the number of cores were left to the individual providers in the community.

In 2009 both trials published their initial results. ERSPC reported it findings after its data monitoring committee found a significant difference in prostate cancer mortality in favor of the screening arm at the time of its third predetermined interim analysis. The publishing of the results for the PLCO trial was done after the safety monitoring committee found a continuing lack of significant difference in the death rates between the two study groups and felt that this presented concerns in regard to public health. The PLCO trial was updated in 2012 with 13-year follow-up between the two arms of the study and continued to show no statistical difference between the intervention arm (organized screening) and the control arm (opportunistic screening) [58]. Recent updates from ERSPC in 2014, now with 13-year follow-up, have continued to show a survival benefit for patients undergoing PSA screening and in fact that benefit has increased modestly [59]. Their findings reported a significant 21 % relative reduction in prostate cancer in intention to screen analyses, and a 27 % relative reduction in men who actually had screening. These recent updates showed an improved benefit of PSA screening with longer follow-up demonstrated by the number needed to screen and number needed to be diagnosed with prostate cancer to prevent one prostate cancer death. As seen in the table below,

Table 1.1 Trending the number needed to screen and diagnose with ERSPC updates

ERSPC follow-up data	Number needed to be screened (per 1000 patients)	Number needed to be diagnosed (per 1000 patients)
9 years	1410	48
11 years	979	35
13 years	781	27

Table 1.1, both numbers in the case of the ERSPC trial have become substantially lower in their most recent follow-up data at 13 years compared to the numbers reported at 11 years and 9 years of follow-up [60]. For reference, the number needed to be screened with digital mammography to save one life from breast cancer was reported as 1339 (CI: 322–7455) and 377 (CI 230 to 1050) in women aged 50–59 years old and 60–69 years old, respectively [61]. Similarly the reported number needed to screen for colorectal cancer with fecal occult blood testing is 1176 [62]. The Göteborg screening trial, which was comprised of a significant number of patients who were enrolled in the ERSPC trial, also further supported these findings and reported a number of approximately 300 patients needing to be screened to prevent one death from prostate cancer at 14 years [63]. In contrast a study that looked at the largest center that participated in ERSPC, Finland, which by itself had a larger number of study patients than PLCO, showed only a non-statistically significant benefit in prostate cancer mortality among patients in the screening arm of the study [64]. This finding along with treatment patterns favoring men in the screened arm continues to cause concern about the real benefit of PSA-based screening.

Several other groups have used modeling data to estimate the improved benefits of PSA screening with longer follow-up. Gulati et al. projected 25-year estimates of the number needed to screen and to treat to prevent one prostate cancer death for men aged 55–69 years at diagnosis using data from ERSPC and PLCO [65]. They reported that in Europe, the number needed to screen was 262 and number needed to treat was nine after 25 years. Attempting to control for rates of overdiagnosis in the USA, they reported the number needed to screen was 186–220 and number needed to treat being 2–5. These statistics are markedly lower than the most recent 13-year follow-up data from the ERSPC.

We strongly encourage the reader to become familiar with both trials as the debate regarding their results and their impact on PSA screening is likely to continue for years to come. The results of future studies, particularly the Comparison Arm for Prostate Testing for Cancer and Treatment trial (CAP/ProtecT) of 450,000 men from the United Kingdom, will likely add to our current data on the use of PSA screening and prostate cancer [66].

At the center of the PSA screening debate is the attempt to realize the beneficial and adverse effects of screening. Finding the equilibrium between these two results is unlikely to be found in the scientific or medical literature but must be valued within the political and social systems in which screening is practiced.

The Effects of Screening with PSA and Overdiagnosis

Some of the issues surrounding screening with PSA revolve around the risk of over-treatment for low grade and low-risk prostate cancer patients. With the influx of new cases in the early 1990s after the integration of regular PSA screening, there was also a natural increase in the number of patient undergoing definitive treatment. Concerns about the long-term effects of these treatments, especially those patients that are younger and those with low-risk disease, gave rise to an emerging field of study in prostate cancer, cancer survivorship. The product of early screening and treatment along with the frequency and high survival rates of prostate cancer patients has created a growing population of prostate cancer survivors [67]. Both the American Cancer Society and a recent study by Mariotto et al. estimate that there are now more than two million prostate cancer survivors living in the USA and that number is expected to climb [68, 69].

Recently several groups have published long-term data regarding the effects of prostate cancer treatment [70]. One of the largest populations that have been reported on for these effects is the Prostate Cancer Outcomes Study (PCOS) which follows 1164 men who underwent treatment with surgery and 491 who had radiotherapy. The study assessed functional status immediately after treatment and at 2, 5, and 15 years after diagnosis. Resnick et al. reported data for this group at 15 years and found the prevalence of erectile dysfunction was very high, affecting 87.0 % of men in the prostatectomy group and 93.9 % of those in the radiotherapy group [71]. This study was somewhat limited by the lack of a control group (e.g., active surveillance) and reliable pretreatment baseline data. Regardless this study and others have placed a spotlight on the long-term effects of invasive procedures needed to treat and cure prostate cancer.

Dealing with the sequelae of prostate cancer treatment, especially long-term survivors, can place a significant burden on patients, both financially and in terms of time and efforts. De Oliveria et al. looked at a population of prostate cancer survivors in Canada and found higher total health care expenses among younger patients, metastatic patients, and those who underwent treatment with surgery [72]. They also found lower costs in patients with better urinary function. Similar findings in a study of prostate cancer patients in the USA who were recently diagnosed, within 1–3 years, found total out of pocket expenses and overall costs were inversely related to most of the commonly employed prostate-specific health-related quality of life survey scores [73].

The long-term effects of prostate cancer treatment are not limited to those undergoing surgery or radiation. Morgans et al. showed that in patients undergoing prolonged androgen deprivation the risk of developing comorbidities, specifically diabetes and cardiovascular disease, is increased well above those of age matched controls [74]. This risk was especially high among those patients who already had significant comorbidities prior to treatment.

The risks of long-term morbidity from prostate cancer treatment need to be considered by both the physician and patient prior to initiating screening. Several

Table 1.2 Risk of mortality from causes other than prostate cancer

	Comorbidity count			
Age	0	1	2	3+
Under 60 (%)	9	19	30	35
60–70 (%)	26	26	48	53
Older than 70 (%)	49	57	66	74

Comorbidity counts were calculated using the Charlson comorbidity index. Other cause mortality at 14 years [77]

groups have attempted to better define those patients suitable for treatment and screening. Using data from the PCOS, Daskivich et al. have published their findings in an attempt to better understand competing risk for mortality in patients with prostate cancer [75]. The cumulative incidence of other cause mortality at 14 years was modeled based on comorbidities (Table 1.2). Prostate cancer mortality at 14 years using the same analysis was 5, 8, and 23 % for men with low-, intermediate-, and high-risk disease respectively using the D'Amico classification [76].

The Evolution of Prostate Tumor Markers

While the exact role for PSA, especially in regard to screening, continues to evolve, the ongoing development of even more specific and ideally more applicable tumor markers for prostate cancer continues to progress. Many of these improvements surround PSA itself. Of these, the prostate health index, which is an assay using the concentration of a molecular isoform of free PSA, total PSA, and proPSA, has a greater specificity than total PSA or percentage-free PSA in select patients [78]. Addition of the four kallikrein protein assay has shown promise in being able to discriminate patients at risk for high grade prostate cancer [79]. Many of these assays are being introduced and appear to be making a clinical impact in the management and diagnosis of prostate cancer patients with a particular focus on their integration into screening algorithms. How they will compare to the current methods for screening and diagnosis will need to be investigated in randomized trials [80].

References

1. Gutman AB, Gutman EB. An acid phosphatase occurring in the serum of patients with metastasizing carcinoma of the prostate gland. J Clin Invest. 1938;17(1):473–9.
2. Huggins HR, Hodges CV. Studies on prostatic cancer: the effects of castration of estrogen and of androgen injection on serum phosphatases on metastatic carcinoma of the prostate. Cancer Res. 1941;1(1):293–7.
3. Fishman WH, Lerner F. A method for estimating serum acid phosphatase of prostatic origin. J Biol Chem. 1953;200(1):89–97.

4. Griffiths JC. Prostate-specific acid phosphatase: re-evaluation of radioimmunoassay in diagnosing prostatic disease. Clin Chem. 1980;26(3):433–6.

5. Li CY, Chuda RA, Lam WK, Yam LT. Acid phosphatases in human plasma. J Lab Clin Med. 1973;82(3):446–60.

6. Flocks R, Urich V, Patel C, Opitz J. Studies on the antigenic properties of prostatic tissue. J Urol. 1960;84:134–43.

7. Hara M, Koyanagi Y, Inoue T, Fukuyama T. Some physico-chemical characteristics of " -seminoprotein", an antigenic component specific for human seminal plasma. Forensic immunological study of body fluids and secretion. VII. Nihon Hoigaku Zasshi. 1971;25(4):322–4. Japanese.

8. Li TS, Beling CG. Isolation and characterization of two specific antigens of human seminal plasma. Fertil Steril. 1973;24(2):134–44.

9. Sensabaugh GF. Isolation and characterization of a semen-specific protein from human seminal plasma: a potential new marker for semen identification. J Forensic Sci. 1978;23(1):106–15.

10. Wang MC, Valenzuela LA, Murphy GP, Chu TM. Tissue specific and tumor specific antigens in human prostate. Fed Proc. 1977;36:1254.

11. Papsidero LD, Wang MC, Valenzuela LA, Murphy GP, Chu TM. A prostate antigen in sera of prostatic cancer patients. Cancer Res. 1980;40(7):2428–32.

12. Ablin RJ, Bronson P, Soanes WA, Witebsky E. Tissue- and species-specific antigens of normal human prostatic tissue. J Immunol. 1970;104(6):1329–39.

13. Ablin RJ, Soanes WA, Bronson P, Witebsky E. Precipitating antigens of the normal human prostate. J Reprod Fertil. 1970;22(3):573–4.

14. Wang MC, Valenzuela LA, Murphy GP, Chu TM. Purification of a human prostate specific antigen. Invest Urol. 1979;17(2):159–63.

15. Stamey TA, Yang N, Hay AR, McNeal JE, Freiha FS, Redwine E. Prostate-specific antigen as a serum marker for adenocarcinoma of the prostate. N Engl J Med. 1987;317:909–16.

16. Sokoll LJ, Chan DW. Prostate-specific antigen. Its discovery and biochemical characteristics. Urol Clin North Am. 1997;24(2):253–9. Review.

17. Ban Y, Wang MC, Watt KW, Loor R, Chu TM. The proteolytic activity of human prostate-specific antigen. Biochem Biophys Res Commun. 1984;123(2):482–8.

18. Lilja H. A kallikrein-like serine protease in prostatic fluid cleaves the predominant seminal vesicle protein. J Clin Invest. 1985;76(5):1899–903.

19. Lilja H. Structure and function of prostatic- and seminal vesicle-secreted proteins involved in the gelation and liquefaction of human semen. Scand J Clin Lab Invest Suppl. 1988;191:13–20.

20. Berg T, Bradshaw RA, Carretero OA, Chao J, Chao L, Clements JA, et al. A common nomenclature for members of the tissue (glandular) kallikrein gene families. Agents Actions Suppl. 1992;38(Pt 1):19–25.

21. Borgoño CA, Michael IP, Diamandis EP. Human tissue kallikreins: physiologic roles and applications in cancer. Mol Cancer Res. 2004;2(5):257–80. Review.

22. De Angelis G, Rittenhouse HG, Mikolajczyk SD, Blair Shamel L, Semjonow A. Twenty years of PSA: from prostate antigen to tumor marker. Rev Urol. 2007;9(3):113–23. Summer.

23. Mikolajczyk SD, Millar LS, Marker KM, Grauer LS, Goel A, Cass MM, et al. Ala217 is important for the catalytic function and autoactivation of prostate-specific human kallikrein 2. Eur J Biochem. 1997;246(2):440–6.

24. Stenman UH, Leinonen J, Alfthan H, Rannikko S, Tuhkanen K, Alfthan O. A complex between prostate-specific antigen and alpha 1-antichymotrypsin is the major form of prostate-specific antigen in serum of patients with prostatic cancer: assay of the complex improves clinical sensitivity for cancer. Cancer Res. 1991;51(1):222–6.

25. Lilja H, Christensson A, Dahlén U, Matikainen MT, Nilsson O, Pettersson K, et al. Prostate-specific antigen in serum occurs predominantly in complex with alpha 1-antichymotrypsin. Clin Chem. 1991;37(9):1618–25.

26. Chen Z, Chen H, Stamey TA. Prostate specific antigen in benign prostatic hyperplasia: purification and characterization. J Urol. 1997;157(6):2166–70.
27. Toubert ME, Guillet J, Chiron M, Meria P, Role C, Schlageter MH, et al. Percentage of free serum prostate-specific antigen: a new tool in the early diagnosis of prostatic cancer. Eur J Cancer. 1996;32A(12):2088–93.
28. Oesterling JE, Chan DW, Epstein JI, Kimball Jr AW, Bruzek DJ, Rock RC, et al. Prostate specific antigen in the preoperative and postoperative evaluation of localized prostatic cancer treated with radical prostatectomy. J Urol. 1988;139(4):766–72.
29. Myrtle JF, Klimley PG, Ivor LP, Brun JF. Clinical utility of prostate-specific antigen (PSA) in the management of prostate cancer. Advances in Cancer Diagnosis. Hybritech. 1986.
30. Kane RA, Littrup PJ, Babaian R, Drago JR, Lee F, Chesley A, et al. Prostate-specific antigen levels in 1695 men without evidence of prostate cancer. Findings of the American Cancer Society National Prostate Cancer Detection Project. Cancer. 1992;69(5):1201–7.
31. Dalkin BL, Ahmann FR, Kopp JB. Prostate specific antigen levels in men older than 50 years without clinical evidence of prostatic carcinoma. J Urol. 1993;150(6):1837–9.
32. Catalona WJ, Smith DS, Ratliff TL, Dodds KM, Coplen DE, Yuan JJ, et al. Measurement of prostate-specific antigen in serum as a screening test for prostate cancer. N Engl J Med. 1991;324(17):1156–61. Erratum in: N Engl J Med 1991 Oct 31;325(18):1324.
33. Catalona WJ, Smith DS, Ratliff TL, Basler JW. Detection of organ-confined prostate cancer is increased through prostate-specific antigen-based screening. JAMA. 1993;270(8):948–54.
34. Dalkin BL, Ahmann FR, Kopp JB, Catalona WJ, Ratliff TL, Hudson MA, et al. Derivation and application of upper limits for prostate specific antigen in men aged 50-74 years with no clinical evidence of prostatic carcinoma. Br J Urol. 1995;76(3):346–50.
35. Catalona WJ, Richie JP, Ahmann FR, Hudson MA, Scardino PT, Flanigan RC, et al. Comparison of digital rectal examination and serum prostate specific antigen in the early detection of prostate cancer: results of a multicenter clinical trial of 6,630 men. J Urol. 1994;151(5):1283–90.
36. Graves HC, Wehner N, Stamey TA. Comparison of a polyclonal and monoclonal immunoassay for PSA: need for an international antigen standard. J Urol. 1990;144(6):1516–22.
37. Punglia RS, D'Amico AV, Catalona WJ, Roehl KA, Kuntz KM. Effect of verification bias on screening for prostate cancer by measurement of prostate-specific antigen. N Engl J Med. 2003;349(4):335–42.
38. Cooner WH, Mosley BR, Rutherford Jr CL, Beard JH, Pond HS, Terry WJ, et al. Prostate cancer detection in a clinical urological practice by ultrasonography, digital rectal examination and prostate specific antigen. J Urol. 1990;143(6):1146–52. discussion 1152-4.
39. Brawer MK. Prostate specific antigen. New York, NY: Marcel Dekker; 2001.
40. Brawer MK, Chetner MP, Beatie J, Buchner DM, Vessella RL, Lange PH. Screening for prostatic carcinoma with prostate specific antigen. J Urol. 1992;147(3 Pt 2):841–5.
41. Carter HB, Pearson JD, Metter EJ, Brant LJ, Chan DW, Andres R, et al. Longitudinal evaluation of prostate-specific antigen levels in men with and without prostate disease. JAMA. 1992;267(16):2215–20.
42. Gann PH, Hennekens CH, Stampfer MJ. A prospective evaluation of plasma prostate-specific antigen for detection of prostatic cancer. JAMA. 1995;273(4):289–94.
43. Carter HB, Ferrucci L, Kettermann A, Landis P, Wright EJ, Epstein JI, et al. Detection of life-threatening prostate cancer with prostate-specific antigen velocity during a window of curability. J Natl Cancer Inst. 2006;98(21):1521–7.
44. Potosky AL, Miller BA, Albertsen PC, Kramer BS. The role of increasing detection in the rising incidence of prostate cancer. JAMA. 1995;273(7):548–52.
45. Plawker MW, Fleisher JM, Vapnek EM, Macchia RJ. Current trends in prostate cancer diagnosis and staging among United States urologists. J Urol. 1997;158(5):1853–8.
46. Sun L, Gancarczyk K, Paquette EL, McLeod DG, Kane C, Kusuda L, et al. Introduction to Department of Defense Center for Prostate Disease Research Multicenter National Prostate Cancer Database, and analysis of changes in the PSA-era. Urol Oncol. 2001;6(5):203–9.

47. Hankey BF, Feuer EJ, Clegg LX, Hayes RB, Legler JM, Prorok PC, et al. Cancer surveillance series: interpreting trends in prostate cancer--part I: evidence of the effects of screening in recent prostate cancer incidence, mortality, and survival rates. J Natl Cancer Inst. 1999;91(12):1017–24.
48. Etzioni R, Legler JM, Feuer EJ, Merrill RM, Cronin KA, Hankey BF. Cancer surveillance series: interpreting trends in prostate cancer – part III: quantifying the link between population prostate-specific antigen testing and recent declines in prostate cancer mortality. J Natl Cancer Inst. 1999;91(12):1033–9.
49. Albertsen PC, Fryback DG, Storer BE, Kolon TF, Fine J. Long-term survival among men with conservatively treated localized prostate cancer. JAMA. 1995;274(8):626–31.
50. Andriole GL, Crawford ED, Grubb 3rd RL, Buys SS, Chia D, Church TR, et al. Mortality results from a randomized prostate-cancer screening trial. N Engl J Med. 2009;360(13):1310–9.
51. Schröder FH, Hugosson J, Roobol MJ, Tammela TL, Ciatto S, Nelen V, et al. Screening and prostate-cancer mortality in a randomized European study. N Engl J Med. 2009;360(13):1320–8.
52. Wilt TJ, Brawer MK, Jones KM, Barry MJ, Aronson WJ, Fox S, et al. Radical prostatectomy versus observation for localized prostate cancer. N Engl J Med. 2012;367(3):203–13.
53. Thompson IM, Goodman PJ, Tangen CM, Lucia MS, Miller GJ, Ford LG, et al. The influence of finasteride on the development of prostate cancer. N Engl J Med. 2003;349(3):215–24.
54. Andriole GL, Bostwick DG, Brawley OW, Gomella LG, Marberger M, Montorsi F, REDUCE Study Group, et al. Effect of dutasteride on the risk of prostate cancer. N Engl J Med. 2010;362(13):1192–202.
55. Pinsky PF, Black A, Kramer BS, Miller A, Prorok PC, Berg C. Assessing contamination and compliance in the prostate component of the Prostate, Lung, Colorectal, and Ovarian (PLCO) cancer screening trial. Clin Trials. 2010;7(4):303–11.
56. Roobol MJ, Kerkhof M, Schröder FH, Cuzick J, Sasieni P, Hakama M, et al. Prostate cancer mortality reduction by prostate-specific antigen-based screening adjusted for nonattendance and contamination in the European Randomised Study of Screening for Prostate Cancer (ERSPC). Eur Urol. 2009;56(4):584–91.
57. Schröder FH, Roobol MJ. ERSPC and PLCO prostate cancer screening studies: what are the differences? Eur Urol. 2010;58(1):46–52.
58. Andriole GL, Crawford ED, Grubb 3rd RL, Buys SS, Chia D, Church TR, et al. Prostate cancer screening in the randomized prostate, lung, colorectal, and ovarian cancer screening trial: mortality results after 13 years of follow-up. J Natl Cancer Inst. 2012;104(2):125–32.
59. Schröder FH, Hugosson J, Roobol MJ, Tammela TL, Zappa M, Nelen V, et al. Screening and prostate cancer mortality: results of the European Randomised Study of Screening for Prostate Cancer (ERSPC) at 13 years of follow-up. Lancet. 2014;384(9959):2027–35.
60. Schröder FH, Hugosson J, Roobol MJ, Tammela TL, Ciatto S, Nelen V, et al. Prostate-cancer mortality at 11 years of follow-up. N Engl J Med. 2012;366(11):981–90.
61. US Preventive Services Task Force. Screening for breast cancer: U.S. Preventive Services Task Force recommendation statement. Ann Intern Med. 2009;151(10):716–26, W-236.
62. Hewitson P, Glasziou P, Irwig L, Towler B, Watson E. Screening for colorectal cancer using the faecal occult blood test. Hemoccult. Cochrane Database Syst Rev. 2007;1, CD001216. Review.
63. Hugosson J, Carlsson S, Aus G, Bergdahl S, Khatami A, Lodding P, et al. Mortality results from the Göteborg randomised population-based prostate-cancer screening trial. Lancet Oncol. 2010;11(8):725–32.
64. Kilpeläinen TP, Tammela TL, Malila N, Hakama M, Santti H, Määttänen L, et al. Prostate cancer mortality in the Finnish randomized screening trial. J Natl Cancer Inst. 2013;105(10):719–25.
65. Gulati R, Mariotto AB, Chen S, Gore JL, Etzioni R. Long-term projections of the harm-benefit trade-off in prostate cancer screening are more favorable than previous short-term estimates. J Clin Epidemiol. 2011;64(12):1412–7.

66. Lane JA, Donovan JL, Davis M, Walsh E, Dedman D, Down L, ProtecT study group, et al. Active monitoring, radical prostatectomy, or radiotherapy for localised prostate cancer: study design and diagnostic and baseline results of the ProtecT randomised phase 3 trial. Lancet Oncol. 2014;15(10):1109–18.

67. Heijnsdijk EA, Wever EM, Auvinen A, Hugosson J, Ciatto S, Nelen V, et al. Quality-of-life effects of prostate-specific antigen screening. N Engl J Med. 2012;367(7):595–605.

68. American Cancer Society: What is prostate cancer?. http://www.cancer.org/cancer/prostatecancer/. Accessed 28 Nov 2014.

69. Mariotto AB, Yabroff KR, Shao Y, Feuer EJ, Brown ML. Projections of the cost of cancer care in the United States: 2010-2020. J Natl Cancer Inst. 2011;103(2):117–28.

70. Taylor KL, Luta G, Miller AB, Church TR, Kelly SP, Muenz LR, et al. Long-term disease-specific functioning among prostate cancer survivors and noncancer controls in the prostate, lung, colorectal and ovarian cancer screening trial. J Clin Oncol. 2012;30(22):2768–75.

71. Resnick MJ, Koyama T, Fan KH, Albertsen PC, Goodman M, Hamilton AS, et al. Long-term functional outcomes after treatment for localized prostate cancer. N Engl J Med. 2013;368(5):436–45.

72. de Oliveira C, Bremner KE, Ni A, Alibhai SM, Laporte A, Krahn MD. Patient time and out-of-pocket costs for long-term prostate cancer survivors in Ontario, Canada. J Cancer Surviv. 2014;8(1):9–20.

73. Jayadevappa R, Schwartz JS, Chhatre S, Gallo JJ, Wein AJ, Malkowicz SB. The burden of out-of-pocket and indirect costs of prostate cancer. Prostate. 2010;70(11):1255–64.

74. Morgans AK, Fan KH, Koyama T, Albertsen PC, Goodman M, Hamilton AS, et al. Influence of age on incident diabetes and cardiovascular disease among prostate cancer survivors receiving androgen deprivation therapy. J Urol. 2014;pii: S0022–5347(14)04835–6.

75. Daskivich TJ, Fan KH, Koyama T, Albertsen PC, Goodman M, Hamilton AS, et al. Prediction of long-term other-cause mortality in men with early-stage prostate cancer: results from the Prostate Cancer Outcomes Study. Urology. 2015;85(1):92–100.

76. D'Amico AV, Whittington R, Malkowicz SB, Schultz D, Blank K, et al. Biochemical outcome after radical prostatectomy, external beam radiation therapy, or interstitial radiation therapy for clinically localized prostate cancer. JAMA. 1998;280(11):969–74.

77. Charlson ME, Pompei P, Ales KL, MacKenzie CR. A new method of classifying prognostic comorbidity in longitudinal studies: development and validation. J Chronic Dis. 1987;40(5):373–83.

78. Loeb S, Sanda MG, Broyles DL, Shin SS, Bangma CH, Wei JT, et al. The Prostate Health Index (phi) selectively identifies clinically-significant prostate cancer. J Urol. 2014;pii: S0022–5347(14)04900–3.

79. Carlsson S, Maschino A, Schröder F, Bangma C, Steyerberg EW, van der Kwast T, et al. Predictive value of four kallikrein markers for pathologically insignificant compared with aggressive prostate cancer in radical prostatectomy specimens: results from the European Randomized Study of Screening for Prostate Cancer section Rotterdam. Eur Urol. 2013;64(5):693–9.

80. Nordström T, Vickers A, Assel M, Lilja H, Grönberg H, Eklund M. Comparison between the four-kallikrein panel and Prostate Health Index for predicting prostate cancer. Eur Urol. 2014;pii: S0302–2838(14)00752–0.

Chapter 2
Pathology of Prostate Cancer: What Has Changed in the Last 30 Years

M. Scott Lucia

Introduction

Thirty years have brought about enormous growth in our understanding of the pathobiology of prostate cancer. For instance, while it was known that prostate cancer development and growth is dependent on androgens since the groundbreaking work of Huggins and Hodges [1], more data is surfacing on the importance of androgen receptor (AR) signaling in prostate cancer progression and the role of genetic variants of AR in resistance to hormone therapy [2, 3]. A number of key molecular abnormalities have been identified that occur with high frequency in prostate cancer including loss of the tumor suppressor PTEN, amplification of the oncogene cMYC, and TMPRSS2:ETS translocations [4, 5]. Evidence of a role for chronic inflammation and oxidative stress in the development and progression of prostate cancer is emerging [6–8]. The last 30 years have also seen striking advancements in the manner in which we diagnose and manage prostate cancer.

The identification of prostate-specific antigen (PSA), and the recognition that increases in serum levels of PSA portend an increased risk of prostate cancer, heralded an era of widespread prostate cancer screening in the United States and a dramatic rise in the number of men diagnosed with prostate cancer in the 1990s [9]. During this time, as more men were diagnosed earlier in the natural history of prostate cancer, there was a marked shift in stage towards clinically localized disease [9–12]. Whereas tumors removed by prostatectomy in the pre-PSA era tended to be large, occupying the majority of the prostate volume, often with extensive extraprostatic extension, more tumors seen today are smaller in volume, more often organ-confined, and associated with improved therapeutic outcomes [11, 12]. It is now clear that the natural history of prostate cancer is quite variable [13]. While a

M.S. Lucia, M.D. (✉)
Anatomic Pathology, Department of Pathology, University of Colorado School of Medicine, 12801 East 17th Avenue, Mail Stop 8104, Aurora, CO, USA
e-mail: Scott.Lucia@ucdenver.edu

© Springer International Publishing Switzerland 2016
N.N. Stone, E.D. Crawford (eds.), *The Prostate Cancer Dilemma*,
DOI 10.1007/978-3-319-21485-6_2

small subset of cancers are highly aggressive and progress rapidly, the majority of cancers have a more protracted course over many years. Some cancers may never become life threatening during the expected lifetime of the patient. Thus, more men die *with* prostate cancer than *of* prostate cancer. Concern now arises that we are detecting many small, slow-growing cancers that would otherwise not be a health threat to the patient. Such tumors could be managed expectantly and monitored rather than treated radically to reduce the overall morbidity associated with therapy. The key to appropriate therapeutic decision-making lies in the ability of pathological examination of prostate biopsy tissue to accurately identify those cancers that are of low risk to progress from those that are potentially lethal. The evolution of new management strategies including active surveillance and targeted focal therapy necessitates greater emphasis in assessing the biological aggressiveness and extent of the tumor from the prostate needle biopsy. Herein we review the advancements made over the last few decades in the pathological examination and reporting of prostate cancer.

Histopathology of Prostate Cancer and Evolving Concepts in Grading

The vast majority of prostate cancers are adenocarcinomas composed of glandular cells exhibiting variable degrees of differentiation into glandular acini that infiltrate the fibromuscular stroma of the prostate gland. The degree of differentiation can range from tumors with well-formed glandular acini to poorly formed ragged appearing acini to sheets, cords, or even single infiltrating cells without true acinar formations (Fig. 2.1). The morphologic or cytologic differentiation of a tumor reflects its

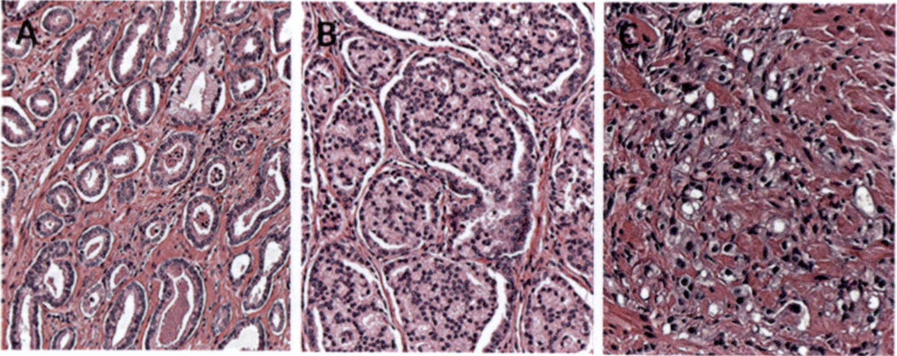

Fig. 2.1 The architectural patterns of prostate cancer reflect the biological aggressiveness of the tumor. (**a**) Low-grade cancers are composed of well-formed, discrete glandular acini that are distributed within the fibromuscular stroma. The tumor in (**a**) depicts Gleason pattern 3 (H&E, 200×). (**b**, **c**) High-grade cancer patterns show variable degrees of glandular fusion and poorly formed acini. The tumor in (**b**) (H&E, 200×) shows glandular fusion (Gleason grade pattern 4), while the tumor in (**c**) (H&E, 400×) shows absence of well-formed acini with tumor cells infiltrating as cords (Gleason pattern 5)

biologic aggressiveness. In general, the more poorly differentiated the tumor, the more aggressive is its behavior. Much of what we have learned regarding tumor biology and natural history comes from the pathological analyses of prostatectomy specimens. In 1966, Donald Gleason described the varied architectural appearances of a large number of prostatic adenocarcinomas and demonstrated that the degree of glandular differentiation and infiltration of the surrounding stroma by tumor cells reflected the biology of the tumor [14]. Those tumors that displayed well-formed acinar structures had favorable outcomes compared with those that had progressively more poorly formed acini. Those tumors that formed only sheets, cords, or single cell arrangements behaved aggressively and were often lethal. These observations formed the basis for the Gleason grading system that has been the most important and widely used grading system for prostate cancer since his landmark publication.

The Gleason grading system contains five tiers or grade ranks and categorizes tumors by their architectural pattern of growth rather than cytologic features. Individual tumors often display more than one pattern. This was addressed by Gleason by adding the most prevalent pattern (the primary pattern) with the second most prevalent pattern (the secondary pattern) to obtain a Gleason "score." If only one pattern was present, then the pattern rank was doubled to result in Gleason scores for each tumor ranging from 2 (grade 1 + grade 1) to 10 (grade 5 + grade 5). The higher the score, the more aggressive is the tumor. Tumors do not necessarily progress from low grade (patterns 1–3) to high grade (patterns 4–5) during their natural course. Tumors can arise as high grade or may remain as low-grade tumors [15, 16].

Over time, the Gleason system has undergone a number of modifications by Gleason and others [17, 18]. The basis for these modifications comes from years of experience with prostate cancer grading on biopsy and prostatectomy specimens by academic pathologists and a plethora of studies relating Gleason grade to disease outcomes and responses to therapy. In 2005, 80 genitourinary pathologists from around the world as members of the International Society of Urologic Pathologists (ISUP) participated in a survey of practice patterns and a consensus conference to document and assess cancer grading trends and refine the guidelines for Gleason grading [18]. Most notable among the items addressed by the ISUP were (1) restrictions on assigning very low-grade patterns (grades 1 and 2) on biopsy specimens, (2) refining the separation between patterns 3 and 4, (3) assigning grade to cribriform patterns of cancer, and (4) scoring biopsies that contain minor amounts of high-grade patterns or tertiary-grade patterns.

Gleason's original work in developing the grading system was based upon examination of prostatectomy specimens, transurethral resections, and large caliber needle biopsies. Contemporary needle biopsies are thin (~18 gauge) and relatively short producing core fragments that average ~1.5 cm in length and 0.6 mm in thickness. Thus, tumor sampling is limited and, as discussed further below, this has an impact on the accuracy of Gleason grading when compared to subsequent prostatectomy specimens. Because of this, assigning grades of 1 or 2 on needle biopsies usually results in upgrading at prostatectomy [19, 21]. In addition, most tumors that would have been graded as 1 + 1 (score = 2) in the past would today be recognized as benign adenoses with the use of basal cell markers. This trend was noted in studies looking

Fig. 2.2 Cribriform cancer
showing nests of cells with
distinctive sharply outlined
holes

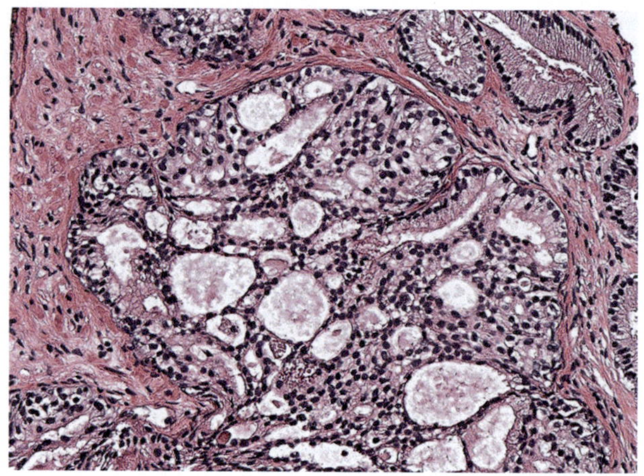

at grading trends over time [20, 21]. Gleason scores of 2–4 represented 21 % of cases diagnosed on prostatectomy and TURP specimens between 1983 and 1984 but only 11 % of cases diagnosed in 1992–1993 [20]. By 2001, the number had fallen to less than 5 % [21]. Therefore, the ISUP recommended that Gleason grades 1 and 2 rarely if ever be used on biopsies.

In contrast, the most important grade patterns to recognize on needle biopsies are the high-grade patterns 4 and 5. Tumors that contain even small amounts of pattern 4 or 5 (corresponding to Gleason scores of 7–10 depending on the relative amount of pattern 3) behave more aggressively than those graded with Gleason scores of 2–6 [22, 23]. Thus, it is important to be able to separate architectural patterns that behave more aggressively than typical grade 3 patterns and include them as pattern 4 or 5 appropriately. Unlike the original Gleason system, it was recommended by the ISUP that ill-defined acini with poorly formed lumens and tumors containing single cells should not be allowed within Gleason pattern 3. Single cells represent pattern 5, while poorly formed glands represent pattern 4. Pattern 3 is reserved for tumors with discrete, well-formed acini with prominent lumens and separated by variable amounts of stroma. When holding to this standard, the outcomes for Gleason score 3 + 3 tumors are very favorable [24, 25].

More problematic is what to do with tumors that display cribriform morphology (Fig. 2.2). In the original Gleason system, these were grouped within grade 3. The ISUP consensus was that cribriform cancers represent a mixed bag of tumor aggressiveness. Most cribriform tumors behave similar to tumors with pattern 4 and therefore should be graded as pattern 4. Only tumors with small, well-rounded arrangements should warrant the designation of pattern 3. However, more recently this notion has been challenged [26, 27]. In our experience, all cribriform cancers behave aggressively regardless of the size or shape of the cribriform structures [27].

Lastly, the 2005 ISUP Consensus Group recommended modifications as to assigning Gleason scores on prostate biopsies. It was recommended that any amount of high-grade patterns seen on a biopsy be recorded as part of the Gleason score even if it was not the primary or secondary grade pattern present or represented less than

5 % of the tumor. In the classic Gleason system, tumor patterns that represented less than 5 % of the tumor or were a tertiary pattern were ignored. For example, a tumor that consists of 75 % pattern 3, >20 % pattern 4, and <5 % pattern 5 would be scored as 3 + 5 under the 2005 recommendations but 3 + 4 using the classic Gleason system. These modifications were recommended to attempt to reduce the number of cancers that would otherwise be upgraded upon prostatectomy, a situation that unfortunately occurs frequently when comparing the Gleason grade on presurgical biopsies with the subsequent prostatectomy [28, 29]. However, applying these modifications also resulted in a shift towards higher Gleason scores reported on biopsies in some studies [30, 31]. Nevertheless, the recommendations documented in the 2005 ISUP Consensus Conference report represent a synthesis of grading practices by leading genitourinary pathologists around the world rather than a new grading scheme per se.

Despite the 2005 ISUP modifications, there are still problems associated with the Gleason grading of biopsies that impact patient care. Since Gleason patterns 1 and 2 are not usually reported on biopsies, the lowest Gleason grade typically assigned to a biopsy is 3 + 3 (score = 6). Gleason score 6 lies halfway between Gleason score 2 and 10; therefore, patients may perceive a Gleason score 6 tumor as being intermediate in aggressiveness. Large population studies clearly indicate that Gleason score 6 tumors have an excellent prognosis, and patients with such tumors represent good candidates for active surveillance [13]. Patients may be reluctant to choose active surveillance if they perceive their cancer to be in the middle of the grading scale. Furthermore, data suggest that the amount of tumor that displays high-grade features is most important prognostically [22, 27, 32]. Classifying a tumor as 3 + 4 versus 4 + 3 may indicate that the latter has relatively more pattern 4 than the former on a particular biopsy, but since both are Gleason scores of 7, it does not really convey prognostic information in a clear way. In 2013, Epstein and colleagues from the Johns Hopkins Medical Center reviewed prognostic variables in the biopsies of 7869 men that underwent radical prostatectomy at their institution [25]. They found that meaningful stratification of biochemical-free survival by Kaplan–Meier analysis was achieved by amalgamating Gleason scores into 5 prognostic groups. Group 1 was composed of tumors with biopsy Gleason score ≤3 + 3. This group had the best overall biochemical-free survival at 5 years (94.6 %). Groups 2 (Gleason score 3 + 4), 3 (Gleason score 4 + 3), and 4 (Gleason score 8) had 5-year biochemical-free survivals of 82.7, 65.1, and 63.1 % respectively. The worst biochemical-free survival (34.5 %) was seen in Group 5 (Gleason score 9–10). By defining Prognostic Group 1 as the group with the most favorable prognosis, they emphasize a patient population that could be the ideal candidates for active surveillance. The other prognostic groups indicate categorically greater relative amounts of the high-grade patterns 4 and 5 that impact treatment outcomes. From these data, a new grading scheme, based upon the architectural features inherent in the Gleason grades, has been proposed to classify tumors by the amount of high-grade patterns that make up the tumor. Table 2.1 compares this new grading scheme with the classic Gleason system and 2005 ISUP Gleason modifications. This concept was presented to 85 pathologists from 17 countries in November 2014 and endorsed by the ISUP. It is anticipated that the new scheme will eventually replace Gleason scoring within the next 5–10 years.

Table 2.1 Comparison of the classical, ISUP modified Gleason grading systems, and proposed new system

Classical Gleason system (1977)	2005 ISUP modified Gleason system	2014 Proposed grading system
Pattern 1: Small, uniform, and closely packed acini in tight circumscribed masses	*Pattern 1*: Closely packed, separate, uniform round–oval, medium-sized acini in circumscribed nodules	*Grade 1*: Tumor purely composed of individual separate well-formed acini
Pattern 2: Mild-moderate variation in size and shape of acini and some cellular atypia; acini more loosely packed than pattern 1, but still relatively circumscribed	*Pattern 2*: Mild acinar irregularity with minimal infiltration at edges of tumor nodule; more loosely packed than pattern 1	*Grade 2*: Tumor with predominantly well-formed individual acini with lesser component of poorly formed, fused or cribriform acini
Pattern 3: Small infiltrating acini with irregularity of size and shape; individual cells invading stroma away from circumscribed glandular masses; papillary and cribriform arrangements ranging from small to large with smooth rounded edges	*Pattern 3*: Small infiltrative individual glandular acini with marked variation in size and shape; smoothly circumscribed small cribriform cellular structures	*Grade 3*: Tumor with predominantly poorly formed, fused or cribriform acini with lesser component of well-formed acini
Pattern 4: Infiltrating fused acini that coalesce and branch (no longer single and separate); acini with large clear cells resembling hypernephroma	*Pattern 4*: Fused microacini and ill-defined acini with poorly formed luminae; cribriform structures that are large or have irregular borders; ductal or hypernephromatoid tumors	*Grade 4*: Tumor composed of only poorly formed, fused or cribriform acini; tumor with predominantly well-formed acini but with lesser component lacking acini
Pattern 5: Poorly differentiated cells infiltrating in solid or diffuse masses; individual cells with essentially no acinar differentiation; Signet ring cells; comedocarcinoma with central necrosis	*Pattern 5*: Infiltrating cells with essentially no acinar differentiation arranged in solid sheets, cords, or single cells; comedocarcinoma with central necrosis	*Grade 5*: Tumor formed of cells lacking any acinar formations (e.g., cords or single cells) with or without component of poorly formed, fused or cribriform acini; comedonecrosis
Gleason scoring:		
Gleason score: add together the most prominent pattern (primary) with the second most prominent pattern (secondary)	Prostatectomy: add together the most prominent pattern (primary) with the second most prominent pattern (secondary)	Gleason scoring not necessary
Same scoring method used for prostatectomy and biopsy	Biopsies: add together the most prominent pattern (primary) with the highest remaining grade pattern regardless of amount: Gleason scores 2–4 should rarely (if ever) be assigned	

Multifocality and Heterogeneity

Although prostate cancers can arise anywhere within the prostate, most (70–80 %) arise in the peripheral lobe [33]. However, in the mid-1990s, it was recognized that prostate cancer often has multiple foci of discrete tumors in surgical prostatectomy specimens. Using computer-assisted three-dimensional reconstructions of prostatectomy specimens obtained from 1987 to 1991, Miller and Cygan found multifocal cancer in more than half of all cases, and concluded that most cases in which the prostate only contained one tumor resulted from the assimilation of multiple smaller tumors when they grew to confluence [15]. As more patients are now diagnosed earlier in the course of the disease, multifocal disease is now seen in over 64–87 % of cases [34] supporting the conclusions of Miller and Cygan. In our database of over 300 prostates that have been whole-mount processed and reconstructed since 2005, multifocal tumor is present in >70 % while the average tumor volume has decreased from over 6 cm^3 in the early 1990s to approximately 2 cm^3. Individual tumor foci are somatically independent and display differences in the degree of differentiation (grade), molecular characteristics, and DNA ploidy [35–37]. These differences do not just exist between separate tumor foci, but even between different regions within an individual tumor focus. Figure 2.3 depicts a representative prostate from our database that has been three-dimensionally reconstructed. Panel (a) shows the intact prostate while in Panel (b) the benign prostate has been stripped away leaving multiple discrete tumor foci. The different colors correspond to the different Gleason grade patterns present. It has also become apparent that tumors can arise deep in the anterior portion of the prostate in either the transition zone or anterior horns of the peripheral zone where they become difficult to detect by digital rectal examination (DRE) or routine prostate needle biopsy protocols. Such anterior

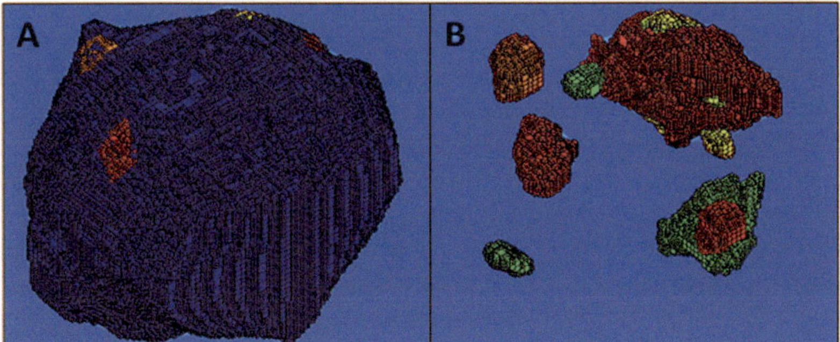

Fig. 2.3 Three-dimensional reconstruction of prostate containing multiple tumor foci. (**a**) Whole-mount reconstruction showing benign prostate (*dark blue*) and colored foci of tumor extending to surface. (**b**) Prostate from (**a**) with benign prostate removed to demonstrate multiple tumor foci. The different *colors* indicate areas with different Gleason grade patterns (*Red*=pattern 3, *Green*=pattern 4, *orange*=pattern 5) and prostatic intraepithelial neoplasia (PIN-*yellow*)

tumors appear similar to tumors arising in the posterior periphery and may attain relatively large size and potentially more advanced stage before being detected [33, 38]. The orange tumor in Fig. 2.3b is an anterior tumor that is high grade (Gleason pattern 5) and present at the resection margin.

The Role of Pathological Examination of the Prostate Biopsy in Management Decisions

The role of the pathologist in the examination of prostate biopsies is to (1) establish the presence or absence of cancer, (2) determine the expected biologic aggressiveness of the tumor, and (3) estimate the extent of the tumor present. Our ability to provide this information is complicated by the nature of the prostate biopsy itself.

Before the advent of PSA screening, most prostate cancers, due to their relatively large volume, were discovered by DRE with subsequent directed biopsy. Now with PSA screening, the majority of prostate cancers are diagnosed when serum elevations in PSA prompt a prostate biopsy. Since most of these tumors are not palpable and, as noted above, are smaller and multifocal making them difficult to image, a series of individual prostate needle biopsies are taken transrectally using transrectal ultrasound (TRUS) guidance in a systematic but largely random manner from the left and right sides of the prostate fanning from apex to base. The manner in which these biopsies are taken has undergone a number of changes over the last few decades. For years obtaining six biopsy cores, three on each side, was routine. As it became increasingly clear that cancers were often missed, biopsy schemes were extended to 10, 12, or even more cores and concentrated on sampling the lateral portions of the gland [39, 40]. While these modifications have increased the sensitivity for diagnosing prostate cancer, extended biopsy protocols can still miss cancer foci [39, 40]. Consequently, many men undergo repeated biopsy after a negative biopsy due to concerns that they might have a cancer that was simply missed on the first biopsy. When a cancer is detected on a needle biopsy, the pathologist gives the tumor a Gleason score, and some measure of extent is provided such as the number of cores positive for cancer and the percent (or millimeter extent) the tumor encompasses on each core. Unfortunately, this critical information is also affected by biopsy sampling. For example, the biopsy may not sample the highest grade of tumor present. It has been shown that the Gleason score of the cancer on subsequent prostatectomy often is one, two, or even three grades higher than the presurgical biopsy specimen [28, 29]. The primary reason is that the biopsy needle only sampled a portion of the tumor and missed foci of high-grade tumor readily apparent when the entire gland was examined. Moreover, a biopsy is a poor staging tool, and although the number of cores positive for cancer in a given set of biopsy cores correlates with tumor volume, the finding of a small amount of tumor on a single biopsy core does not necessarily indicate a clinically inconsequential tumor will be found on the subsequent prostatectomy [41].

Table 2.2 Pathological and clinical features at time of biopsy used to predict potentially limited tumor of prostate and determine eligibility for active surveillance protocols

Reference	Clinical stage	PSA[a] (ng/ml)	PSAD[b] (ng/ml/g)	Gleason score	No. of cores positive	Core[c] percent positive
Epstein 1994 [45]	T1c	NS[d]	≤0.15	≤3+3	≤2	<50 %
Van den Bergh 2009 [46]	T1c/2	≤10	<0.2	≤3+3	≤2	NS
Soloway 2010 [47]	T1/2	≤10	NS	≤3+3	≤2	≤20 %
Adamy 2011 [48]	T1/2a	≤10	NS	≤3+3	≤3	≤50 %
Whitson 2011 [49]	T1c/2	≤10	NS	≤3+3	≤33 %	≤50 %

[a]PSA = prostate-specific antigen
[b]PSAD = PSA density
[c]Core percent positive = percent linear extent of any core
[d]NS = not stated

These sampling issues are particularly problematic when considering active surveillance or targeted focal therapy as management options. Thirty years ago when treatment options were limited, merely rendering a diagnosis of cancer on prostate biopsy or transurethral resection led to radical definitive therapy. In contemporary practice, patients with low-grade, low volume organ-confined tumors may be candidates for active surveillance or targeted focal therapy. The most commonly used definition of a low-risk tumor is a tumor of <0.5 cm^3 (some have expanded this to 1.3 cm^3) that is confined to the prostate and has a Gleason score of 6 or less (no pattern 4 or 5) at prostatectomy [42–44]. A number of investigators have attempted to predict such low-risk tumors by defining thresholds on the grade and extent of disease present on the biopsy, and then using these criteria for active surveillance protocols (Table 2.2) [45–49]. Perhaps the most stringent and accepted definition is that of Epstein and colleagues which defines a tumor as "potentially insignificant" if the following criteria are met: (1) clinical stage T1c, (2) PSA density of <0.15 ng/ml/gm as calculated by TRUS, (3) biopsy Gleason score ≤6 (no pattern 4 or 5), and (4) tumor involving less than three cores with no core containing more than 50 % linear involvement [45]. Unfortunately, attempts to predict low volume, low-grade organ-confined tumor using these biopsy criteria are imperfect. The performance of the active surveillance protocols as defined in Table 2.2 was compared on common patient cohorts [50, 51] and demonstrated upgrading to Gleason scores of 7 or greater anywhere from 42 to 51 % of cases, while upstaging to non-organ-confined disease was reported in 5–9 % of cases [50]. Sensitivities for predicting insignificant tumors ranged from 45 to 83 % with specificities of 39–82 % [51]. Sensitivities for just predicting organ-confined, low-grade tumors at prostatectomy ranged from 34 to 73 % with specificities of 39–83 % [51].

The biologic aggressiveness of a tumor combined with its volume or extent of spread determines the outcome for a patient following treatment. Therefore, accurate assessment of biologic potential and tumor extent at the time of biopsy is crucial in order to identify those tumors that should be treated aggressively from those

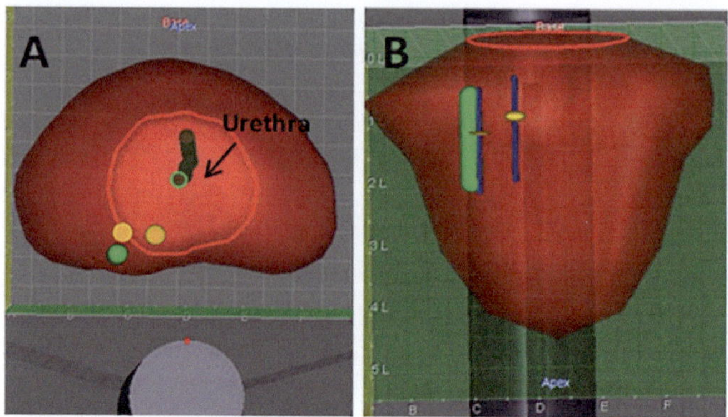

Fig. 2.4 Ultrasound image of prostate fused with transperineal mapping biopsy results. (**a**) views the prostate from the apex. (**b**) views the prostate from above. A cluster of three positive biopsies is present in left posterior base of the prostate. The positive needle locations (represented in *blue*) show foci of 3 + 3 cancer, shown in *yellow* indicating the amount of the core positive for tumor, and 3 + 4 cancer, shown in *green* with the amount of core represented by the *length of the bar.*

tumors that could be focally ablated or be monitored by active surveillance. Due to the limited tumor sampling inherent with current TRUS biopsy methods, accurate identification of tumors that can be assured not to progress remains a challenge. Physicians are faced with uncertainty as to whether or not the tumor biology is accurately captured in the biopsy sample taken, the true volume of tumor present, and whether or not there are additional foci of tumor, particularly in anterior portions of the prostate, that may have been missed. To better address these issues, a recent approach that has been used by us and others is to "map" the prostate for areas of cancer using a transperineal template-guided method with biopsies taken at regular intervals across all three dimensions of the prostate [52, 53]. Each core is separately graded, measured for extent, and then grid-mapped to produce a three-dimensional representation of the prostate with all tumor foci (Fig. 2.4). This method requires a relatively large number of biopsies to completely map a prostate, but results in improved grade accuracy when compared to TRUS-guided transrectal biopsies upon subsequent prostatectomy. Comparison of TRUS-guided transrectal biopsy (TRB) with three-dimensional template-guided transperineal mapping biopsies (TPMB) in 215 patients undergoing both procedures showed Gleason score ≤6 tumor in the TRB of 73 % of the patients, but in only 50 % of TPMB [53]. Upgrading to Gleason score 7 or higher from TRB to TPMB occurred in 27 %, while 46 % of tumors were upstaged on TPMB compared to TRB. In 25 patients that underwent prostatectomy after having both TRB and TPMB, the tumors were upgraded from the TRB in 52 % of cases, but upgraded from the TPMB in only 12 % of the cases [54]. This method also allows for improved determination of the location of all tumor foci which is necessary for proper targeting for focal ablation. Efforts to improve the precision of this approach and reduce the labor-intensiveness are underway to promote wider acceptance for patients considering active surveillance or targeted focal therapy.

Advances in Molecular Pathology: The New Frontier

While the grade of a tumor reflects its biologic aggressiveness, the mechanistic basis for a tumor's biology lies at the molecular level. A thorough understanding of the molecular events that lead to the aggressive cancer phenotype has been elusive. This is due in part to the heterogeneity of prostate cancer. Compounding the problem has been the difficulty in obtaining sufficient quantities of fresh cancerous tissue from surgical specimens and biopsies for analyses. Recent advances in technology have largely overcome this barrier allowing for robust analysis of progressively smaller quantities of DNA and RNA even from formalin-fixed and paraffin-embedded (FFPE) pathological specimens. This has led to the identification of a number of genetic abnormalities associated with prostate cancer including alterations in PTEN, cMyc, and the TMPRSS2:ETS gene fusions found in many prostate cancers [4, 5]. However, the utility of these abnormalities as prognostic or predictive markers has not been proven. More progress has been made in the development of gene expression assays on RNA isolated from FFPE biopsy tissue as prognostic markers for prostate cancer.

Commercially offered gene expression assays are now available for use on as little as 1 mm of tumor on prostate needle biopsies. For example, one such assay determines a cell cycle progression (CCP) score derived from 31 genes across the spectrum of the cell proliferation cycle normalized to 15 reference housekeeping genes (Prolaris®, Myriad Genetics, Salt lake City, UT). In a cohort of 349 men conservatively managed following prostate biopsy, the CCP score was independently predictive of cancer-specific mortality within 10 years and showed additive value when combined with Gleason score and PSA [55]. In patients treated with prostatectomy, the CCP score as calculated from the pretreatment needle biopsy was a strong predictor of biochemical recurrence and metastasis-free survival [56]. Thus, combining the CCP score with other pathological prognostic variables such as grade and number of cores positive may better identify patients who would be the ideal candidates for active surveillance from those requiring definitive treatment. However, most prostate cancers are heterogeneous not only in grade but also in terms of genetic abnormalities and molecular expression [35–37], and concern remains as to how sampling bias for such prostate cancers affects the results for individual patients. In this context, mapping biopsies may help to improve the performance of molecular tissue biomarkers by limiting the impact of tumor heterogeneity and sampling.

Another commercially available prognostic gene expression assay was recently developed specifically to address the concerns regarding tumor heterogeneity and under-sampling. This assay (Onco*type* DX®, Genomic Health, Inc., Redwood City, CA) calculates a genomic prostate score (GPS) using a 17-gene expression panel including 5 reference genes and 12 genes across multiple molecular pathways that have been shown to be predictive of metastasis and death in prostatectomy tissue while also being predictive of having high-grade or advanced stage cancer of the prostate regardless of the grade of tumor sampled [57, 58]. The gene expression panel covers pathways associated with poor outcomes (e.g., stromal response and proliferation genes) as well as favorable outcomes (e.g., androgen signaling and cellular organization genes). The assay was validated on a set of men who were considered by National Comprehensive Cancer Network (NCCN) criteria to be very low risk (Stage T1c, PSA density ≤0.15, Gleason score ≤3+3, <3 cores positive with no core having ≥50 % tumor involvement; n=37), low risk (stage T1-T2a, PSA<10 ng/ml, Gleason score ≤3+3; $n=191$), or intermediate risk (stage T2b/c or Gleason score 7 or PSA 10–20 ng/ml; n=160). For each risk group, the GPS added independent prognostic value and identified men whose scores indicated a more favorable prognosis and also men whose scores indicated a less favorable prognosis than expected for their NCCN risk group, thereby providing improved discriminatory power for selecting men who could be managed conservatively versus those who would benefit best from definitive therapy [58].

The examples of gene expression assays described above represent some of the first generation of molecular tests that serve as adjuncts to traditional pathology. It is anticipated that continuing advances in technology will ultimately better define the aggressive phenotype for prostate cancer at the molecular level improving our ability to predict tumor behavior and grant the clinician more tools to guide treatment strategies for individual patients in the new era of precision medicine.

Conclusion

The last 30 years has given us a better understanding of the biology of prostate cancer. We now know that not all tumors are destined to be life threatening, and defined a subset of tumors from a pathologic basis that could be better managed conservatively. We have also refined our ability to predict the aggressiveness and extent of tumors at the time of biopsy using traditional pathologic features and the development of newer molecular investigations. However, our ability to do so accurately for every patient at the time of biopsy is still hampered by limitations in the amount of information that can be obtained from routine prostate biopsies. While the process of carcinogenesis and cancer progression evolves over time, a biopsy can only capture a glimpse of the tumor at a single time point. Maximizing the amount of information that can be gleaned from the biopsy is paramount in order to identify those patients that may be candidates for active surveillance or targeted focal therapy. Continued refinements in our ability to recognize the histologic and molecular features of cancer that contribute to its aggressiveness will ultimately improve the predictive accuracy of prostate biopsies.

References

1. Huggins C, Hodges CV. Studies on prostatic cancer. I. The effect of castration, of estrogen and androgen injection on serum phosphatases in metastatic carcinoma of the prostate. CA Cancer J Clin. 1972;22:232–40.

2. Lonergan PE, Tindall DJ. Androgen receptor signaling in prostate cancer development and progression. J Carcinog. 2011;10:20. Epub 2011 August 23.
3. Antonarakis ES, Lu C, Wang H, Luber B, Nakazawa M, Roeser JC, Chen Y, Mohammad TA, Chen Y, Fedor HL, Lotan TL, Zheng Q, De Marzo AM, Isaacs JT, Isaacs WB, Nadal R, Paller CJ, Denmeade SR, Carducci MA, Eisenberger MA, Luo J. AR-V7 and resistance to enzalutamide and abiraterone in prostate cancer. N Engl J Med. 2014;371(11):1028–38.
4. Gurel B, Iwata T, Koh CM, Yegnasubramanian S, Nelson WG, De Marzo AM. Molecular alterations in prostate cancer as diagnostic, prognostic, and therapeutic targets. Adv Anat Pathol. 2008;15:319–31.
5. Barbieri CE, Tomlins SA. The prostate cancer genome: perspectives and potential. Urol Oncol 2014;32(1):53.e15-22.
6. Koul HK, Kumar B, Koul S, Deb AA, Hwa JS, Maroni P, van Bokhoven A, Lucia MS, Kim FJ, Meacham RB. The role of inflammation and infection in prostate cancer: importance in prevention, diagnosis and treatment. Drugs Today (Barc). 2010;46:929–43.
7. Lucia MS, Lambert JR, Platz EA, De Marzo AM. Inflammation as a target in prostate cancer. In: Figg WD, Chau CH, Small EJ, editors. Drug management of prostate cancer. New York, NY: Springer; 2010. p. 375–86.
8. Paschos A, Pandya R, Duivenvoorden WC, Pinthus JH. Oxidative stress in prostate cancer: changing research concepts towards a novel paradigm for prevention and therapeutics. Prostate Cancer Prostatic Dis. 2013;16:217–25.
9. Crawford ED. Epidemiology of prostate cancer. Urology. 2003;62(6 Suppl 1):3–12.
10. Stephenson RA. Population-based prostate cancer trends in the PSA era: data from the Surveillance, Epidemiology, and End Results (SEER) Program. Monogr Urol. 1998;19:3–19.
11. Falzarano SM, Magi–Galluzzi C. Prostate cancer staging and grading at radical prostatectomy over time. Adv Anat Pathol. 2011;18(2):159–64.
12. Moul JW, Wu H, Sun L, et al. Epidemiology of radical prostatectomy for localized prostate cancer in the era of prostate-specific antigen: an overview of the Department of Defense Center for Prostate Disease Research national database. Surgery. 2002;132(2):213–9.
13. Eggener SE, Scardino PT, Walsh PC, Han M, Partin AW, Trock BJ, Feng Z, Wood DP, Eastham JA, Yossepowitch O, Rabah DM, Kattan MW, Yu C, Klein EA, Stephenson AJ. Predicting 15-year prostate cancer specific mortality after radical prostatectomy. J Urol. 2011;185:869–75.
14. Gleason DF. Classification of prostatic carcinomas. Cancer Chemother Rep. 1966;50(3): 125–8.
15. Miller GJ, Cygan JM. Morphology of prostate cancer: the effects of multifocality on histological grade, tumor volume and capsule penetration. J Urol. 1994;152(5 Pt 2):1709–13.
16. Klotz L. Active surveillance for prostate cancer: a review. Curr Urol Rep. 2010;11(3): 165–71.
17. Gleason DF. Histological grading and clinical staging of prostatic carcinoma. In: Tannenbaum M, editor. Urologic pathology: the prostate. Philadelphia, PA: Lea & Febiger; 1977. p. 171–98.
18. Epstein JI, Allsbrook Jr WC, Amin MB, Egevad LL, ISUP Grading Committee. The 2005 International Society of Urological Pathology (ISUP) consensus conference on gleason grading of prostatic carcinoma. Am J Surg Pathol. 2005;29(9):1228–42.
19. Epstein JI. Gleason score 2-4 adenocarcinoma of the prostate on needle biopsy: a diagnosis that should not be made. Am J Surg Pathol. 2000;24(4):477–8.
20. Gilliland FD, Gleason DF, Hunt WC, Stone N, Harlan LC, Key CR. Trends in Gleason score for prostate cancer diagnosed between 1983 and 1993. J Urol. 2001;165:846–50.
21. Ghani KR, Grigor K, Tulloch DN, Bollina PR, McNeal SA. Trends in reporting Gleason score 1991 to 2001: changes in the pathologist's practice. Eur Urol. 2005;47:196–201.
22. Pan CC, Potter SR, Partin AW, Epstein JI. The prognostic significance of tertiary Gleason patterns of higher grade in radical prostatectomy specimens. A proposal to modify the Gleason grading system. Am J Surg Pathol. 2000;24:563–9.
23. Servoll E, Saeter T, Vlatkovic L, Lund T, Nesland J, Waaler G, Axcrona K, Beisland HO. Impact of a tertiary Gleason pattern 4 or 5 on clinical failure and mortality after radical prostatectomy for clinically localised prostate cancer. BJU Int. 2012;109(10):1489–94.

24. Miyamoto H, Hernandez DJ, Epstein JI. A pathological reassessment of organ-confined, Gleason score 6 prostatic adenocarcinomas that progress after radical prostatectomy. Hum Pathol. 2009;40(12):1693–8.
25. Pierorazio PM, Walsh PC, Partin AW, Epstein JI. Prognostic Gleason grade grouping: data based on the modified Gleason scoring system. BJU Int. 2013;111:753–60.
26. Sarbay BC, Kir G, Topal CS, Gumus E. Significance of the cribriform pattern in prostatic adenocarcinomas. Pathol Res Pract. 2014;210(9):554–7.
27. Iczkowski KA, Torkko KC, Kotnis GR, Wilson RS, Huang W, Wheeler TM, Abeyta AM, La Rosa FG, Cook S, Werahera PN, Lucia MS. Digital quantification of five high-grade prostate cancer patterns, including the cribriform pattern, and their association with adverse outcome. Am J Clin Pathol. 2011;136:98–107.
28. Sved PD, Gomez P, Manoharan M, Kim SS, Soloway MS. Limitations of biopsy Gleason grade: implications for counseling patients with biopsy Gleason score 6 prostate cancer. J Urol. 2004;172(1):98–102.
29. King CR, McNeal JE, Gill H, Presti Jr JC. Extended prostate biopsy scheme improves reliability of Gleason grading: implications for radiotherapy patients. Int J Radiat Oncol Biol Phys. 2004;59(2):386–91.
30. Guimaraes MS, Billis A, Quintal MM, et al. The impact of the 2005 International Society of Urological Pathology (ISUP) consensus conference on standard Gleason grading of prostatic carcinoma. Mod Pathol. 2006;19:139A.
31. Zareba P, Zhang J, Yilmaz A, Trpkov K. The impact of the 2005 International Society of Urological Pathology (ISUP) consensus on Gleason grading in contemporary practice. Histopathology. 2009;55:384–91.
32. Stamey TA, McNeal JE, Yemoto CM, Sigal BM, Johnstone IM. Biological determinants of cancer progression in men with prostate cancer. JAMA. 1999;281:1395–400.
33. Jack GS, Cookson MS, Coffey CS, Vader V, Roberts RL, Chang SS, Smith Jr JA, Shappell SB. Pathological parameters of radical prostatectomy for clinical stages T1c versus T2 adenocarcinoma: decreased pathological stage and increased detection of transition zone tumors. J Urol. 2002;168:519–24.
34. Algaba F, Montironi R. Impact of prostate cancer multifocality on its biology and treatment. J Endourol. 2010;24(5):799–804.
35. Karavitakis M, Ahmed HU, Abel PD, Hazell S, Winkler M. Tumor focality in prostate cancer: implications for focal therapy. Nat Rev Clin Oncol. 2011;8(1):48–55.
36. Liu J, Lau SK, Varma VA, Moffitt RA, Caldwell M, Liu T, Young AN, Petros JA, Osunkoya AO, Krogstad T, Leyland-Jones B, Wang MD, Nie S. Molecular mapping of tumor heterogeneity on clinical tissue specimens with multiplexed quantum dots. ACS Nano. 2010;4:2755–65.
37. Lindberg J, Klevebring D, Liu W, Neiman M, Wiklund F, Mills IG, Egevad L, Gronberg H. Exome sequencing of prostate cancer supports the hypothesis of independent tumour origins. Eur Urol. 2013;63:347–53.
38. Sundi D, Kryvenko ON, Carter HB, Ross AE, Epstein JI, Schaeffer EM. Pathological examination of radical prostatectomy specimens in men with very low risk disease at biopsy reveals distinct zonal distribution of cancer in black American men. J Urol. 2014;191(1):60–7.
39. Presti JC. Prostate biopsy: current status and limitations. Rev Urol. 2007;9(3):93–8.
40. Raja J, Ramachandran N, Munneke G, Patel U. Current status of transrectal ultrasound-guided prostate biopsy in the diagnosis of prostate cancer. Clin Radiol. 2006;61(2):142–53.
41. Quann P, Jarrard DF, Huang W. Current prostate biopsy protocols cannot reliably identify patients for focal therapy: correlation of low-risk prostate cancer on biopsy with radical prostatectomy findings. Int J Clin Exp Pathol. 2010;3(4):401–7.
42. Stamey TA, Freiha FS, McNeal JE, Redwine EA, Whittemore AS, Schmid HP. Localized prostate cancer: relationship of tumor volume to clinical significance for treatment of prostate cancer. Cancer. 1993;71(3 Suppl):933–8.
43. Epstein JI, Chan DW, Sokoll LJ, Walsh PC, Cox JL, Rittenhouse H, Wolfert R, Carter HB. Nonpalpable stage T1c prostate cancer: prediction of insignificant disease using free/total prostate specific antigen levels and needle biopsy findings. J Urol. 1998;160(6 Pt 2):2407–11.

44. Sengupta S, Blute ML, Bagniewski SM, Inman B, Leibovich BC, Slezak JM, Myers RP, Zincke H. After radical retropubic prostatectomy 'insignificant' prostate cancer has a risk of progression similar to low-risk 'significant' cancer. BJU Int. 2008;101(2):170–4.
45. Epstein JI, Walsh PC, Carmichael M, Brendler CB. Pathologic and clinical findings to predict tumor extent of nonpalpable (stage T1c) prostate cancer. JAMA. 1994;271(5):368–74.
46. Van den Bergh RC, Roemeling S, Roobol MJ, Aus G, Hugosson J, Rannikko AS, Tammela TL, Bangma CH, Schroder FH. Outcomes of men with screen-detected prostate cancer eligible for active surveillance who were managed expectantly. Eur Urol. 2009;55:1–8.
47. Soloway MS, Soloway CT, Eldefrawy A, Acosta K, Kava B, Manoharan M. Careful selection and close monitoring of low-risk prostate cancer patients on active surveillance minimizes the need for treatment. Eur Urol. 2010;58:831–5.
48. Adamy A, Yee DS, Matsushita K, Maschino A, Cronin A, Vickers A, Guillonneau B, Scardino PT, Eastham JA. Role of prostate specific antigen and immediate confirmatory biopsy in predicting progression during active surveillance for low risk prostate cancer. J Urol. 2011;185:477–82.
49. Whitson JM, Porten SP, Hilton JF, Cowan JE, Perez N, Cooperberg MR, Greene KL, Meng MV, Simko JP, Shinohara K, Carroll PR. The relationship between prostate specific antigen change and biopsy progression in patients on active surveillance for prostate cancer. J Urol. 2011;185:1656–60.
50. Kim TH, Jeon HG, Choo SH, Jeong BC, Seo SI, Jeon SS, Choi HY, Lee HM. Pathological upgrading and upstaging of patients eligible for active surveillance according to currently used protocols. Int J Urol. 2014;21:377–81.
51. Iremashvili V, Pelaez L, Manoharan M, Jorda M, Rosenberg DL, Soloway MS. Pathologic cancer characteristics in patients eligible for active surveillance: a head-to-head comparison of contemporary protocols. Eur Urol. 2012;62:462–8.
52. Crawford ED, Wilson SS, Torkko KC, Hirano D, Stewart JS, Brammell C, Wilson RS, Kawata N, Sullivan H, Lucia MS, Werahera PN. Clinical staging of prostate cancer: a computer-simulated study of transperineal prostate biopsy. BJU Int. 2005;96:999–1004.
53. Barqawi AB, Rove KO, Gholizadeh S, O'Donnell CI, Koul H, Crawford ED. The role of 3-dimensional mapping biopsy in decision making for treatment of apparent early stage prostate cancer. J Urol. 2011;186:80–5.
54. Crawford ED, Rove KO, Barqawi AB, Maroni PD, Werahera PN, Baer CA, Koul HK, Rove CA, Lucia MS, La Rosa FG. Clinical-pathologic correlation between transperineal mapping biopsies of the prostate and three-dimensional reconstruction of prostatectomy specimens. Prostate. 2013;73:778–87.
55. Cuzick J, Berney DM, Fisher G, Mesher D, Moller H, Reid JE, Perry M, Park J, Younus A, Gutin A, Foster CS, Scardino P, Lanchbury JS, Stone S, Transatlantic Prostate Group. Prognostic value of a cell cycle progression signature for prostate cancer death in a conservatively managed needle biopsy cohort. Br J Cancer. 2012;106:1095–9.
56. Bishoff JT, Freedland SJ, Gerber L, Tennstedt P, Reid J, Welbourn W, Graefen M, Sangale Z, Tikishvili E, Park J, Younus A, Gutin A, Lanchbury JS, Sauter G, Brawer M, Stone S, Schlomm T. Prognostic utility of the cell cycle progression score generated from biopsy in men treated with prostatectomy. J Urol. 2014;192:409–14.
57. Knezevic D, Goddard AD, Natraj N, Cherbavaz DB, Clark-Langone KM, Snable J, Watson D, Falzarano SM, Magi–Galluzzi C, Klein EA, Quale C. Analytical validation of the oncotype DX prostate cancer assay – a clinical RT-PCR assay optimized for prostate needle biopsies. BMC Genomics. 2013;14:690.
58. Klein EA, Cooperberg MR, Magi–Galluzzi C, Simko JP, Falzarano SM, Maddala T, Chan JM, Li J, Cowan JE, Tsiatis A, Cherbavaz DB, Pelham RJ, Tenggara-Hunter I, Baehner FL, Knezevic D, Febbo PG, Shak S, Kattan MW, Lee M, Carroll PR. A 17-gene assay to predict prostate cancer aggressiveness in the context of Gleason grade heterogeneity, tumor mulitfocality, and biopsy undersampling. Eur Urol. 2014;66:550–60.

Chapter 3
Clinical Risk Prediction Tools for Prostate Cancer: TNM to CAPRA—Should Risk Be Redefined?

Michael S. Leapman and Matthew R. Cooperberg

Introduction: Rationale for Consistent Risk Stratification in Research and Clinical Practice

Prostate cancer is a remarkably heterogeneous disease, ranging from a slow-growing, organ-confined tumor to an aggressive malignancy capable of metastasis and death [1]. Uniform treatment of all individuals with newly diagnosed prostate cancer each year—some 240,000 men in the United States alone—would expose many with indolent tumors to the morbidities of treatment and would not effect cure for many with aggressive disease [2, 3]. From this vantage, accurate risk stratification—approximating extant disease and future behavior—is of clear importance: clinicians may tailor the method and intensity of treatment and provide patients useful prognostic information during counseling. Those with a sufficiently high probability of favorable risk profiles may opt for surveillance strategies, while those at higher risk can be guided towards a growing array of interventions, perhaps applied in combination as appropriate.

The value of accurate risk prediction tools applies to both clinical decision making and in the design and interpretation of research studies. Given the biological basis for variable clinical phenotypes it is critically important that accurate methods are used to stratify study subjects, thereby delineating participants by disease status.

M.S. Leapman, M.D.
Department of Urology, University of California, San Francisco,
550 16th Street, 6th Floor, Box 1695, San Francisco, CA 94109, USA

M.R. Cooperberg, M.D., M.P.H. (✉)
Department of Epidemiology, University of California, San Francisco,
550 16th Street, 6th Floor, Box 1695, San Francisco, CA 94109, USA

Epidemiology & Biostatistics, University of California, San Francisco,
550 16th Street, 6th Floor, Box 1695, San Francisco, CA 94109, USA
e-mail: Matthew.cooperberg@ucsf.edu

N.N. Stone, E.D. Crawford (eds.), *The Prostate Cancer Dilemma*,
DOI 10.1007/978-3-319-21485-6_3

Beyond limiting the heterogeneity within research cohorts and offering "apples to apples" comparisons, consistency in risk assessment is increasingly important for optimal interpretation of the many emerging prognostic assays which are intended to be interpreted within the context of standard clinical risk assessment.

Paralleling our understanding of the complexity of prostate cancer outcomes, an expanding selection of tools have been developed that enable researchers and clinicians to stratify men with prostate cancer, or at risk for its diagnosis. These range from classically utilized staging tools including digital rectal examination (DRE), biopsy histopathology (Gleason score), and serum assays (prostate-specific antigen, PSA) to modern iterations of biomarkers (e.g., Kallikrein-related peptidase 2, and [-2]proPSA), tissue-based gene expression tests, and advanced imaging. A clear benefit exists in the integration of multiple clinically relevant factors that function to offer improvements in risk estimation that surpass single variables alone.

As a result, a trove of clinical risk prediction tools has been presented in the urological literature. In 2008 Shariat and colleagues published a compendium of 111 prediction models relating to prostate cancer outcomes [4], and this number has grown considerably since that time; a conservative estimate may be obtained from a PubMed search for "prostate cancer nomogram" which offers over several hundred articles addressing risk prediction. These include tools to stratify individuals in numerous disease contexts including pathological outcomes at surgery, likelihood of biochemical recurrence (BCR) or mortality following treatment, to functional recovery after definitive intervention. In this chapter we will review the trajectory of risk prediction tools in prostate cancer, from early clinical staging schema, to the integration of multivariate models and novel assays receiving present-day assessment and clinical utilization. We argue that while risk classification systems like the D'Amico/AUA/NCCN risk groups are still widely used, they are inadequate for use in contemporary practice for a variety of reasons and should be replaced with validated, multivariable risk stratification tools.

Principles of Instrument Evaluation

Risk prediction tools reflect the population from which they are derived. The criteria used to evaluate these instruments relate to the characteristics of their development, observed performance, and ease of use. These considerations are therefore relevant to their utilization, in that one must consider whether a clinical or research context maintains a meaningful resemblance to the conditions under which a risk stratification tool was devised. Properties of risk instruments used in their critical appraisal include *discrimination*, *calibration*, *applicability*, *validation*, and *parsimony*.

The *discrimination* of a particular risk assessment tool refers to its accuracy in the prediction of a specified endpoint. This may be seen as a statistical measure of the likelihood of experiencing a particular clinical outcome. Naturally, a perfect model would offer 100 % accuracy; it would predict the result in all instances (sensitivity) without incorrectly identifying negative results as positive (specificity). Overall discriminatory ability reflects the likelihood of predicting an event across all risk thresholds and may be nonuniform among lower and higher risk patients, for example [5]. Common measures of discrimination include receiver operating characteristic (ROC) curve analysis for binary outcomes (e.g., does a diagnostic test identify the cancer) and Harrell's concordance (c) index for survival analysis analyzing outcomes over time.

Calibration refers to an objective assessment of observed versus predicted outcomes based on a model, offering a valuable indication of performance in various settings. Calibration plots can be generated that depict predicted and observed frequencies among training or discovery cohorts as well as external validation populations. A given instrument might have high discrimination in that it will consistently identify which man in a pair is more likely to have an adverse outcome—but simultaneously poor calibration if it is consistently over-optimistic or under-optimistic across a range of risk strata.

Standard metrics of discrimination (ROC or c-index) that provide an aggregate measure of a risk instrument's ability to predict a desired outcome may be alone inadequate to gauge the broader implications of its clinical implementation. Management decisions vary considerably by perceived disease risk level, in addition to other factors including age, comorbid conditions, and patient preference. Therefore, the true performance of a risk prediction model may best be viewed as dynamic, and varying by risk and benefit levels. The decision curve analysis (DCA) method has been advanced as a statistical means to evaluate the benefit of a particular test in influencing decision making across a spectrum of hypothetical probability thresholds [6]. This modeling approach was initially conceived for the evaluation of prediction models and has since been applied to numerous diagnostic and prognostic schema. Applied to newly diagnosed prostate cancer, *net benefit* reflects the difference between anticipated benefit (treatment efficacy) and anticipated harm (cost, morbidity, inconvenience), while *probability thresholds* represent a scaled probability of predictive accuracy of a particular instrument that may lead to treatment. DCA curves offer an opportunity to graphically compare risk prediction tools, plotting *net benefit* on the *Y*-axis, and *probability threshold* on the *X*-axis [7]. In comparison, an instrument of superior performance will possess the highest net benefit across a range of probabilities; some may demonstrate greater value in all situations, while others may appear advantageous within particular thresholds of probability.

Applicability refers to the generalizability of an instrument to other study populations or samples. Because prostate cancer incidence, treatment, and outcomes vary considerably among various factors including year of diagnosis, patient age, and race, one must also therefore be mindful of the population from which a particular risk prediction instrument is derived [8, 9]. For example, models drawn from patients in the pre-PSA era may not perform equally well today, where early detection has driven a migration in favor of earlier stage disease. The same is true for many clinical risk tools that were created in academic institutions and draw from high-volume centers that may not apply equally in clinical practice. Because nonuniformity among various populations must be expected, the evaluation of clinical instruments should occur in an initial development or training set that reflects the initial test population and should be also evaluated in an external *validation* study. Such measures ensure that the findings of a discovery phase are not limited to the circumstances and particularities of that population and serve to provide an evaluation of the viability of the instrument, as well a secondary assessment of applicability.

The *parsimony* of a particular test is a qualitative judgment of its complexity in practical application. Seen from the perspective of real-world utilization, it is important that the number of variables entered and the interpretation of these factors are not overly cumbersome. In the research setting, intricate models may not appear as limiting as their computation may be performed by most statistical platforms used in clinical research—though even in research, a cumbersome or opaque instrument may be difficult to validate, reproduce, or apply in other settings. However, in the attempt to provide crossover to clinical practice, complex instruments that require the iterative performance of calculations for individual patient will likely not see uptake in the face of simpler methods. Increasingly, as a function of the diffusion of handheld devices, prostate cancer nomograms have been offered on smartphone devices that seek to offer added convenience and portability—but even using such an application may still be seen as a break in the clinic workflow, depending on the speed and performance of the software. As such, a balance is to be struck between accounting maximally for all clinically relevant variables that may offer value in predicting an outcome while simultaneously providing a nimble and intuitive system that will enjoy broad appeal.

TNM Staging

Early attempts at estimating prognosis were performed on the basis of clinical stage and histological grade [10, 11]. The 1992 American Joint Committee on Cancer (AJCC) tumor, lymph node, metastasis (TNM) staging classification was updated from the 1987 system which grouped prostate cancer histologic diagnosis by T1a versus T1b: greater than or less than three microscopic foci, and T2a versus 2b based on size threshold of 1.5 cm (Table 3.1) [12]. The 1992 update (since modified in 2002 and most recently in 2010) categorizes nonpalpable/nonvisible lesions as T1, and palpable/visible lesions as T2. It is important to stress that subdividing stage T2 is based on physical exam and imaging, not biopsy findings. It is common for stage to be misreported, for example, as T2c based on the bilateral presence of disease on biopsy, when in fact this designation actually requires visible or palpable disease on both sides of the prostate [13]. In any event, clinical stage has proved a relatively unimportant prognostic factor, compared to PSA, Gleason grade, and measures of tumor burden which are better proxies for tumor volume than clinical stage [14].

Table 3.1 Comparison of the American Joint Commission on Cancer Tumor, Lymph Node, Metastasis (TNM) clinical staging systems

1987		1992, 2002, 2010	
T1	Incidental histologic finding	T1	Clinically unapparent; tumor not palpable or visible by imaging
T1a	$\leq$3 microscopic foci	T1a	Incidental finding $\leq$5 % of tissue resected
T1b	>3 microscopic foci	T1b	Incidental finding in >5 % of tissue resected
T2	Palpable tumor, limited to the gland	T1c	Tumor identified by needle biopsy (e.g., because of elevated PSA)
T2a	Tumor $\leq$1.5 cm	T2	Tumor confined within prostate (palpable or visible on TRUS)
T2b	Tumor >1.5 cm or in more than one lobe	T2a	Involves half of a lobe or less
T3	Tumor invades apex, into or beyond capsule, bladder neck, or seminal vesicle	T2b	Involves more than half of a lobe but not both lobes
		T2c	Tumor involves both lobes
		T3	Tumor extends through prostatic capsule
		T3a	Unilateral extracapsular extension
		T3b	Bilateral extracapsular extension
		T3c	Tumor invades seminal vesicle(s)

Used with permission of the American Joint Committee on Cancer (AJCC), Chicago, Illinois. The original and primary source for this information is the AJCC Cancer Staging Manual, Seventh Edition (2010) published by Springer Science+Business Media

Epstein Criteria

The Epstein criteria, described initially in 1994, remain a commonly utilized rubric for defining "insignificant" prostate cancer, specifying tumor volume <0.2 cm^3, absent Gleason pattern 4 or 5, and clinically organ-confined disease (<cT3) as insignificant, and tumors between 0.2 and 0.5 cm^3 as minimally significant. This framework was developed by Epstein and colleagues from patients with nonpalpable ($\leq$T1c) prostate cancer treated with prostatectomy at the Johns Hopkins Medical Center, where tumor volume estimates were derived from observational studies of palpable tumors without extraprostatic extension or BCR at 5-year follow-up [15–17]. Many have argued that these criteria are too restrictive, and that tumors of larger volume, if low grade and organ confined, may be equally indolent as those under 0.5 cc [18, 19].

The Johns Hopkins investigators have also proposed an expanded criteria including: PSA density <0.15 ng/mL, Gleason score <7, fewer than two cores positive for tumor, no single core with >50 % prostate cancer involvement, and clinically organ-confined ($\leq$cT2) disease. This model was evaluated in a case series of 157 men with

T1c disease, where the positive predictive and negative predictive values were 95 and 66 %, respectively. Overall, the yield for prediction of insignificant and minimal cancer was 73 % [20]. A clear advantage of such criteria is the ability to render a dichotomous judgment based on intuitive and easy to mobilize clinical variables. However, these are also very restrictive criteria, and in longitudinal assessment, the Epstein criteria have been questioned in their ability to predict more meaningful prostate cancer endpoints beyond pathological stage alone [21].

Risk Groupings

Many of the commonly utilized pretreatment risk groupings offer easy to conceptualize (and to calculate) classification schemes that broadly distinguish patients with Prostate cancer on empiric clinical criteria. The rationale for their development reflects the integration of PSA testing as well as the ascendency and standardization of the Gleason histological classification schemes. These schemata include the D'Amico classification, and its modifications reflected in the American Urological Association (AUA) and National Comprehensive Caner Network (NCCN) risk classifications.

D'Amico

The D'Amico classification system was initially proposed in 1998 as a means to stratify patients according to risk of BCR following treatment with radical prostatectomy, external beam radiotherapy, or brachytherapy. These groupings are defined on the basis of biopsy Gleason score, categorical PSA, and clinical stage. Low risk includes individuals with PSA $\leq$10ng/mL, stage $\leq$cT2a, *and* Gleason $\leq 3+3$; intermediate risk includes those with stage T2b, PSA >10 and $\leq$20 ng/ml, *or* Gleason 7; and high risk includes those with stage $\geq$T2c, PSA >20, *or* Gleason score $\geq$8 [22]. A subsequent validation study was performed in a cohort of 1100 patients treated at Brigham and Women's Hospital with radical prostatectomy. In a Cox regression model, the relative risk for biochemical failure after treatment was 3.3 for intermediate versus low disease, and 6.3 for high versus low categories [23]. Numerous additional studies have emerged in recent years that demonstrate a consistent and statistically significant stratification among group, though reflect the well-known stage migration associated with early detection and efficacious treatment [24–26].

   In a critical appraisal, the D'Amico risk groups are clearly exemplary in their ease of use and parsimony. The initial groupings require no calculation to be performed and can readily be recalled by providers in a clinical context. Yet while validation studies have demonstrated that separation of outcomes does indeed exist, the discriminative ability and accuracy of this three-tiered scheme is suboptimal due to the heterogeneity within these groupings. This effect, termed spectrum bias, is illustrated by Pierorazio et al., among others, who demonstrated that among patients meeting D'Amico criteria for high-risk disease, there is considerable variability in outcomes determined by the number of criteria that are possessed [27–30]. There are multiple reasons for this: the classification over-weights T-stage which, as noted above, is frequently inaccurate. It also fails to distinguish Gleason 3 + 4 from 4 + 3 disease; if anything Gleason 7 disease should be considered at even more granular levels [31]. Most importantly, the risk groupings do not comprise a true multivariable model. A patient with a Gleason 3 + 4, PSA 4.1, cT2a tumor and one with a Gleason 4 + 3, PSA 18.3, cT2b tumor are both classified as "intermediate" risk.

Moreover, it has become clear that other pretreatment factors add additional value in the prediction of prostate cancer outcome. Lee et al. reported on the presence of >50 % positive biopsies for cancer as associated with pathologic upgrading at surgery and poorer BCR free survival outcomes among a concordance testing of 427 patients treated with RP within the low-risk category [32]. Further refinements to this classification scheme based on tumor volume within low and intermediate categories based on tumor volume were also made based on data from prostatectomy patients [33].

AUA and NCCN Risk Groupings

Risk groupings in the style of the D'Amico classification are employed by the American Urological Association (AUA) and National Comprehensive Cancer Network (NCCN) Guidelines for prostate cancer [34, 35]. The AUA and NCCN provide risk groupings in the context of management guidelines and differ from the D'Amico classification in that the systems were not subject to validation within a training or external dataset. Thus, the rationale by which the clinical criteria were selected reflects a consensus of relevant variables but was not derived from a multivariate model attuned to a particular endpoint. One important difference is that stage T2c is not assigned to high risk under the NCCN or AUA classifications. Updates to the NCCN Guidelines for Prostate Cancer Initial Clinical Assessment and Staging Evaluation seek to add discrimination between categories and specify five groupings: very low, low, intermediate, high, and very high risk. These groupings incorporate numerous clinical criteria derived from individual variables that bear prognostic significance, yet are not shared among all categories.

This is perhaps best illustrated by examining the distinction between very low- and low-risk disease, where "very low risk" is specified by men possessing *all of the following*: clinical stage T1c, biopsy Gleason score ≤6, PSA <10 ng/mL, less than three biopsy cores with disease, ≤50 % prostate cancer in any single core, and PSA density <0.15 ng/ml/g. In contrast, low-risk patients are defined as clinical T1–T2a, Gleason ≤6, PSA <10 without a designation of tumor volume or PSA density [36]. These criteria are similar to the Epstein "insignificant disease" criteria discussed above, but have not been externally validated. While the rationale for these groupings is individually evidence based, an important caveat must be applied for the use of these groupings to generate probabilistic determinations of outcome, be they for the purposes of clinical counseling or research. It is critical to emphasize that while these risk classification systems are still widely used, they ultimately are inadequate for all the reasons delineated above, and going forward, prostate cancer risk really must be considered and assessed using a true multivariable instrument.

Nomograms

In this context of prediction instruments, a *nomogram* refers to a graphic depiction of a risk calculation formula that is typically derived from multivariate models yielding quantitative estimates of a proposed outcome. As a result, such tools provide a clear benefit over risk groupings in the prediction of treatment outcomes after surgery or radiotherapy and have been used to predict BCR, metastatic progression, and cancer-specific mortality (CSM). They are usually generated from time-dependent survival models (e.g., Cox proportional hazards) or statistical classification models (e.g., logistic regression), as appropriate. The consequence of incorporating *continuous* variables is that nomograms limit spectrum bias by accounting for the contribution of variables along a range of values, as opposed to groupings where values are dichotomized.

In 1998 Kattan and colleagues reported on a nomogram to predict biochemical recurrence 5 years following radical prostatectomy. The authors evaluated clinical data associated with BCR in a Cox proportional hazards model comprised of 983 men treated with RP for clinically localized prostate cancer between 1983 and 1996 including 196 experiencing PSA failure, yielding an area under the ROC curve (AUC) of 0.79 [37]. This initial model incorporated PSA (scaled 0.1–110), clinical stage, and biopsy Gleason score and has since received external validation in various settings [38]. In these assessments, the Kattan nomogram has demonstrated robust performance as a risk prediction instrument in the academic setting, with slightly lower discrimination in a community-based cohort (c-index = 0.68), potentially reflecting bias within the training set from which it was derived [39, 40].

A multitude of nomograms have since emerged in the style of Kattan, often applying a similar methodology to other prostate cancer endpoints including likelihood of seminal vesicle or lymph node invasion at prostatectomy, BCR, and metastatic progression after radiation therapy or surgery [41–45]. A plain benefit to the use of nomograms is the ability to offer a visual depiction of generated risk scores as well as an appreciation for the constituent components of the model. Moreover, nomograms clearly represent a step forward as compared with risk groupings with respect to methodology and discrimination. Ultimately, though, nomograms have not gained widespread acceptance in clinical practice, an observation that may be attributable to their requirement of a multi-step paper instrument or computer software, as well as the necessity of obtaining abstruse code for large-scale calculations in an academic setting, since the regression equations underlying the nomograms are rarely published.

Because they are usually derived from high-volume academic cohorts, nomograms tend to calibrate suboptimally—specifically they tend to be over-optimistic in their predictions for any given outcome when validated in a community-based setting [46]. The other problem is that nomogram generation has become very simple, requiring no more than a single command issued to standard statistical software following a regression procedure. This phenomenon has fed a proliferation of nomograms, most of which are never validated, and very few of which actually find their way into either clinical practice or subsequent research studies.

UCSF-CAPRA Score

In 2005, the Cancer of the Prostate Risk Assessment (CAPRA) Score was developed at the University of California San Francisco (UCSF) in response to the growing appreciation of an unmet need for a risk prediction instrument that offers robust performance, yet can be applied without the necessity of a drawn paper tool or online calculator. The cohort used for initial development set was the Cancer of the Prostate Strategic Urologic Research Endeavor (CaPSURE), a community practice database drawing from over 40 US sites with longitudinal follow-up. This initial cohort included 1439 men diagnosed with prostate cancer between 1992 and 2001 who received treatment with radical prostatectomy without neoadjuvant or adjuvant radiation therapy or hormonal therapy. Significant clinical factors associated with BCR or secondary treatment in a Cox proportional hazards regression model included age, pretreatment PSA, Gleason score, percentage of biopsy cores positive for cancer, and clinical stage. The resulting 10-point system, designed to provide an approximate doubling of risk with every 2-point increase in the total score, is derived from logarithmic parameter estimates yielded in the final Cox model. The final system is detailed in Table 3.2. Strong correlations were seen between the UCSF-CAPRA score and the D'Amico and Kattan tools, and the c-index appeared comparable for all: CAPRA (0.66), D'Amico (0.63), and Kattan nomogram (0.65) [47].

Several external validations of the CAPRA score have been performed to date. Among a racially diverse Veterans Affairs and military population of 1346 men, the c-index for the prediction of clinical recurrence after RP was 0.68 [48]. The CAPRA score has performed slightly better in external validation studies from academic institutions (c-index 0.76–0.81), a finding that appears to invert the findings of nomograms derived from academic cohorts in community-based populations [40, 49–51]. It should also be stressed, with respect to calibration, that the CAPRA score is intended to indicate *relative* rather than *absolute* risk. For example, a patient with a CAPRA score of 4 or 2 may have better outcomes in a high-volume academic center than in a lower volume community context, but a patient with the score of 4 will always have higher risk of recurrence and progression than a patient with the score of 2.

In addition, the CAPRA score has been externally evaluated in international populations (Table 3.3) [50, 52]. Beyond BCR, the CAPRA score has also been validated to predict pathological stage, as well as significant oncological endpoints including metastatic progression and prostate cancer mortality (PCSM) following treatment [53]. The CAPRA score is also one of the only risk stratification systems

Table 3.2 PScoring systems for the Cancer of the Prostate Risk Assessment (CAPRA), CAPRA-S, and J-CAPRA tools

CAPRA		CAPRA-S		J-CAPRA	
Variable	*Points*	*Variable*	*Points*	*Variable*	*Points*
Age (years)		*Margin status*		*Biopsy Gleason score*	
<50	0	Negative	0	3+3	0
≥50	1	Positive	2	3+4/4+3	1
				8–10	2
PSA (ng/mL)		*PSA (ng/mL)*		*PSA (ng/mL)*	
<6	0	0–6	0	0–20	0
6.1–10	1	6.01–10	1	>20–100	1
10.1–20	2	10.01–20	2	>100–500	2
20.1–30	3	>20	3	>500	3
>30	4				
Biopsy Gleason score		*Pathologic Gleason score*		*T-stage*	
1–3/1–3	0	2–6	0	≤T2a	0
1–3/4–5	1	3+4	1	≤T3a	1
4–5/1–5	3	4+3	2	T3b	2
		8–10	3	T4	3
Percent of biopsy cores positive for cancer		*Seminal vesicle invasion*		*N-stage*	
<34 %	0	No	0	N1	1
≥34 %	1	Yes	2		
T-stage		*Extracapsular extension*		*M-stage*	
T1/T2	0	No	0	M1	3
≥T3a	1	Yes	1		
		Lymph node invasion			
		No	0		
		Yes	1		
Sum of all points	/10		/12		/12

to have been evaluated successfully following prostatectomy, radiation therapy, hormonal therapy, and other management approaches [48, 54–56].

A 2013 meta-analysis of seven studies evaluating the prediction of risk among trichotomized categories—low risk (0–2), intermediate risk (3–5), and high risk (6–10)—recapitulated the ability of the CAPRA score to predict clinical recurrence after RP, though appeared to suggest an underprediction of risk at 5 years [57]. It should be noted though that while these risk groupings represent validated compressions, the CAPRA score represents a *near continuous* risk prediction model and the meta-analysis did not look at these groupings. Variability in the performance among cohorts may also be related to the quality of the clinical data utilized in the model, considerations which are less of an issue for variables that are reliably *measured* (i.e., age, PSA) a significant factor to consider with respect to Gleason score,

Table 3.3 External validation studies of the UCSF CAPRA, CAPRA-S, and J-CAPRA risk assessment instruments

Instrument	Author, year	Country	N	Setting	Endpoint	Performance
CAPRA	Coopberberg [48], 2006	USA	1346	Veterans affairs/ SEARCH	BCR after RP	c-index 0.68
	May [50], 2007	Germany	1296	Academic	BCR after RP	c-index 0.81 (7-grouped CAPRA score); 0.78, three-tiered CAPRA score[a]
	Zhao [49], 2008	USA	6737	Academic	BCR after RP	c-index 0.78
	Lughezzani [52], 2010	Germany	1976	Academic	BCR after RP	3- and 5-year c-index 0.743, 0.729 respectively
	Halverson [56], 2011	USA	612	Academic	5-year BCR after EBRT	c-index 0.69
	Ishizaki [73], 2011	Japan	211	Academic	5-year BCR after RP	c-index 0.755
	Tamblyn [74], 2011	Australia	635	Academic	BCR after RP	c-index 0.787
	Budäus [75], 2012	Germany	2937	Academic	BCR, MR after RP	BCRFS: c-index 0.762; MR: c-index 0.785
	Yoshida [76], 2012	Japan	503	Academic	5-year BCR after RP	BCRFS: c-index 0.673
	Krishnan [55], 2014	Canada	345	Academic	BCR after EBRT or LDR BT	HR per continuous CAPRA score 1.37 (95 % CI 1.10–1.72, $p=0.006$)
	Seo [77], 2014	Korea	115	Academic	BCR after RP	3- and 5-year: c-index 0.74, 0.77, respectively
	Delouya [54], 2014	Canada	744	Academic	BCR after EBRT or BT	AUC 3-year BCRFS 0.66; 5-year, 0.62
CAPRA-S	Seong [78], 2013	Korea	134	Academic	5-year BCRFS	c-index 0.776
	Punnen [46], 2014	USA	2670	Veterans Affairs/ SEARCH	5-year BCR, CSM after RP	c-index, BCR 0.73; CSM, 0.85
	Cooperberg [79], 2014	USA	1010	Academic	PCSM	c-index 0.75
	Tilki [62], 2014	Germany	14,532	Academic	5-year BCR, metastasis, mortality	c-index, BCR: 0.80; metastasis: 0.85; CSM: 0.88

(continued)

Table 3.3 (continued)

Instrument	Author, year	Country	N	Setting	Endpoint	Performance
J-CAPRA	Seo [80], 2014	Korea	130	Academic	5-year PFS	c-index 0.80
	Kitagawa [81], 2013	Japan	319	Academic	PFS, PCSM	c-index CSS 0.833; OS, 0.665
	Akakura [82], 2014	Japan	426	Academic	10-year PFS, PCSM	Categories 1–2 (75.6, 98.9 %) versus 3–6 (52.6, 93.1 %), $p<0.001$ and $p=0.044$
	Shiota [83], 2015	Japan	248	Academic	PFS, PCSM, OS	c-index PFS 0.890; PCSM 0.836; OS 0.700
	Yamaguchi [84], 2015	Japan	255	Academic	PFS, PCSM, OS	c-index PFS 0.847; PCSM 0.820; OS 0.669

PSM positive surgical margins, *RFS* recurrence free survival, *c-index* concordance index, *RP* radical prostatectomy, *RARP* robotic assisted radical prostatectomy, *MR* metastatic recurrence, *BT* brachytherapy, *EBRT* external beam radiation therapy, *PCSM* prostate cancer-specific mortality, *SEARCH* Shared Equal Access Regional Cancer Hospital
[a]Three-tiered CAPRA score (0–2 = low risk; 3–5 = intermediate risk; 6–10 = high risk)

clinical stage, and the percentage of biopsy cores positive which are subject to interpretation by clinicians [58].

The CAPRA score was designed to perform in research and clinical settings, and has been reflected in a system that can be calculated rapidly, without pen, paper, or computer, and may be committed to memory with relative ease, while functioning on par with other risk assessment instruments. Beyond calibration alone, prognostic tests are practically held to a standard that is proportional to their clinical value. Such insights may be appreciated by examining the DCA comparison of prostate cancer risk assessment tools. Lughezzani et al. compared calibration and DCA models among the D'Amico, Stephenson, and CAPRA instruments among 1976 patients among a European RP cohort. While the CAPRA and Stephenson systems demonstrated c-indices of 72.9 and 73.5 %, respectively, a benefit was seen with the CAPRA score, implying a potential advantage in clinical performance [52].

CAPRA-S

Following radical prostatectomy, the enhanced pathological staging information offered by surgery may often inform further management decisions based on the risk for recurrence or other ensuing events. The value of this new information has been previously incorporated in nomograms tailored to the post-RP setting [59, 60]. Kattan et al. first described a postoperative nomogram for disease recurrence derived from a

Cox proportional hazards regression analysis from a cohort of 996 men treated with RP [61]. The performance of this nomogram was excellent, with an AUC in an initial separate validation cohort of 332 men of 0.89, yet is subject to the same limitations in utilization and scalability that affect nomograms in the pretreatment setting.

The postsurgical CAPRA-S score was developed and published in 2011 as an analogous model to CAPRA that can be readily calculated on-demand, based largely on pathological data. Like CAPRA, the training set used for the development of CAPRA-S was a cohort of 3837 men from the CaPSURE database, where putative clinical and pathological variables were entered into a multivariate Cox proportional hazards model. These included categorical preoperative PSA (0–6; 6.01–10; 10.01–20; >20), pathological Gleason score (3+3; 3+4; 4+3; 8–10), as well the presence or absence of seminal vesicle invasive, positive surgical margins, extracapsular extension (pT3a), or lymph node positivity. The point values obtained for the final model were derived from the log hazard ratio parameter estimates, yielding a theoretical maximum of 12-point scale, though very few patients fall above 10, allowing scores ≥9 to be grouped together (Table 3.3). Within the initial analytic CaPSURE cohort, the bootstrap corrected c-index was 0.77 (95 % CI 0.75–0.79).

The CAPRA-S score has since been externally validated in US and international populations (Table 3.3). Punnen et al. performed a multi-institutional validation in the VA SEARCH database comprising 2670 with complete data and median follow-up of 58 months. In this ethnically diverse population, including 42 % non-Caucasians, the c-index for BCR was 0.73. In a DCA comparison to the Stephenson nomogram, the CAPRA-S demonstrated greater net benefit, particularly in situations of threshold probabilities >40 % [46]. The CAPRA-S score has also demonstrated robust performance in the prediction of downstream oncologic endpoints. Within the original validation set the sub-hazard ratio for PCSM per unit-increase in CAPRA-S was 1.42 (95 % CI 1.27–1.60); when applied to a European population, the c-index for BCR was 0.80, systemic progression (c-index 0.85), and for PCSM, 0.88 [62].

J-CAPRA

Prostate cancer screening has catalyzed a shift in the nature of disease at presentation, favoring the detection of clinically localized disease [63]. However, for patients with metastatic or locally advanced disease at presentation—accounting for approximately one-fifth of new diagnoses in Japan—treatment is initially approached with androgen deprivation therapy (ADT). While this approach is not endorsed by Western guidelines, it is endorsed and widely practiced in Asia. The J-CAPRA score was developed from data including CaPSURE and the Japan Study Group of Prostate Cancer (J-CaP) registries to offer risk estimation for patients receiving primary ADT, capturing nearly half of all Japanese men diagnosed with prostate cancer during the study period, as well as nearly *all* patients treated with ADT. The J-CAPRA score was derived from a Cox proportional hazards regression model of *progression free survival* (PFS). The J-CAPRA was thereby rendered using the following variables: Gleason score, PSA, T-stage, N-stage, and M-stage. The c-index for PFS was 0.71 in J-CaP; and 0.84 for PCSM among CaPSURE patients. A summary of J-CAPRA validation studies is presented in Table 3.3.

Future Directions: Novel Biomarkers, Gene Expression Testing, Advanced Imaging

Advances in the molecular and genetic characterization of prostate cancer have recently paid dividends in the form of novel assays that offer risk prediction in various settings. The pace of innovation appears to reflect an appreciation for the limitations of even the highest performing risk prediction instruments derived from standard clinical variables to accurately characterize all patients. To this end, progress has been seen on several fronts, including the nomination and assessment of new biomarkers that aim to mitigate the vaunted over-detection and over-treatment associated with contemporary PSA screening. Following diagnosis, opportunities exist to better characterize disease across risk spectra utilizing prostate magnetic resonance imaging (MRI) and tissue-based assays evaluating unique genomic signatures.

Prostate magnetic resonance imaging (MRI) interrogating multiple parameters including T2 intensity, dynamic contrast enhancement (DCE), diffusion weighted sequences, and magnetic resonance spectroscopy also represents a powerful tool for risk prognostication. The ability of baseline prostate MRI to predict non-organ-confined disease (pT3a) has been extensively studied and is subject to issues of nonstandardization relating to technology (3 Tesla versus 1.5 Tesla), interobserver variability, and sequences performed. Nomograms incorporating MRI and MRSI have demonstrated improved performance when compared to standard clinical models. Among 181 low D'Amico risk patients, the incorporation of MR findings into a basic clinical model consisting only of PSA, clinical stage, and biopsy Gleason score resulted in a significantly improved performance; however these differences were not maintained among a more sophisticated clinical model inclusive of the percentage of biopsy cores positive [64]. mpMRI has also demonstrated considerable potential to change risk prediction at the time of detection by facilitating MR-ultrasound fusion biopsy. This modality has shown improved detection of Gleason ≥ 7 tumors at biopsy though the optimal manner in which to incorporate the pathological data from these high-probability biopsies in existing risk prediction instruments remains to be determined [65, 66].

Tissue-based gene expression assays derived from genes highly associated with prostate cancer aggressiveness have also been developed that can assist in the prognostication of extant disease in various contexts including from prostate biopsy specimens or radical prostatectomy tissue. Central to the evaluation of these promising new tools is the benchmark for comparison where new assays are tasked to offer an improvement in risk assessment over currently available clinical instruments. Therefore, in the development and validation phases of study, it is particularly critical that subjects are appropriately stratified by the nature of their presumed risk.

A putative marker that merely associates with known risk factors may be interesting from a scientific standpoint but will have little clinical value; what is needed is tests that *improve* over a multivariable gold standard in terms of discrimination and/or calibration.

The Prolaris assay (Myriad Genetics, Salt Lake City, UT) generates a cell cycle progression score (CCP) derived from a 31 gene signature associated with prostate cancer outcome. In validation studies derived from archival biopsy radical prostatectomy specimens, the CCP score was associated with adverse outcomes after prostatectomy including BCR and metastatic progression [67, 68]. The importance of accurate clinical assessment is underscored in the evaluation of this assay, where the predictive performance was assessed in relation to CAPRA-S score. While the CCP score alone was not superior to the clinical model, a composite score (derived from a weighting of CAPRA-S and CCP) demonstrated improved performance across risk spectra, a benefit that was maintained as well for low-risk patients [69].

Decipher (GenomeDX Biosciences, San Diego, CA), a genomic classifier (GC) comprised of 22 genes highly associated with prostate cancer aggressiveness, developed from high density transcriptosome-wide microarrays and has been validated in a high-risk cohort for the prediction of metastatic progression after RP (AUC 0.79) [70]. In a subset of 185 high-risk patients from a cohort utilized for discovery and validation, CAPRA-S and the GC were independent predictors of PCMS (c-indices 0.75 and 0.78 respectively). While the combination of the two did not improve the AUC for predicting PCSM, the GC was able to further sub-stratify clinically high-risk men (CAPRA-S $\geq$6, $p<0.001$) as well as CAPRA-S to re-stratify high GC scores (>0.6, $p=0.005$) [71]. The findings gleaned from the Prolaris and Decipher studies serve to illustrate the value of improved methods to predict risk in the post-treatment setting where considerable heterogeneity in outcomes exists, even among patients with high-risk features by clinical criteria.

The Onco*type* DX Genomic Prostate Score (GPS) assay (Genomic Health, Redwood City, CA) utilizes a 17-gene signature, including 12 genes highly associated with prostate cancer outcome along four biological pathways. Amplification of minute tumor volumes (1 mm) yield quantitative gene expression levels that are calculated into a scaled (0–100) GPS score. In a validation study of 395 patients with CAPRA <5 disease and biopsy Gleason pattern $\leq$3+4, GPS score was compared against CAPRA score for the prediction of favorable pathology at radical prostatectomy (defined as Gleason pattern <4+3, and pathological stage <pT3a). The AUC for this endpoint was 0.63 for CAPRA alone, and improves to 0.67 in a model incorporating both GPS and CAPRA [72].

Tumor-based gene expression tests represent a new frontier for risk assessment in prostate cancer and have been adapted at all stages of disease, including clinically localized to locally advanced. While offering new insights, these do not supplant existing clinical models which appear to perform *nearly* as well, though net benefits have been projected in DCA modeling studies. One must also be mindful of the growing complexity and health care infrastructure expense that is associated with their development and widespread integration. Just as overly complex clinical models that offer strong predictive performance may not meet universal clinical utilization such considerations also apply to emerging biomarkers and tissue expression assays. Thus, while numerous platforms may seek to exist within these clinical spaces, those that offer strong clinical performance, parsimony, and intuitive use may be best suited to enjoy empiric success.

Conclusion

Clinical staging of prostate cancer is complex, reflecting the shifting sands of disease epidemiology, therapeutics, and an ever-expanding armamentarium of tools with which to estimate risk at various junctures of clinical impact. From early risk estimation models, relying on relatively crude means of digital rectal examination alone, to the integration of histopathology and biomarkers (PSA), risk prediction has evolved past risk groups to multivariable instruments integrating all known clinical information, with some models like the CAPRA score nearly as easy to apply as the risk groups. A new era of advancement, heralded by innovative leaps in biomarker validation, advanced imaging, and cancer genomics, is positioned to add predictive accuracy to clinical models and may deliver higher degrees of predictive certainty at several intersections of prostate cancer decision making.

References

1. Wyatt AW, Mo F, Wang K, et al. Heterogeneity in the inter-tumor transcriptome of high risk prostate cancer. Genome Biol. 2014;15(8):426.
2. Siegel R, Ma J, Zou Z, Jemal A. Cancer statistics, 2015. CA Cancer J Clin. 2015;65(1):5–29.
3. Resnick MJ, Koyama T, Fan KH, et al. Long-term functional outcomes after treatment for localized prostate cancer. N Engl J Med. 2013;368(5):436–45.
4. Shariat SF, Karakiewicz PI, Roehrborn CG, Kattan MW. An updated catalog of prostate cancer predictive tools. Cancer. 2008;113:3075–99.
5. Shariat SF, Karakiewicz PI, Margulis V, Kattan MW. Inventory of prostate cancer predictive tools. Curr Opin Urol. 2008;18(3):279–96.
6. Vickers AJ, Elkin EB. Decision curve analysis: a novel method for evaluating prediction models. Med Decis Making. 2006;26(6):565–74.
7. Fitzgerald M, Saville BR, Lewis RJ, et al. Decision curve analysis. JAMA. 2015;313(4):409–10.
8. Chu DI, Moreira DM, Gerber L, et al. Effect of race and socioeconomic status on surgical margins and biochemical outcomes in an equal-access health care setting: results from the Shared Equal Access Regional Cancer Hospital (SEARCH) database. Cancer. 2012;118(20):4999–5007.
9. Kattan MW. Comparison of Cox regression with other methods for determining prediction models and nomograms. J Urol. 2003;170(6 pt 2):S6–S9; discussion S10.
10. Gleason DF, Mellinger GT. Prediction of prognosis for prostatic adenocarcinoma by combined histological grading and clinical staging. J Urol. 1974;111(1):58–64.
11. Spigelman SS, McNeal JE, Freiha FS, Stamey TA. Rectal examination in volume determination of carcinoma of the prostate: clinical and anatomical correlations. J Urol. 1986;136(6):1228–30.

12. Edge S, Byrd DR, Compton CC, et al. American Joint Committee on Cancer staging manual. 7th ed. New York, NY: Springer; 2010.
13. Reese AC, Sadetsky N, Carroll PR, et al. Inaccuracies in assignment of clinical stage for localized prostate cancer. Cancer. 2011;117(2):283–9.
14. Reese AC, Cooperberg MR, Carroll PR. Minimal impact of clinical stage on prostate cancer prognosis among contemporary patients with clinically localized disease. J Urol. 2010;184(1):114–9.
15. Epstein JI, Pizov G, Walsh PC. Correlation of pathologic findings with progression following radical retropubic prostatectomy. Cancer. 1993;71:3582–93.
16. Bastian PJ, Mangold LA, Epstein JI, Partin AW. Characteristics of insignificant clinical T1c prostate tumors: a contemporary analysis. Cancer. 2004;101:2001–5.
17. Epstein JI, Carmichael M, Partin AW, Walsh PC. Is tumor volume an independent predictor of progression following radical prostatectomy? A multivariate analysis of 185 clinical stage B adenocarcinomas of the prostate with five years follow-up. J Urol. 1993;149:1478–81.
18. Wolters T, Roobol MJ, van Leeuwen PJ, et al. A critical analysis of the tumor volume threshold for clinically insignificant prostate cancer using a data set of a randomized screening trial. J Urol. 2011;185(1):121–5.
19. Porten SP, Cooperberg MR, Carroll PR. The independent value of tumour volume in a contemporary cohort of men treated with radical prostatectomy for clinically localized disease. BJU Int. 2010;105(4):472–5.
20. Epstein JI, Walsh PC, Carmichael M, Brendler CB. Pathologic and clinical findings to predict tumor extent of nonpalpable (stage T1c) prostate cancer. JAMA. 1994;271:368–74.
21. Lee MC, Dong F, Stephenson AJ, et al. The Epstein criteria predict for organ-confined but not insignificant disease and a high likelihood of cure at radical prostatectomy. Eur Urol. 2010;58(1):90–5.
22. D'Amico AV, Whittington R, Malkowicz SB, et al. Biochemical outcome after radical prostatectomy, external beam radiation therapy, or interstitial radiation therapy for clinically localized prostate cancer. JAMA. 1998;280:969–74.
23. D'Amico AV, Whittington R, Malkowicz SB, et al. Predicting prostate specific antigen outcome preoperatively in the prostate specific antigen era. J Urol. 2001;166:2185–8.
24. Boorjian SA, Karnes RJ, Rangel LJ. Mayo Clinic validation of the D'amico risk group classification for predicting survival following radical prostatectomy. J Urol. 2008;179(4):1354–60. discussion 1360-1.
25. Hernandez DJ, Nielsen ME, Han M, Partin AW. Contemporary evaluation of the D'amico risk classification of prostate cancer. Urology. 2007;70(5):931–5.
26. D'Amico AV, Whittington R, Malkowicz SB, et al. Pretreatment nomogram for prostate-specific antigen recurrence after radical prostatectomy or external-beam radiation therapy for clinically localized prostate cancer. J Clin Oncol. 1999;17(1):168–72.
27. Shariat SF, Karakiewicz PI, Suardi N, et al. Comparison of nomograms with other methods for predicting outcomes in prostate cancer: a critical analysis of the literature. Clin Cancer Res. 2008;14(14):4400–7.
28. Kattan MW. Nomograms. Introduction. Semin Urol Oncol. 2002;20:79–81.
29. Mitchell JA, Cooperberg MR, Elkin EP, et al. Ability of 2 pretreatment risk assessment methods to predict prostate cancer recurrence after radical prostatectomy: data from CaPSURE. J Urol. 2005;173(4):1126–31.
30. Pierorazio PM, Ross AE, Han M, et al. Evolution of the clinical presentation of men undergoing radical prostatectomy for high-risk prostate cancer. BJU Int. 2012;109(7):988–93.
31. Reese AC, Cowan JE, Brajtbord JS, et al. The quantitative Gleason score improves prostate cancer risk assessment. Cancer. 2012;118(24):6046–54.
32. Lee AK, Schultz D, Renshaw AA, et al. Optimizing patient selection for prostate monotherapy. Int J Radiat Oncol Biol Phys. 2001;49(3):673–7.
33. Lieberfarb ME, Schultz D, Whittington R, et al. Using PSA, biopsy Gleason score, clinical stage, and the percentage of positive biopsies to identify optimal candidates for prostate-only radiation therapy. Int J Radiat Oncol Biol Phys. 2002;53(4):898–903.

34. Mohler JL, Kantoff PW, Armstrong AJ, et al. Prostate cancer, version 2.2014. J Natl Compr Canc Netw. 2014;12(5):686–718.
35. American Urological Association Education and Research, Inc. (AUA). Guideline for the management of clinically localized prostate cancer: AUA guideline. Linthicum, MD: American Urological Association Education and Research, Inc.; 2007.
36. Reese AC, Pierorazio PM, Han M, Partin AW. Contemporary evaluation of the National Comprehensive Cancer Network prostate cancer risk classification system. Urology. 2012;80:1075–9.
37. Kattan MW, Eastham JA, Stapleton AM, et al. A preoperative nomogram for disease recurrence following radical prostatectomy for prostate cancer. J Natl Cancer Inst. 1998;90(10):766–71.
38. Graefen M, Karakiewicz PI, Cagiannos I, et al. A validation of two preoperative nomograms predicting recurrence following radical prostatectomy in a cohort of European men. Urol Oncol. 2002;7(4):141–6.
39. Graefen M, Karakiewicz PI, Cagiannos I, et al. International validation of a preoperative nomogram for prostate cancer recurrence after radical prostatectomy. J Clin Oncol. 2002;20:3206–12.
40. Greene KL, Meng MV, Elkin EP, et al. Validation of the Kattan preoperative nomogram for prostate cancer recurrence using a community based cohort: results from Cancer of the Prostate Strategic Urological Research Endeavor (CaPSURE). J Urol. 2004;171(6 Pt 1):2255–9.
41. Stephenson AJ, Scarcino PT, Eastham JA, et al. Preoperative nomogram predicting the 10-year probability of prostate cancer recurrence after radical prostatectomy. J Natl Cancer Inst. 2006;98:715–7.
42. Dotan ZA, Bianco Jr JF, Rabbani F, et al. Pattern of prostate-specific antigen (PSA) failure dictates the probability of a positive bone scan in patients with an increasing PSA after radical prostatectomy. J Clin Oncol. 2005;23:1962–8.
43. Briganti A, Chun FK, Salonia A, et al. Validation of a nomogram predicting the probability of lymph node invasion among patients undergoing radical prostatectomy and an extended pelvic lymphadenectomy. Eur Urol. 2006;49(6):1019–26. discussion 1026-7.
44. Kattan MW, Potters L, Blasko JC, et al. Pretreatment nomogram for predicting freedom from recurrence after permanent prostate brachytherapy in prostate cancer. Urology. 2001;58(3):393–9.
45. Koh H, Kattan MW, Scardino PT, et al. A nomogram to predict seminal vesicle invasion by the extent and location of cancer in systematic biopsy results. J Urol. 2003;170(4 pt 1):1203–8.
46. Punnen S, Freedland SJ, Presti Jr JC, et al. Multi-institutional validation of the CAPRA-S score to predict disease recurrence and mortality after radical prostatectomy. Eur Urol. 2014;65(6):1171–7.
47. Cooperberg MR, Pasta DJ, Elkin EP, et al. The University of California, San Francisco Cancer of the Prostate Risk Assessment score: a straightforward and reliable preoperative predictor of disease recurrence after radical prostatectomy. J Urol. 2005;173(6):1938–42.
48. Cooperberg MR, Freedland SJ, Pasta DJ, et al. Multiinstitutional validation of the UCSF cancer of the prostate risk assessment for prediction of recurrence after radical prostatectomy. Cancer. 2006;107(10):2384–91.
49. Zhao KH, Hernandez DJ, Han M, Humphreys EB, Mangold LA, Partin AW. External validation of University of California, San Francisco, Cancer of the Prostate Risk Assessment score. Urology. 2008;72:396–400.
50. May M, Knoll N, Siegsmund M, et al. Validity of the CAPRA score to predict biochemical recurrence-free survival after radical prostatectomy. Results from a European multicenter survey of 1296 patients. J Urol. 2007;178:1957–62.
51. Loeb S, Carvalhal GF, Kan D, et al. External validation of the cancer of the prostate risk assessment (CAPRA) score in a single-surgeon radical prostatectomy series. Urol Oncol. 2012;30(5):584–9.
52. Lughezzani G, Budäus L, Isbarn H, et al. Head-to-head comparison of the three most commonly used preoperative models for prediction of biochemical recurrence after radical prostatectomy. Eur Urol. 2010;57(4):562–8.

53. Cooperberg M, Broering J, Carroll P. Risk assessment for prostate cancer metastasis and mortality at the time of diagnosis. J Natl Cancer Inst. 2009;101:878–87.
54. Delouya G, Krishnan V, Bahary JP, et al. Analysis of the Cancer of the Prostate Risk Assessment to predict for biochemical failure after external beam radiotherapy or prostate seed brachytherapy. Urology. 2014;84(3):629–33.
55. Krishnan V, Delouya G, Bahary JP, et al. The Cancer of the Prostate Risk Assessment (CAPRA) score predicts biochemical recurrence in intermediate-risk prostate cancer treated with external beam radiotherapy (EBRT) dose escalation or low-dose rate (LDR) brachytherapy. BJU Int. 2014;114(6):865–71.
56. Halverson S, Schipper M, Blas K, et al. The Cancer of the Prostate Risk Assessment (CAPRA) in patients treated with external beam radiation therapy: evaluation and optimization in patients at higher risk of relapse. Radiother Oncol. 2011;101:513–20.
57. Meurs P, Galvin R, Fanning DM, Fahey T. Prognostic value of the CAPRA clinical prediction rule: a systematic review and meta-analysis. BJU Int. 2013;111(3):427–36.
58. Goodman M, Ward KC, Osunkoya AO, et al. Frequency and determinants of disagreement and error in Gleason scores: a population-based study of prostate cancer. Prostate. 2012;72(13):1389–98.
59. Bauer JJ, Connelly RR, Seterhenn IA, et al. Biostatistical modeling using traditional preoperative and pathological prognostic variables in the selection of men at high risk for disease recurrence after radical prostatectomy for prostate cancer. J Urol. 1998;159:929–33.
60. Stephenson AJ, Scardino PT, Eastham JA, et al. Postoperative nomogram predicting the 10-year probability of prostate cancer recurrence after radical prostatectomy. J Clin Oncol. 2005;23:7005–12.
61. Kattan MW, Wheeler TM, Scardino PT. Postoperative nomogram for disease recurrence after radical prostatectomy for prostate cancer. J Clin Oncol. 1999;17(5):1499–507.
62. Tilki D, Mandel P, Schlomm T et al. External validation of the CAPRA-S score to predict biochemical recurrence, metastasis and mortality after radical prostatectomy in a European cohort. J Urol. 2014;pii: S0022–5347(14)05061–7. doi: 10.1016/j.juro.2014.12.020. [Epub ahead of print].
63. Siegel R, Ma J, Zou Z, Jemal A. Cancer statistics, 2014. CA Cancer J Clin. 2014;64(1):9–29.
64. Shukla-Dave A, Hricak H, Akin O, et al. Preoperative nomograms incorporating magnetic resonance imaging and spectroscopy for prediction of insignificant prostate cancer. BJU Int. 2012;109(9):1315–22.
65. Siddiqui MM, Rais-Bahrami S, Truong H, et al. Magnetic resonance imaging/ultrasound-fusion biopsy significantly upgrades prostate cancer versus systematic 12-core transrectal ultrasound biopsy. Eur Urol. 2013;64(5):713–9.
66. Wysock JS, Rosenkrantz AB, Huang WC, et al. A prospective, blinded comparison of Magnetic Resonance (MR) imaging-ultrasound fusion and visual estimation in the performance of MR-targeted prostate biopsy: the PROFUS trial. Eur Urol. 2014;66(2):343–51.
67. Cuzick J, Swanson GP, Fisher G, et al. Prognostic value of an RNA expression signature derived from cell cycle proliferation genes in patients with prostate cancer: a retrospective study. Lancet Oncol. 2011;12(3):245–55.
68. Bishoff JT, Freedland SJ, Gerber L, et al. Prognostic utility of the cell cycle progression score generated from biopsy in men treated with prostatectomy. J Urol. 2014;192(2):409–14.
69. Cooperberg MR, Simko JP, Cowan JE, et al. Validation of a cell-cycle progression gene panel to improve risk stratification in a contemporary prostatectomy cohort. J Clin Oncol. 2013;31(11):1428–34.
70. Karnes RJ, Bergstralh EJ, Davicioni E, et al. Validation of a genomic classifier that predicts metastasis following radical prostatectomy in an at risk patient population. J Urol. 2013;190(6):2047–53.
71. Cooperberg MR, Davicioni E, Crisan A, et al. Combined value of validated clinical and genomic risk stratification tools for predicting prostate cancer mortality in a high-risk prostatectomy cohort. Eur Urol. 2015;67(2):326–33.
72. Klein EA, Cooperberg MR, Magi-Galluzzi C, et al. A 17-gene assay to predict prostate cancer aggressiveness in the context of gleason grade heterogeneity, tumor multifocality, and biopsy undersampling. Eur Urol. 2014;66(3):550–60.

73. Ishizaki F, Hoque MA, Nishiyama T, et al. External validation of the UCSF-CAPRA (University of California, San Francisco, Cancer of the Prostate Risk Assessment) in Japanese patients receiving radical prostatectomy. Jpn J Clin Oncol. 2011;41(11):1259–64.
74. Tamblyn DJ, Chopra S, Yu C, et al. Comparative analysis of three risk assessment tools in Australian patients with prostate cancer. BJU Int. 2011;108 Suppl 2:51–6.
75. Budäus L, Isbarn H, Tennstedt P, et al. Risk assessment of metastatic recurrence in patients with prostate cancer by using the Cancer of the Prostate Risk Assessment score: results from 2937 European patients. BJU Int. 2012;110(11):1714–20.
76. Yoshida T, Nakayama M, Takeda K, et al. External validation of the cancer of the prostate risk assessment score to predict biochemical relapse after radical prostatectomy for prostate cancer in Japanese patients. Urol Int. 2012;89(1):45–51.
77. Seo WI, Kang PM, Chung JI. Predictive value of the cancer of the prostate risk assessment score for recurrence-free survival after radical prostatectomy in Korea: a single-surgeon series. Korean J Urol. 2014;55(5):321–6.
78. Seong KT, Lim JH, Park CM, et al. External validation of the cancer of the prostate risk assess-ment-s score in Koreans undergoing radical prostatectomy. Korean J Urol. 2013;54(7):433–6.
79. Cooperberg MR, Davicioni E, Crisan A et al. Combined value of validated clinical and genomic risk stratification tools for predicting prostate cancer mortality in a high-risk prosta-tectomy cohort. Eur Urol. 2014; pii: S0302–2838(14)00521–1. doi: 10.1016/j.eururo.2014.05.039. [Epub ahead of print].
80. Seo WI, Kang PM, Kang DI, et al. Cancer of the Prostate Risk Assessment (CAPRA) Preoperative Score Versus Postoperative Score (CAPRA-S): ability to predict cancer progres-sion and decision-making regarding adjuvant therapy after radical prostatectomy. J Korean Med Sci. 2014;29(9):1212–6.
81. Kitagawa Y, Hinotsu S, Shigehara K, et al. Japan Cancer of the Prostate Risk Assessment for combined androgen blockade including bicalutamide: clinical application and validation. Int J Urol. 2013;20(7):708–14.
82. Akakura K, Tsuji H, Suzuki H, et al. Usefulness of J-CAPRA score for high-risk prostate cancer patients treated with carbon ion radiotherapy plus androgen deprivation therapy. Jpn J Clin Oncol. 2014;44(4):360–5.
83. Shiota M, Yokomizo A, Takeuchi A, et al. The oncological outcome and validation of Japan Cancer of the Prostate Risk Assessment score among men treated with primary androgen-deprivation therapy. J Cancer Res Clin Oncol. 2015;141(3):495–503.
84. Yamaguchi Y, Hayashi Y, Ishizuya Y, et al. A single-center study on predicting outcomes of primary androgen deprivation therapy for prostate cancer using the Japan Cancer of the Prostate Risk Assessment (J-CAPRA) score. Jpn J Clin Oncol. 2015;45(2):197–201.

Chapter 4
TRUS Biopsy: Is There Still a Role?

Michael S. Leapman and Katsuto Shinohara

Introduction

Transrectal ultrasound-guided prostate needle biopsy (TRUS-Bx) is the standard for obtaining a histological diagnosis of prostate cancer (PCa) and thereby represents a cornerstone in subsequent treatment planning by dictating Gleason score and measures of tumor volume [1]. Systematic biopsy of the prostate in men with clinical suspicion of PCa has been recognized as a problematic element in the management algorithm due to limitations on two fronts: *undersampling* clinically significant disease in a proportion of patients, and *oversampling* biologically low-risk cancers [2]. Consequential undertreatment and overtreatment have been identified as significant concerns in modern PCa management, driving the development of novel strategies to limit biopsies that may be regarded as *unnecessary* in that they detect tumors with little clinical significance. These concerns, as well as the growing appreciation for biopsy-related complications, and the incorporation of image-targeted biopsy modalities have culminated in the broader questioning of the relevance of TRUS-Bx in the contemporary era [3].

In this chapter, we will address the current role for TRUS-Bx in the initial evaluation of men with clinical suspicion of PCa, giving treatment to issues relating to observed diagnostic performance, and complications associated with its utilization. In addition, we will review current methods under investigation to improve the initial diagnostic accuracy of systematic TRUS-Bx, measures to lowering complication rates, increasing diagnostic yield, patient discomfort, and examine the integration of *hybrid* image-guided techniques exploiting advancements in magnetic resonance imaging (MRI) and TRUS.

M.S. Leapman, M.D. • K. Shinohara, M.D. (✉)
Department of Urology, University of California, San Francisco,
UCSF Box 1695, 550 16th Street, 6th Floor, San Francisco, CA 94143, USA
e-mail: kshinohara@urology.ucsf.edu

© Springer International Publishing Switzerland 2016
N.N. Stone, E.D. Crawford (eds.), *The Prostate Cancer Dilemma*,
DOI 10.1007/978-3-319-21485-6_4

Principles of Evaluation

The performance of a given prostate biopsy strategy may be assessed on several levels. Typically, the principal question to be answered by biopsy is an appraisal of the presence of cancer, its grade, and extent of disease within the prostate, often compared to a gold standard reference of step-sectioned radical prostatectomy specimens. In this context these findings can be regarded in a dichotomous fashion (i.e., upgrading versus downgrading, or significant cancer versus nonclinically significant cancers). *Sensitivity*, a measure of the true positive rate, refers to the statistical likelihood of detecting such an event while *specificity* is a measure of the *true negative rate* that reflects the percentage of negative results which are appropriately identified. Furthermore, the positive predictive value (precision) reflects the proportion of true positives divided by true and false positives and the negative predictive rate reflects the true negatives divided by all negatives. A classification model for a prostate biopsy strategy to predict a dichotomous endpoint may also be represented by the area under the receiver operator characteristic curve (AUC), represented graphically as a plot of true positive rate (Y-axis) by false positive rate (X-axis).

Many initial studies evaluate the performance of a biopsy method in relation to overall cancer yield of any Gleason score or volume. However, in light of the recognition of the variability of cancer-related outcomes and the nearly uniformly favorable longitudinal experience with pathological Gleason $3+3$ disease, an increasing trend towards active surveillance or non-treatment a distinction may be made between significant prostate tumors (regarded to be those possessing a variable component of Gleason 4) and those with limited biological potential [4, 5]. Moreover, given the prevalence of PCa and the associated frequency biopsy, other relevant issues bear consideration on a population scale including healthcare expense, adverse health-related quality of life (HRQOL) outcomes, and procedure-related complications.

Rationale for Systematic Biopsy

By its nature, adenocarcinoma is a multifocal disease within the prostate [6, 7]. On this basis, systematic sampling of the peripheral zone represents a means by which multiple areas may be examined in one setting and offer a broader appreciation for tumor status beyond a targeted palpable or visualized nodule. The sophistication of prostate biopsy techniques has improved dramatically from an initial 1953 report by Grabstald and Elliot in JAMA reporting on 50 cases utilizing a rectal speculum [8]. Early targeted biopsy of palpable lesions has given way to systematic templates incorporating prostate sextants, and ultimately to extended templates offering improved diagnostic yields, and serving as the standard in contemporary clinical practice [9–12].

In a meta-analysis of 20,698 patients derived from 87 studies including 68 studies comparing extended sampling schemes with sextant biopsy, diagnostic yield was improved with the inclusion of additional cores [13]. Moreover, the inclusion of apical and lateral biopsy cores has been associated with the detection of significantly more cancer than central cores [14, 15]. The use of 10–12 core extended sampling methods has been shown to result in improved cancer detection; however initial sampling strategies that extend beyond 12 cores appear to confer little additional value [16, 17]. Moreover, it does not appear that overdetection of clinically insignificant disease is a direct consequence of extended sampling techniques [18].

The superior yield of extended systematic sampling techniques over sextant biopsy has been established, culminating in the majority of guideline statements recommending extended biopsy templates as the approach of choice. The American Urological Association White Paper on "Optimal Techniques of Prostate Biopsy and Specimen Handling" offers an expert recommendation on the use of protocols involved 10–12 cores in men with an abnormal digital rectal examination (DRE) or elevated PSA [19]. The National Comprehensive Cancer Network recommendation panel recommends an extended-pattern biopsy including standard sextants including the peripheral base, mid-gland, apex, as well as directed biopsy of nodules or radiographically suspicious lesions [20].

Sampling Limitations of Systematic Biopsy

A considerable limitation associated with systematic TRUS prostate biopsy relates to mischaracterization of the true grade, stage, and volume of PCa within the gland seen at radical prostatectomy. This discordance in staging is often cited as a justification for early treatment in ostensibly favorable risk disease, and may conversely result in undertreatment for patients who are undersampled [21, 22]. Epstein and colleagues evaluated the concordance between radical prostatectomy specimens and biopsy. Among 7643 men with prostate biopsy specimens evaluated under the rubric of the 2005 modified ISUP Gleason scoring system, 36.3 % with Gleason $\leq$6 tumors were upgraded at surgery. Among biopsy Gleason $3+4=7$ biopsies, 49.7 were concordant at final pathology while 24.4 % were downgraded, and 25.8 % upgraded [23]. From a Surveillance, Epidemiology, and End Results (SEER) study of 10,273 men treated with radical prostatectomy for clinical low-risk disease, upgrading was observed in 44 %, where biopsy core volume was a significant clinical predictor of upgrading [24].

Despite the use of extended biopsy templates, the false negative rate has been reported in the range of 16–41 % seen among men undergoing repeat biopsy [25–28]. In light of the frequency of TRUS-Bx—approximately one million performed annually in the United States—this may be appreciated as a considerable proportion of repeated procedures, with associated costs and morbidity. Therefore, an interest exists in identifying patients in whom an initial negative biopsy result may warrant additional investigation. To this end, clinical risk factors associated with subsequent positive findings have been investigated and include serum PSA, PSA density, and % free PSA and prostate volume [29].

Histological findings within the spectrum of negative pathology have been associated with findings on repeat biopsy. The presence of atypical small acinar proliferation (ASAP) on biopsy has been associated with a likelihood of cancer in nearly one half of repeat biopsies which informs the recommendation to perform repeat sampling within 1 year [30, 31]. High-grade prostatic intraepithelial neoplasia (HGPIN), a pathological diagnosis given to structurally benign prostatic glands that are lined by atypical cells believed to be a precursor for adenocarcinoma, has been associated with a variable detection rate of PCa on subsequent biopsy [32, 33].

Procedure-Related Complications

TRUS biopsy is associated with a low but non-inconsequential complication rate when considered in aggregate. With biopsy undertaken with such frequency, concerns beyond sampling metrics are relevant to the discussion. While many biopsy-related complications are rare, or transient, taken in aggregate they represent a significant potential burden [34]. Infectious complications following TRUS biopsy occur in a rate of 1–10 %. Loeb et al. recently conducted a comprehensive analysis of reported complications following TRUS-Bx identifying a range of reported incidences. A study from the Rotterdam section of the European Randomized Study of Prostate Cancer indicated a 4.2 % rate of febrile episodes among 10,474 biopsies, where risk factors for infection included diabetes and larger prostates. Most patients who experience an infection were treated with an outpatient course of antibiotics; however severe sepsis requiring hospitalization was reported in less than 1 % of procedures [35]. Fluoroquinolone use and resistance is a commonly recognized risk factor for infectious complications following biopsy [36, 37]. As a result, many authors advocate consulting a hospital or local antibiogram to assess patterns of antibiotic resistance patterns to better direct prophylaxis.

The association between repeat TRUS biopsy and erectile dysfunction has been explored. Fujita and colleagues examined urinary and sexual quality of life functional scores among 231 men with PCa managed with active surveillance (AS) at Johns Hopkins. Decreased Sexual Health Inventory for Men (SHIM) scores were observed in men receiving three or greater biopsies when compared with men receiving two or fewer ($p = 0.02$); however when stratified by baseline erectile function increasing number of biopsies trended towards but did not reach statistical significance [38]. A UCSF study of 427 men with PCa managed with AS receiving multiple prostate biopsies however demonstrated a considerable variation in sexual activity within AS cohorts, with no association between erectile dysfunction and prostate biopsy exposure when adjusting for clinical factors including age, sexual activity, clinical stage, and diagnostic period [39]. Such findings have been supported by other studies suggesting a small decrease in erectile function over time and increased use of PDE5 inhibitors in this demographic which may be in part attributable to the aging process [40].

Patient anxiety discomfort during biopsy is an important consideration particularly for men facing repeat biopsies. Factors associated with reported levels of pain also appear to include pre-biopsy anxiety state, use of local anesthetic, and prostate size [41, 42]. Among one study 289 men administered a visual analog questionnaire prior to ten core biopsy, 47.6 % reported the procedure as painful [43]. Moreover, a subset of patients report pain or discomfort limiting enough that they would not accept a second biopsy [44]. Measures to mitigate procedural discomfort have been examined, including the addition of diclofenac suppositories to periprostatic nerve blockade. In 2005 Ragayan et al. reported on 65 patients receiving 12-core biopsy, demonstrating that the combination of suppository provided a modest improvement in procedural pain compared to lidocaine block alone (pain scores of 1.8/10 on a visual analog scale compared with 1.95 for lidocaine alone) without added risk of bleeding complications [45]. However, a randomized trial of 96 patients comparing lidocaine periprostatic block with or without combined diclofenac suppositories found no significant benefit to pain levels or tolerability [46]. Other well-reported sequelae of TRUS-Bx include urinary retention, hematuria, and hematospermia [47]. Urinary retention has been noted in a small percentage (<2 %) and does not appear to correlate with number of cores sampled, though a saturation techniques may reasonably pose a greater risk than very limited sampling [48]. Gross hematuria following TRUS-Bx represents a common entity that has been reported in between 8.1 % and 8.4 % of patients [49]. Incidence rates were compared among men undergoing 12 vs. 18 vs. more than 24-core biopsies, where rates of hematuria were 8.1, 9.7, and 10.4 % respectively with the majority being self-limiting and not requiring hospitalization.

Measures to Improve Biopsy

Rectal Swab Cultures

In response to an increasing appreciation for antibiotic resistance among patients receiving TRUS-Bx, publications have examined the use routine rectal swab cultures from patients to guide prophylaxis [50]. In a study of 457 men undergoing TRUS prostate biopsy, antibiotic selection derived from rectal swab cultures to examine fluoroquinolone resistance. Of 112 patients receiving targeted antimicrobial prophylaxis experienced no infectious complications were observed, compared with nine among men treated with empirical ciprofloxacin therapy; however these differences did not reach statistical significance ($p = 0.12$) [51]. In a randomized prospective trial of preprocedural povidone-iodine rectal cleansing consisting of 885 patients, patients in the intervention group had a slight, though nonstatistically significant reduction in the percentage of infectious complications (3.5 % vs. 4.5 %) [52].

Refined Selection

Improved methods for selecting men for initial prostate biopsy are a promising means to reduce the number of unnecessary biopsies. Pre-biopsy nomograms have been developed using PSA screening data to predict the likelihood of cancer on biopsy, thereby allowing greater ability to select patients for biopsy beyond dichotomous PSA thresholds alone. For example, the Prostate Cancer Prevention Trial (PCPT) Risk Calculator is a validated and widely used risk prediction instrument derived from 5088 men within the PCPT study for men who are aged 55 and older, have no prior history of prostate cancer, and have PSA and DRE results within 1 year [53]. The nomogram utilizes the following variables: race, age, PSA level, family history of prostate cancer, DRE findings, and status of prior prostate biopsy. Additional calculators have been generated that incorporate other clinical characteristics including BMI, finasteride usage, and AUA symptom score [54, 55]. Other factors including % free PSA and [-2]proPSA have also been incorporated. In an external validation study derived from 446 men undergoing TRUS-Bx from the San Antonio Center of Biomarkers of Risk for Prostate Cancer (SABOR) cohort, the AUC for detection of PCa was 65.5 % (95 % CI 60.2–70.8 %, $p < 0.0001$) [56]. In a larger cohort of 3482 men receiving an extended biopsy scheme, the AUC for cancer detection appeared more modest: 0.57 for any tumor, and 0.60 for Gleason ≥ 7 [57].

Biomarkers for Biopsy Selection

Biomarkers with improved sensitivity and specificity for PCa including the 4-Kallikrein panel (4Kscore) offer promise for the detection of significant PCas while potentially limiting overdetection of lower grade disease. This assay includes measurement of free PSA, total PSA, intact PSA, and human kallikrein 2 (hK2) in addition to clinical staging risk factors associated with risk of PCa (age, digital rectal examination, and prior biopsy status) to generate a numerical likelihood of significant PCa. Among 1012 men prospectively scheduled for prostate biopsy, the 4Kscore yielded an AUC of 0.82 for the detection of Gleason ≥ 7 disease, and outperformed the multivariable Prostate Cancer Prevention Trial Risk Calculator in decision curve analysis [58, 59]. The Prostate Health Index (PHI) is another assay calculated from multiple serum markers: [-2]proPSA, free and total PSA that has been examined in independent prospective cohorts of biopsy naïve men. In a multicenter evaluation of 956 total patients, the AUC for detection of Gleason ≥ 7 prostate cancer was 0.815 [60]. These tools hold promise in assessing risk of significant disease prior to biopsy with improved accuracy and may potentially refine the subsequent path to biopsy, diagnosis, and treatment in these individuals. Future studies are warranted to determine how these novel biomarkers add to clinical risk prediction of oncological events beyond the detection of disease.

Improved US Imaging Techniques

Power Doppler Ultrasound

The use of power Doppler enhanced TRUS to guide biopsy has also been evaluated in the setting of initial diagnosis. Power Doppler Imaging generates a visual depiction of total signal and is believed to allow for improved detection of tumor vascularity that may not be appreciated on conventional color Doppler studies [61, 62]. In a study of 136 patients with initial PSA between 2.5 and 10 ng/mL, the sensitivity and specificity for PCa detection was 82.8 and 78.8 % for PDI-TRUS [63]. Sauvain et al. evaluated 243 patients undergoing PDI-TRUS with a 4-tier grading system of vascularity in which normal Doppler signal was strongly associated with the likelihood of detecting favorable risk PCa [64].

Contrast-Enhanced Ultrasound

Prostatic tumors appear as hypoechoic lesions on TRUS examination, though the predictive value of biopsy targeted of these lesions has been suboptimal in most series [65, 66]. In terms of staging, B-mode TRUS has been shown to offer similarly favorable abilities at staging when compared with T2-MRI [67]. Interest has emerged in enhancing TRUS imaging using additional imaging modalities. Contrast agents for ultrasound imaging have been devised using micrometer scale bubbles (MB) arranged in a concentric fashion around high density compounds including perfluorocarbon and sulfur hexafluoride that are delivered intravascularly [68–71]. In a randomized, blinded, placebo-controlled trial of oral dutasteride pretreatment 272 total patients underwent a systematic and targeted biopsy following contrast administration using liposome encapsulated perfluoropropane microbubbles. The area under the ROC curve for the detection of any cancer was 0.60 for TRUS alone imaging compared with 0.64 following contrast enhancement, and 0.74 and 0.80, respectively, for the detection of Gleason score ≥ 7 [72]. The potential to add ligand specificity for microbubble contrast agents has been explored with PSMA monoclonal antibodies targeting nanoscale MBs that appear to bind PCa cells with high specificity [73].

Elastography

Ultrasound elastography exploits differences in stiffness between benign and malignant tissue that can be visually depicted on an elastogram wherein regions resisting deformation are represented more darkly, while elastic areas are shown in brighter colors [74–76]. The clinical performance has been assessed in several studies including a prospective study of 353 patients with clinical suspicion for PCa randomized 1:1 to real-time elastography or standard gray-scale TRUS receiving 10-core prostate biopsy with extended targeted biopsy of hypoechoic (gray-scale TRUS) or relatively inelastic (blue) lesions. Elastographic guided approaches detected PCa in 51.1 % compared with 39.4 % ($p = 0.027$), demonstrating sensitivity of 60.8 % and specificity of 68.4 % [77]. The combination of multiple ultrasound parameters has also been examined. Brock et al. examined 86 patients undergoing combined real-time elastography and CE-TRUS, which decreased the false-positive rate of elastography from 34.9 to 10.3 %, and resulted in a positive predictive value of cancer detection of 89.7 % [78].

Improving Negative Predictive Value

Commercial applications have explored the premise that a field effect within histologically benign prostate tissue can identify occult PCa missed due to sampling errors. The confirmMDX assay evaluates epigenetic changes within GSTP1, APC, and RASSF1 and has been examined in two blinded studies of men with negative biopsies [79]. In a study of the methylation assay among 498 European patients with negative biopsies undergoing subsequent repeat biopsy within 30 months, a negative predictive value of 90 % (95 % CI 87–93) was demonstrated where a strong independent association was observed when adjusting for age, PSA, DRE, and histopathological characteristics [80]. Similarly, in a study of 350 patients from five US centers undergoing repeat biopsy within 2 years of a negative study, the negative predictive value of the assay was 88 % (95 % CI 85–91) [81]. The clinical utility of such tools in the translation to reducing subsequent biopsy has also been estimated in an observational study of 138 men with negative assay results in which the repeat biopsy rate was 4 %, an estimated tenfold decrease from previous observed patterns in that setting [82, 83].

MR Fusion Biopsy Techniques

Prostate MRI reflecting multiple imaging parameters is a highly promising means with which to improve on the yield of conventional biopsy by identifying lesions for biopsy with a greater likelihood of harboring significant PCa [84, 85]. Recently, novel techniques have been developed to align previously obtained MR images with real-time TRUS [86]. Improvements in magnetic field strength (a transition from 1.5 to 3 T) have been associated with associated benefits in anatomic resolution on T2 weighted sequences. The integration of multiple imaging parameters including diffusion weighted imaging (DWI), dynamic contrast enhancement (DCE) imaging, and MR-spectroscopy imaging (MRSI) appears to offer additional insights with regard to the detection of intraprostatic tumors [87–89]. Thus, prospectively identified

MR lesions with high suspicion for significant cancer have been proposed as an efficacious means to select lesions for high probability biopsy.

Cognitive biopsy techniques in which lesion location obtained from MR is tracked and targeted with TRUS have represented an early means to integrate on the multiparametric MRI findings within TRUS-Bx. In a study of 95 patients undergoing cognitive versus systematic biopsy, detection of clinically significant PCa was 67 % versus 52 %, respectively ($p=0.0011$). Fusion MR-Ultrasound techniques have been developed which superimpose MR images with TRUS offering electromagnetic tracking that facilitates 3D recognition in space and biopsy (Fig. 4.1) [90, 91].

The comparative performance of systematic biopsy versus MR fusion biopsy has been evaluated in several well-designed studies comparing the two modalities.

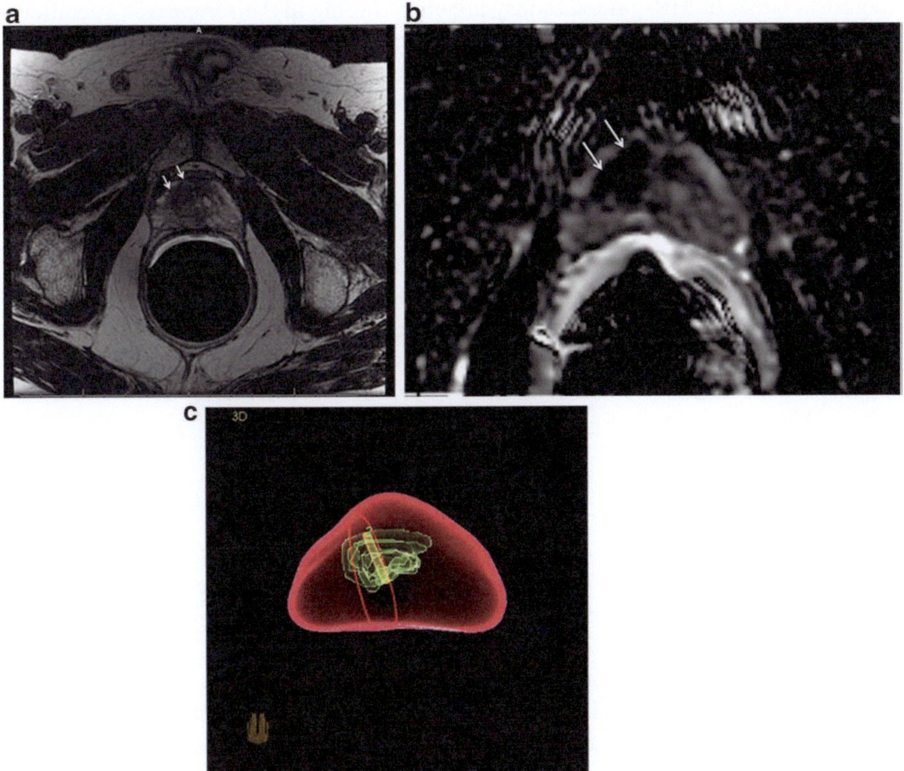

Fig. 4.1 Multiparametric MRI images of a 67-year-old man with Gleason grade 3+3 cancer PSA 5.9 ng/ml on active surveillance. (**a**) T2 weighed image shows a hypo-intense lesion at right anterior mid-gland (*arrows*). (**b**) Average diffusion co-efficiency map shows marked restricted diffusion in the corresponding lesion represented by a *dark area* (*arrows*). (**c**) Diagram of MRI fusion biopsy showing 3D prostate shape in *red*, suspicious lesion in *green line*, and a biopsy tract going through the lesion in *yellow line*. Biopsy revealed Gleason grade 4+3 cancer from the lesion

Siddiqui et al. reported on 1003 men receiving systematic and MR fusion biopsies in the setting of clinical suspicion of PCa. MR fusion biopsy resulted in the detection of 30 % more high-risk tumors than systematic TRUS while missing 17 % fewer low-risk cancers. When compared to radical prostatectomy pathology among 170 men treated surgically, the AUC for detection of high-grade disease was 0.73 for a targeted MR/Ultrasound fusion approach compared with 0.59 for a standard extended template TRUS biopsy, and 0.67 for a combined approach [92].

Future Directions

The optimal sequence and timing of imaging and biopsy in men with clinical suspicion of PCa remains to be definitively determined. While studies addressing the improved diagnostic yield of MR-guided biopsy are encouraging in their improved specificity for high-risk disease, barriers to a widespread pre-biopsy imaging approach do exist that reflect healthcare expenditure, convenience, and patient discomfort. However, if sufficient predictive value can be demonstrated with MR imaging alone, a potential to forego biopsy altogether is particularly enticing, though the viability of such a framework has not yet been empirically demonstrated. In the context of men undergoing AS for clinically favorable PCa who have already received histologic diagnosis via biopsy, the ability to pursue an mpMRI-alone system without routine biopsy has also been proposed [93]. Longitudinal evidence from the Prostate Cancer Research International Active Surveillance (PRIAS) study suggests that MRI positivity may represent a valuable predictor for disease reclassification, and a robust area of future investigation [94].

Conclusions

TRUS-Bx is a highly utilized method for PCa detection and risk assessment, offering multifocal gland sampling in one setting. Despite improvements in diagnostic yield associated with extended biopsy templates, sampling limitations with systematic methods may drive overtreatment of nonlethal disease, or may mischaracterize more significant tumors. Viewed from a population level, relatively infrequent procedure-related complications including pain, infection, and hematuria bear relevance to whole-scale PSA-driven biopsy schema. Measures to improve the performance of TRUS biopsy, including the integration of novel biomarkers to enable better patient selection for biopsy and advancements in ultrasound imaging, may afford improved diagnostic yield. Simultaneously, multiparametric MRI imaging has demonstrated superior detection of clinically significant disease when combined with TRUS localization. With refinements in its application and methodology, TRUS-Bx is poised to receive continued integration in the PCa detection algorithm.

References

1. Dugan JA, Bostwick DG, Myers RP, et al. The definition and preoperative prediction of clinically insignificant prostate cancer. JAMA. 1996;275(4):288–94.
2. Tilki D, Schlenker B, John M, et al. Clinical and pathologic predictors of Gleason sum upgrading in patients after radical prostatectomy: results from a single institution series. Urol Oncol. 2011;29(5):508–14.
3. Ploussard G, de la Taille A. Prostate biopsies: let's move forward. Eur Urol. 2013;64(6): 893–4.
4. Lecornet E, Ahmed HU, Hu Y, et al. The accuracy of different biopsy strategies for the detection of clinically important prostate cancer: a computer simulation. J Urol. 2012;188(3): 974–80.
5. Klotz L, Vesprini D, Sethukavalan P, et al. Long-term follow-up of a large active surveillance cohort of patients with prostate cancer. J Clin Oncol. 2015;33(3):272–7.
6. Swanson GP, Epstein JI, Ha CS, Kryvenko ON. Pathological characteristics of low risk prostate cancer based on totally embedded prostatectomy specimens. Prostate. 2015;75(4):424–9.
7. Miller GJ, Cygan JM. Morphology of prostate cancer: the effects of multifocality on histological grade, tumor volume and capsule penetration. J Urol. 1994;152(5 Pt 2):1709–13.
8. Grabstald H, Elliott JL. Transrectal biopsy of the prostate. JAMA. 1953;153(6): 563–565
9. Hodge KK, McNeal JE, Terris MK, Stamey TA. Random systematic versus directed ultrasound guided transrectal core biopsies of the prostate. J Urol. 1989;142:71.
10. Siu W, Dunn RL, Shah RB, Wei JT. Use of extended pattern technique for initial prostate biopsy. J Urol. 2005;174:505–9.
11. Norberg M, Egevad L, Holmberg L, Sparen P, Norlen BJ, Busch C. The sextant protocol for ultrasound-guided core biopsies of the prostate underestimates the presence of cancer. Urology. 1997;50:562.
12. Hodge KK, McNeal JE, Stamey TA. Ultrasound guided transrectal core biopsies of the palpably abnormal prostate. J Urol. 1989;142(1):66–70.
13. Eichler K, Hempel S, Wilby J, et al. Diagnostic value of systematic biopsy methods in the investigation of prostate cancer: a systematic review. J Urol. 2006;175(5):1605–12.
14. Gore JL, Shariat SF, Miles BJ, et al. Optimal combinations of systematic sextant and laterally directed biopsies for the detection of prostate cancer. J Urol. 2001;165(5):1554–9.
15. Babaian RJ, Toi A, Kamoi K, et al. A comparative analysis of sextant and an extended 11-core multisite directed biopsy strategy. J Urol. 2000;163:152–7.
16. Elabbady AA, Khedr MM. Extended 12-core prostate biopsy increases both the detection of prostate cancer and the accuracy of Gleason score. Eur Urol. 2006;49:49–53.
17. de la Taille A, Antiphon P, Salomon L, et al. Prospective evaluation of a 21-sample needle biopsy procedure designed to improve the prostate cancer detection rate. Urology. 2003;61:1181.
18. Meng MV, Elkin EP, DuChane J, Carroll PR. Impact of increased number of biopsies on the nature of prostate cancer identified. J Urol. 2006;176:63–8.
19. AUA. Optimal Techniques of Prostate Biopsy and Specimen Handling. White Paper. http://www.auanet.org/common/pdf/education/clinical-guidance/Prostate-Biopsy-WhitePaper.pdf. Accessed 22 Feb, 2015.
20. National Comprehensive Cancer Network. NCCN clinical practice guidelines in oncology (NCCN guidelines(r)): prostate cancer early detection. Version 1.2014. http://www.nccn.org/professionals/physician_gls/pdf/prostate_detection.pdf. Accessed 22 Feb 2015.
21. Capitanio U, Karakiewicz PI, Valiquette L, et al. Biopsy core number represents one of foremost predictors of clinically significant gleason sum upgrading in patients with low-risk prostate cancer. Urology. 2009;73(5):1087–91.
22. Chun FK, Steuber T, Erbersdobler A, et al. Development and internal validation of a nomogram predicting the probability of prostate cancer Gleason sum upgrading between biopsy and radical prostatectomy pathology. Eur Urol. 2006;49(5):820–6.

23. Epstein JI, Feng Z, Trock BJ, Pierorazio PM. Upgrading and downgrading of prostate cancer from biopsy to radical prostatectomy: incidence and predictive factors using the modified Gleason grading system and factoring in tertiary Grades. Eur Urol. 2012;61(5):1019–24.
24. Dinh KT, Mahal BA, Ziehr DR et al. Incidence and predictors of upgrading and upstaging among 10,000 contemporary patients with low-risk prostate cancer. J Urol. 2015;pii: S0022–5347(15)00254–2. doi: 10.1016/j.juro.2015.02.015. [Epub ahead of print].
25. Borboroglu PG, Comer SW, Riffenburgh RH, Amling CL. Extensive repeat transrectal ultrasound guided prostate biopsy in patients with previous benign sextant biopsies. J Urol. 2000 Jan;163(1):158–62
26. Serefoglu EC, Altinova S, Ugras NS, et al. How reliable is 12-core prostate biopsy procedure in the detection of prostate cancer? Can Urol Assoc J. 2012;2:1–6.
27. Clyne M. Prostate cancer: does a negative second biopsy give patients false hope? Nat Rev Urol. 2013;10(6):310.
28. Presti Jr JC, O'Dowd GJ, Miller MC, et al. Extended peripheral zone biopsy schemes increase cancer detection rates and minimize variance in prostate specific antigen and age related cancer rates: results of a community multi-practice study. J Urol. 2003;169(1):125–9.
29. Ploussard G, Nicolaiew N, Marchand C, et al. Risk of repeat biopsy and prostate cancer detection after an initial extended negative biopsy: longitudinal follow-up from a prospective trial. BJU Int. 2013;111(6):988–96.
30. Iczkowski KA, MacLennan GT, Bostwick DG. Atypical small acinar proliferation suspicious for malignancy in prostate needle biopsies: clinical significance in 33 cases. Am J Surg Pathol. 1997;21(12):1489–95.
31. Alsikafi NF, Brendler CB, Gerber GS, et al. High-grade prostatic intraepithelial neoplasia with adjacent atypia is associated with a higher incidence of cancer on subsequent needle biopsy than high-grade prostatic intraepithelial neoplasia alone. Urology. 2001;57(2):296–300.
32. Netto GJ, Epstein JI. Widespread high-grade prostatic intraepithelial neoplasia on prostatic needle biopsy: a significant likelihood of subsequently diagnosed adenocarcinoma. Am J Surg Pathol. 2006;30(9):1184–8.
33. Lee MC, Moussa AS, Yu C, et al. Multifocal high grade prostatic intraepithelial neoplasia is a risk factor for subsequent prostate cancer. J Urol. 2010;184(5):1958–62.
34. Raaijmakers R et al. Complication rates and risk factors of 5802 transrectal ultrasound-guided sextant biopsies of the prostate within a population-based screening program. Urology. 2002;60(5):826–30.
35. Loeb S, van den Heuvel S, Zhu X, et al. Infectious complications and hospital admissions after prostate biopsy in a European randomized trial. Eur Urol. 2012;61(6):1110–4.
36. Williamson DA, Masters J, Freeman J, Roberts S. Travel-associated extended-spectrum β-lactamase-producing Escherichia coli bloodstream infection following transrectal ultrasound-guided prostate biopsy. BJU Int. 2012;109(7):E21–2.
37. Dalhoff A. Global fluoroquinolone resistance epidemiology and implications for clinical use. Interdiscip Perspect Infect Dis. 2012;2012:976273.
38. Fujita K, Landis P, McNeil BK. Serial prostate biopsies are associated with an increased risk of erectile dysfunction in men with prostate cancer on active surveillance. J Urol. 2009;182(6):2664–9.
39. Hilton JF, Blaschko SD, Whitson JM, Cowan JE, Carroll PR. The impact of serial prostate biopsies on sexual function in men on active surveillance for prostate cancer. J Urol. 2012;188(4):1252–8.
40. Braun K, Ahallal Y, Sjoberg DD, et al. Effect of repeated prostate biopsies on erectile function in men on active surveillance for prostate cancer. J Urol. 2014;191(3):744–9.
41. Macefield RC, Lane JA, Metcalfe C, et al. Do the risk factors of age, family history of prostate cancer or a higher prostate specific antigen level raise anxiety at prostate biopsy? Eur J Cancer. 2009;45:2569–73.
42. Tekdogan U, Tuncel A, Nalcacioglu V, Kisa C, Aslan Y, Atan A. Is the pain level of patients affected by anxiety during transrectal prostate needle biopsy? Scand J Urol Nephrol. 2008;42:24–8.

43. Peyromaure M, Ravery V, Messas A, Toublanc M, Boccon-Gibod L. Pain and morbidity of an extensive prostate 10-biopsy protocol: a prospective study in 289 patients. J Urol. 2002;167:218–21.
44. Mkinen T, Auvinen A, Hakama M, Stenman UH, Tammela TL. Acceptability and complications of prostate biopsy in population-based PSA screening versus routine clinical practice: a prospective, controlled study. Urology. 2002;60(5):846–50.
45. Ragavan N, Philip J, Balasubramanian SP, et al. A randomized, controlled trial comparing lidocaine periprostatic nerve block, diclofenac suppository and both for transrectal ultrasound guided biopsy of prostate. J Urol. 2005;174(2):510–3. discussion 513.
46. Ooi WL, Hawks C, Tan AH, Hayne D. A randomised controlled trial comparing use of lignocaine periprostatic nerve block alone and combined with diclofenac suppository for patients undergoing transrectal ultrasound (TRUS)-guided prostate biopsy. BJU Int. 2014;114 Suppl 1:45–9.
47. Loeb S, Carter HB, Berndt SI, et al. Complications after prostate biopsy: data from SEER-Medicare. J Urol. 2011;186:1830–4.
48. Berger AP, Gozzi C, Steiner H, et al. Complication rate of transrectal ultrasound guided prostate biopsy: a comparison among 3 protocols with 6, 10 and 15 cores. J Urol. 2004;171(4):1478–80. discussion 1480-1.
49. Loeb S, Vellekoop A, Ahmed HU, et al. Systematic review of complications of prostate biopsy. Eur Urol. 2013;64(6):876–92.
50. Liss MA, Taylor SA, Batura D, et al. Fluoroquinolone resistant rectal colonization predicts risk of complications after transrectal prostate biopsy. J Urol. 2014;192(6):1673–8.
51. Taylor AK, Zembower TR, Nadler RB, et al. Targeted antimicrobial prophylaxis using rectal swab cultures in men undergoing transrectal ultrasound guided prostate biopsy is associated with reduced incidence of postoperative infectious complications and cost of care. J Urol. 2012;187(4):1275–9.
52. Abughosh Z, Margolick J, Goldenberg SL, et al. A prospective randomized trial of povidone-iodine prophylactic cleansing of the rectum before transrectal ultrasound guided prostate biopsy. J Urol. 2013;189(4):1326–31.
53. Prostate Cancer Prevention Trial (PCPT) Prostate Cancer Risk Calculator. Available at http://deb.uthscsa.edu/URORiskCalc/Pages/uroriskcalc.jsp. Accessed 25 Feb, 2015.
54. Thompson IM, Chi C, Ankerst DP, Goodman P, Tangen C, Lippman S, et al. Effect of finasteride on the sensitivity of PSA for detecting prostate cancer. J Natl Cancer Inst. 2006;98:1128–33.
55. Ankerst DP, Till C, Boeck A, Goodman P, Tangen CM, Feng Z, et al. The impact of prostate volume, number of biopsy cores, and AUA symptom score on the sensitivity of cancer detection using the Prostate Cancer Prevention Trial Risk Calculator. J Urol. 2013;190(1):70–6.
56. Parekh DJ, Ankerst DP, Higgins BA, et al. External validation of the Prostate Cancer Prevention Trial risk calculator in a screened population. Urology. 2006;68(6):1152–5.
57. Nguyen CT, Yu C, Moussa A, Kattan MW, Jones JS. Performance of prostate cancer prevention trial risk calculator in a contemporary cohort screened for prostate cancer and diagnosed by extended prostate biopsy. J Urol. 2010;183(2):529–33.
58. Parekh DJ, Punnen S, Sjoberg DD et al. A multi-institutional prospective trial in the USA confirms that the 4Kscore accurately identifies men with high-grade prostate cancer. Eur Urol. 2014;pii: S0302–2838(14)01035–5. doi: 10.1016/j.eururo.2014.10.021. [Epub ahead of print].
59. Vedder MM, de Bekker-Grob EW, Lilja HG, et al. The added value of percentage of free to total prostate-specific antigen, PCA3, and a kallikrein panel to the ERSPC risk calculator for prostate cancer in prescreened men. Eur Urol. 2014;66(6):1109–15.
60. Nordström T, Vickers A, Assel M et al. Comparison between the four-kallikrein panel and prostate health index for predicting prostate cancer. Eur Urol. 2014;pii: S0302–2838(14)00752–0. doi: 10.1016/j.eururo.2014.08.010. [Epub ahead of print].
61. Bilger SA, Deering RE, Brawer MK. Comparison of microscopic vascularity in benign and malignant prostate tissue. Hum Pathol. 1993;24:220–6.
62. Donnelly EF, Geng L, Wojcicki WE, Fleischer AG, Hallahan DE. Quantified power Doppler US of tumor blood flow correlates with microscopic quantification of tumor blood vessels. Radiology. 2001;219:166–70.

63. Remzi M, Dobrovits M, Reissigl A, et al. Can Power Doppler enhanced transrectal ultrasound guided biopsy improve prostate cancer detection on first and repeat prostate biopsy? Eur Urol. 2004;46(4):451–6.
64. Sauvain JL, Sauvain E, Rohmer P, et al. Value of transrectal power Doppler sonography in the detection of low-risk prostate cancers. Diagn Interv Imaging. 2013;94(1):60–7.
65. Rifkin MD, Dahnert W, Kurtz AB. State of the art: endorectal sonography of the prostate gland. AJR Am J Roentgenol. 1990;154:691–700.
66. Engelbrecht MR, Barentsz JO, Jager GJ, et al. Prostate cancer staging using imaging. BJU Int. 2000;86 Suppl 1:123–34.
67. Jung AJ, Coakley FV, Shinohara K, et al. Local staging of prostate cancer: comparative accuracy of T2-weighted endorectal MR imaging and transrectal ultrasound. Clin Imaging. 2012;36(5):547–52.
68. Xie SW, Li HL, Du J, et al. Contrast-enhanced ultrasonography with contrast-tuned imaging technology for the detection of prostate cancer: comparison with conventional ultrasonography. BJU Int. 2012;109:1620–6.
69. Jiang J, Chen YQ, Zhu YK, et al. Factors influencing the degree of enhancement of prostate cancer on contrast-enhanced transrectal ultrasonography: correlation with biopsy and radical prostatectomy specimens. Br J Radiol. 2012;85:e979–86.
70. Sano F, Terao H, Kawahara T, et al. Contrast-enhanced ultrasonography of the prostate: various imaging findings that indicate prostate cancer. BJU Int. 2011;107:1404–10.
71. Cosgrove D. Ultrasound contrast agents: an overview. Eur J Radiol. 2006;60:324–30.
72. Halpern EJ, Gomella LG, Forsberg F, et al. Contrast enhanced transrectal ultrasound for the detection of prostate cancer: a randomized, double blind trial of dutasteride pretreatment. J Urol. 2012;188(5):1739–45.
73. Wang L, Li L, Guo Y, et al. Construction and in vitro/in vivo targeting of PSMA-targeted nanoscale microbubbles in prostate cancer. Prostate. 2013;73(11):1147–58.
74. Barr RG, Memo R, Schaub CR. Shear wave ultrasound elastography of the prostate: initial results. Ultrasound Q. 2012;28:13–20.
75. Salomon G, Köllerman J, Thederan I, et al. Evaluation of prostate cancer detection with ultrasound real-time elastography: a comparison with step section pathological analysis after radical prostatectomy. Eur Urol. 2008;54(6):1354–62.
76. Zhang M, Nigwekar P, Castaneda B, Hoyt K, Joseph JV, di Sant'Agnese A, et al. Quantitative characterization of viscoelastic properties of human prostate correlated with histology. Ultrasound Med Biol. 2008;34:1033–42.
77. Brock M, von Bodman C, Palisaar RJ, et al. The impact of real-time elastography guiding a systematic prostate biopsy to improve cancer detection rate: a prospective study of 353 patients. J Urol. 2012;187(6):2039–43.
78. Brock M, Eggert T, Palisaar RJ, et al. Multiparametric ultrasound of the prostate: adding contrast enhanced ultrasound to real-time elastography to detect histopathologically confirmed cancer. J Urol. 2013;189(1):93–8.
79. Troyer DA, Lucia MS, de Bruine AP, et al. Prostate cancer detected by methylated gene markers in histopathologically cancer-negative tissues from men with subsequent positive biopsies. Cancer Epidemiol Biomark Prev. 2009;18(10):2717–22.
80. Stewart GD, Van Neste L, Delvenne P, et al. Clinical utility of an epigenetic assay to detect occult prostate cancer in histopathologically negative biopsies: results of the MATLOC study. J Urol. 2013;189(3):1110–6.
81. Partin AW, Van Neste L, Klein EA, et al. Clinical validation of an epigenetic assay to predict negative histopathological results in repeat prostate biopsies. J Urol. 2014;192(4):1081–7. doi:10.1016/j.juro.2014.04.013. Epub 2014 Apr 18.
82. Wojno KJ, Costa FJ, Cornell RJ, et al. Reduced rate of repeated prostate biopsies observed in ConfirmMDx Clinical Utility Field Study. Am Health Drug Benefits. 2014;7(3):129–34.
83. Pinsky PF, Crawford ED, Kramer BS, et al. Repeat prostate biopsy in the prostate, lung, colorectal and ovarian cancer screening trial. BJU Int. 2007;99:775–9.

84. Numao N, Yoshida S, Komai Y, et al. Usefulness of prebiopsy multiparametric magnetic resonance imaging and clinical variables to reduce initial prostate biopsy in men with suspected clinically localized prostate cancer. J Urol. 2013;190:502–8.
85. Jambor I, Kahkonen E, Taimen P, et al. Prebiopsy multiparametric 3T prostate MRI in patients with elevated PSA, normal digital rectal examination, and no previous biopsy. J Magn Reson Imaging. 2015;41(5):1394–404.
86. Rastinehad AR, Turkbey B, Salami SS, et al. Improving detection of clinically significant prostate cancer: magnetic resonance imaging/transrectal ultrasound fusion guided prostate biopsy. J Urol. 2014;191(6):1749–54.
87. Oto A, Yang C, Kayhan A, et al. Diffusion-weighted and dynamic contrast-enhanced MRI of prostate cancer: correlation of quantitative MR parameters with Gleason score and tumor angiogenesis. AJR Am J Roentgenol. 2011;197(6):1382–90.
88. Testa C, Schiavina R, Lodi R, et al. Accuracy of MRI/MRSI-based transrectal ultrasound biopsy in peripheral and transition zones of the prostate gland in patients with prior negative biopsy. NMR Biomed. 2010;23(9):1017–26.
89. Donati OF, Mazaheri Y, Afaq A, et al. Prostate cancer aggressiveness: assessment with whole-lesion histogram analysis of the apparent diffusion coefficient. Radiology. 2014;271(1):143–52.
90. Pokorny MR, de Rooij M, Duncan E, et al. Prospective study of diagnostic accuracy comparing prostate cancer detection by transrectal ultrasound-guided biopsy versus magnetic resonance (MR) imaging with subsequent MR-guided biopsy in men without previous prostate biopsies. Eur Urol. 2014;66(1):22–9.
91. Wysock JS, Rosenkrantz AB, Huang WC, et al. A prospective, blinded comparison of magnetic resonance (MR) imaging-ultrasound fusion and visual estimation in the performance of MR-targeted prostate biopsy: the PROFUS trial. Eur Urol. 2014;66(2):343–51.
92. Siddiqui MM, Rais-Bahrami S, Turkbey B, et al. Comparison of MR/ultrasound fusion-guided biopsy with ultrasound-guided biopsy for the diagnosis of prostate cancer. JAMA. 2015;313(4):390–7.
93. Moore CM, Petrides N, Emberton M. Can MRI replace serial biopsies in men on active surveillance for prostate cancer? Curr Opin Urol. 2014;24(3):280–7.
94. Bul M, Zhu X, Valdagni R, et al. Active surveillance for low-risk prostate cancer worldwide: the PRIAS study. Eur Urol. 2013;63:597–603.

Chapter 5
Transperineal Biopsy Technique

Nelson N. Stone, Vassilios M. Skouteris, and E. David Crawford

Abbreviations

AS	Active surveillance
EBRT	External beam irradiation
RP	Radical prostatectomy
TPMB	Transperineal prostate mapping biopsy
TRUS	Transrectal ultrasound

Electronic supplementary material: The online version of this chapter (doi:10.1007/978-3-319-21485-6_5) contains supplementary material, which is available to authorized users. Videos can also be accessed at http://link.springer.com/chapter/10.1007/978-3-319-21485-6_5.

N.N. Stone, M.D. (✉)
Professor of Urology and Radiation Oncology, Department of Urology,
The Icahn School of Medicine at Mount Sinai, 1 Gustave L. Levy Place,
New York, NY 10029, USA

675 Lionshead Place, Unit 622, Vail, CO 81657, USA
e-mail: drnelsonstone@gmail.com

V.M. Skouteris, M.D.
Prostate Brachytherapy Department, Hygeia Hospital, Hygeia Group,
4 Er. Stavrou Str. Kifissias Av., Marousi, Athens 15123, Greece
e-mail: basileskout@hotmail.com

E.D. Crawford, M.D.
Professor of Urology/Surgery, Radiation Oncology, University of Colorado,
Mail Stop # F 710, 6510, Denver, Aurora, CO 80045, USA
e-mail: edc@edavidcrawford.com

© Springer International Publishing Switzerland 2016
N. Stone, E.D. Crawford (eds.), *The Prostate Cancer Dilemma*,
DOI 10.1007/978-3-319-21485-6_5

Introduction

Transrectal ultrasound guided biopsy (TRUS) has been the gold-standard for diagnosing prostate cancer for over 30 years. The introduction of the biplanar ultrasound probe combined with a spring loaded biopsy needle facilitated what was before a painful procedure associated with a high complication rate [1]. Adoption of this technique coincided with the introduction of PSA testing, first identified by immunoperoxidase staining of prostate tissue, its application as a monoclonal antibody test to detect serum levels, and its eventual utility as a screening test for prostate cancer [2–6]. In 1987 the American Cancer Society estimated 96,000 new prostate cancer cases [7]. Coinciding with the widespread application of PSA testing, new cases increased to 165,000 in 1993, 244,000 in 1995 and peaked in 1997 at 334,500 [8–10]. Since then the number of new cases has steady declined and had remained fairly constant at 200,000–250,000 with 2014 projected at 233,000 [8]. In 1987, only 65 % of prostate cancers were considered local at diagnosis compared to 81 % for years 2003–2009 [11–12]. In a report on 226,046 men who attended Prostate Cancer Awareness Weeks 1989–1993, 13.1 % of the attendees had an abnormal digital rectal exam (DRE) and 24.5 % of these were diagnosed with prostate cancer [9]. Today most localized prostate cancers are diagnosed with non-palpable (T1c) disease which is directly related to the widespread application of both PSA testing and TRUS guided biopsy over the last three decades.

The increasing incidence of newly diagnosed non-palpable prostate cancer has made its detection more difficult. Larger lesions were more easily discovered because of their hypoechoic appearance on ultrasound and their predilection within the peripheral zone of the gland (close to the optimal focal point of the transducer). Lesions have dramatically decreased in size without a concomitant reduction in the percent of high grade, potentially lethal cancers. Finding these smaller aggressive lesions, which comprise 20–25 % of newly detected disease, has become a priority. In addition, the 75 % of prostate cancers diagnosed with low grade disease are potential candidates for active surveillance. However, mixed in with these apparent "low risk cancers" are a substantial number of high grade lesions that were "missed" by the TRUS biopsy. The transperineal prostate mapping biopsy (TPMB) presents an opportunity to find these lesions and better stratify patients into active treatment or surveillance.

Transperineal Prostate Mapping Biopsy Technique

The hallmark of the TPMB technique is taking the prostate biopsy by puncture of the skin in the perineum rather than through the anterior rectal wall. When transrectal ultrasound was introduced as an adjunct to prostate biopsy, both techniques were initially described in 1987. Lee described the TRUS approach while Vallancien described a transperineal technique [1, 13]. The TRUS biopsy quickly became the favorite because it could be easily and quickly performed in an office setting without

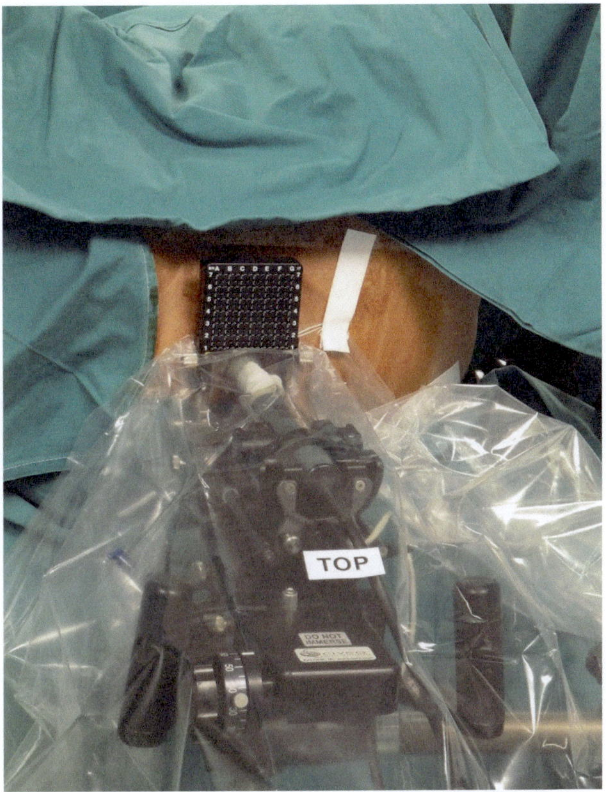

Fig. 5.1 Template setup against perineum. US probe is in rectum

the need for anesthesia which has resulted in over 1,200,000 yearly TRUS biopsies performed in the USA [14]. It is estimated that over 3.7 million TRUS biopsy are performed worldwide.

The TPMB procedure performed today is markedly different from that described by Vallancien. Clinicians utilize a brachytherapy setup and the procedure is performed in the operating theater under general, spinal, or regional anesthesia. The patient is placed in dorsal lithotomy position with the ultrasound probe placed in a stepping device with the template attached and applied to a sterile field (Fig. 5.1). The outer template is aligned to the puncture sites as depicted on the ultrasound image (Fig. 5.2). The urologist starts at the upper left on the template (11 o'clock position on the prostate) and punctures the perineum and pushes the biopsy needle so it is visualized on the axial prostate image (Fig. 5.3). Imaging is switched to sagittal and the needle is pulled back to the apex before it is fired (Fig. 5.4). When sampling longer lengths of the prostate (for example in the midline) the standard TRUS needle is limited to a 17–20 mm core bed. This necessitates re-puncture in the same grid point in order to biopsy from the longitudinal midpoint to the base (Fig. 5.5). In cases of very large prostates this could require 3 or more punctures (17 mm $\times$ 3 = 51 mm prostate length). Re-puncture of the prostate increases error as

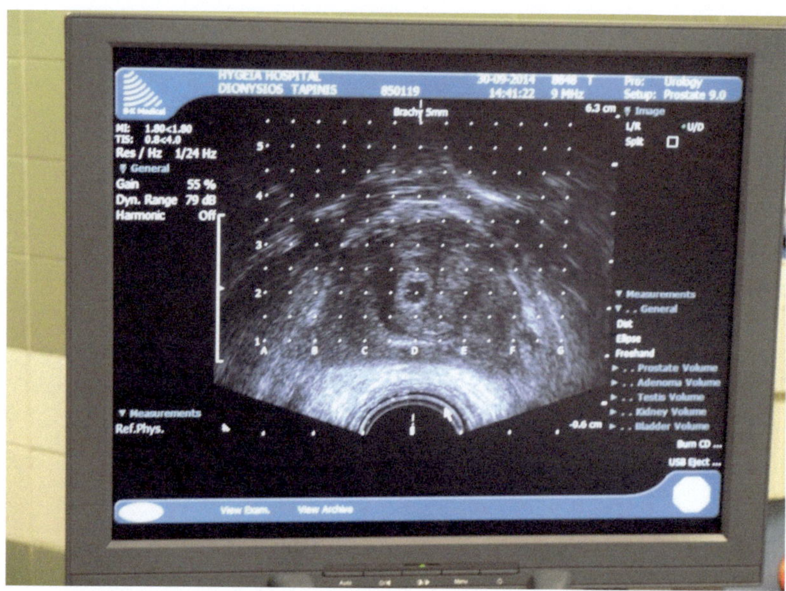

Fig. 5.2 Ultrasound grid is aligned to outer template puncture holes (Fig. 5.1)

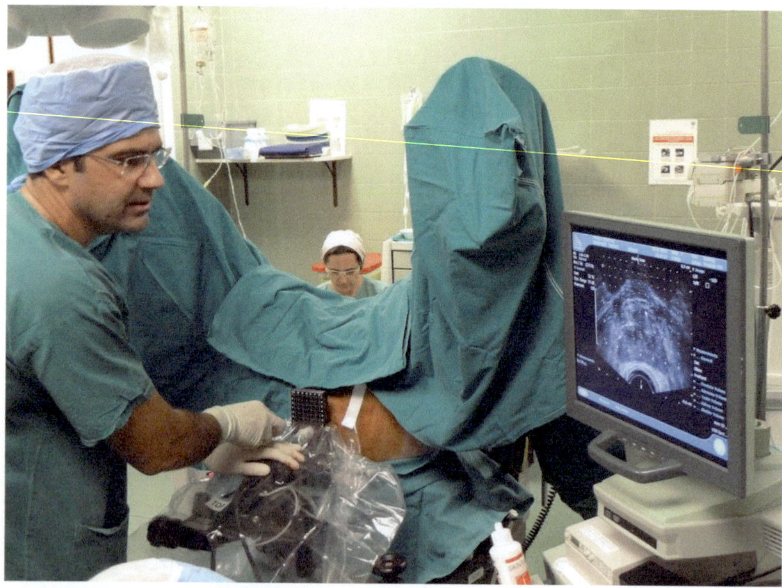

Fig. 5.3 Each 5 mm site is punctured and observed on the US transverse image. The urologist is viewing the needle puncture site at the 11 o'clock position

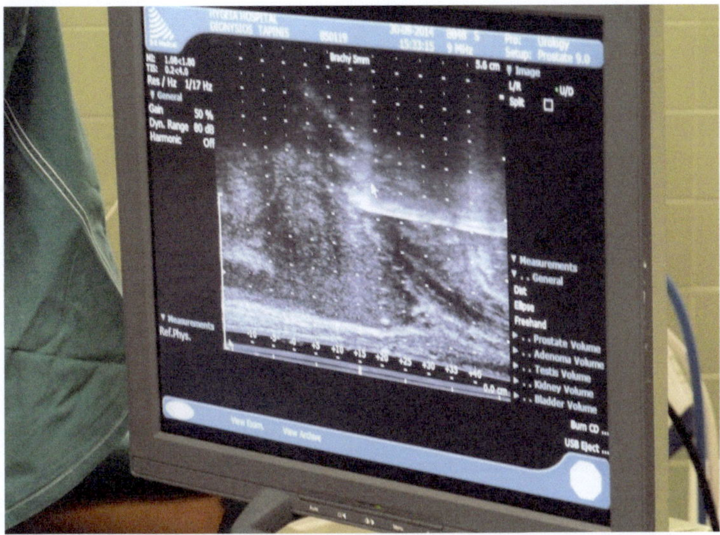

Fig. 5.4 Sagittal image with tip of biopsy needle at apex before it is fired

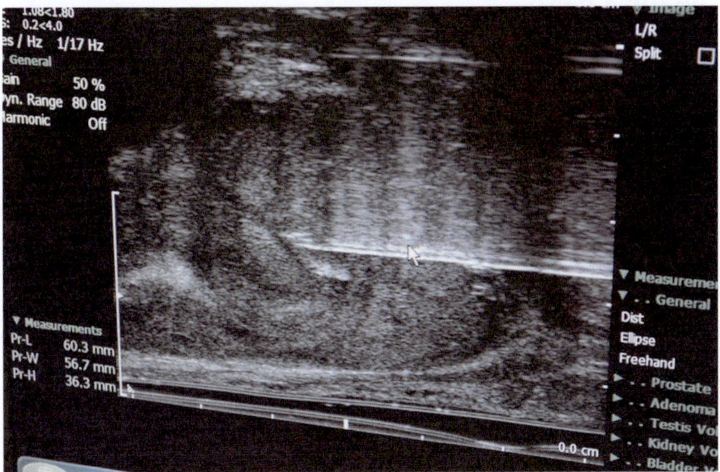

Fig. 5.5 Sagittal image of biopsy needle after firing. The specimen only includes tissue from apex to mid prostate. Another biopsy needle will need to be introduced in same grid point to sample same longitudinal path from mid prostate to base of gland

each reentry results in some drift in the longitudinal plane. Each biopsy specimen is inked at its end and placed in individual vials (Fig. 5.6). A record of lesion location can be used if focal therapy is contemplated. A video of a TPMB procedure is provided (Video 5.1).

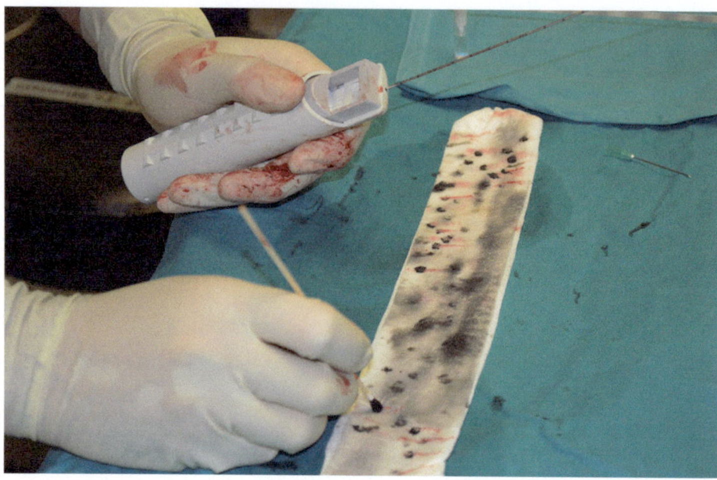

Fig. 5.6 Each specimen is inked and put in individual vials allowing recording of lesion position within the prostate

Rationale for TPMB

Recent data suggests that active surveillance (AS) in low risk patients may offer similar survival advantages as definitive therapy [15]. Selecting candidates most appropriate for surveillance has been an ongoing problem. In the Klotz study more than 1/3 of men went off surveillance or were treated by 10 years [15]. Part of the problem is that prostate cancer is known to be a multifocal disease. Meiers found that more than 2/3 of men undergoing radical prostatectomy had multiple bilateral lesions [16]. A number of studies have reviewed their prostatectomy experiences in men who were AS candidates. Ploussard studied 177 men who underwent a 21-core TRUS biopsy protocol and had less than 3 positive cores and less than 3 mm tumor length or less than 50 % involvement or less than 33 % positive cores [17]. Over 25 % had adverse pathology. In a literature search Shapiro found more than 1/3 men with low risk disease where upgraded on their prostatectomy specimen [18]. In a retrospective analysis of 10,785 consecutive radical prostatectomy performed in 10 university hospitals, Beauval found 919 patients with T1c, PSA <10 ng/mL, a single positive biopsy, tumor length <3 mm, and Gleason score <7 [19]. Only 26 % of patients had "insignificant" tumors and would have been ideal candidates for AS. Thus the data seems to indicate that TRUS biopsy does not properly differentiate low risk patients who would be ideal candidates for AS versus definitive therapy. This statement holds true even when a saturation strategy is utilized with more than 20 biopsies taken [20].

Validation of TPMB as a More Accurate Prostate Cancer Detection Technique

Brede conducted a study to evaluate the reliability of TPMB [21]. They sought to determine if bevel position, tissue deformity and technique affected its accuracy. He noted substantial deviation of the needle which increased at increasing depths and concluded that proper technique was critical to improve accuracy. Huo sought to compare the results of TPMB to 414 RP specimens [22]. The sensitivity and specificity of detecting cancer in all biopsy zones was only 48 % and 84.1 %, respectively. Rather than follow a 5 mm grid plan these authors took an average of 22 biopsies through 12 regions. This study and several others like it reinforce the need to follow a strict sampling plan so all prostate is evaluated. Katz evaluated 17 men who had TPMB then subsequent RP [23]. Sensitivity and specificity for prostate cancer detection was 86 % and 83 %. However, four quadrants negative for cancer on TPMB were positive on prostatectomy, and six positive on TPMB were negative on prostatectomy. Compared to the previous study many more cores were taken (17–114) as well as multiple samples when prostate core length exceeded core bed. Crawford analyzed 64 men who had TPMP followed by RP [24]. The specimens were whole-mounted and reconstructed in 3D. When comparing Gleason score between the two 72 % were identical, 12 % upgraded, and 16 % downgraded. TPMB missed 16/64 lesions but only one was clinically significant.

Comparison of TPMB to TRUS Biopsy

The most common application of TPMB is re-biopsy of patients diagnosed with low risk disease based on TRUS biopsy. There are two basic techniques for TPMB. The prostate is divided into zones and a set number of cores are taken from each one. Alternatively, cores are taken at 5 mm intervals starting at the upper right edge (on axial) of the gland (Table 5.1). Both techniques need to consider that biopsy needle is limited to a maximum of 2 cm of specimen. The zonal approach usually divides the length of the gland into basal and apical zones, whereas the grid approach requires multiple cores through the same puncture site if the gland length exceeds 2 cm at that point.

Symons evaluated 409 men using a 14-region technique [25]. Indications for biopsy included elevated PSA level (75 %, median 6.5 ng/ml), abnormal digital rectal examination (8 %), and active surveillance restaging (18 %). Typically, 22 cores were taken from 14 biopsy locations as designated by a standardized biopsy scheme. Stratified between those having their first TPMB or a repeat procedure (after a previous negative biopsy), the detection rates were 64.4 % and 35.6 %, respectively. Significantly higher detection rates were found in prostates <50 mL in volume than in larger prostates (65.2 % vs. 38.3 %, respectively, $p < 0.001$). Li reported on 303 cases that had an 11-region template-guided transperineal saturation

Table 5.1 Prostate cancer detection rates following transperineal prostate mapping biopsy (TPMB)

Study	Technique	Number patients	Number cores [mean]	Detection rate as initial biopsy (%)	Detection rate as repeat biopsy (%)	Overall detection rate (%)	Gleason score ≥ 7 (%)
Symons [25]	Zonal	409	22	64.4	35.6	56.7	74
Li [26]	Zonal	303	23.7	37.6		37.6	66.4
Moran [27]	Zonal	180	NS	–	38	38	31
Novara [28]	Zonal	143	24	–	26	26	25
Pal [29]	Zonal	40	36	–	68	68	40.7
Pinkstaff [30]	Zonal	210	21.2	–	37	37	45
Taira [31]	Zonal	373	54	75.9	46.9	69.7	55.5

biopsy of the prostate as their first biopsy [26]. The inclusion criteria included a PSA ≥ 4.0 ng/ml (median 13.7), suspicious findings on the digital rectal examination, or abnormal prostate gland findings on ultrasonography, computed tomography, or magnetic resonance imaging. A mean of 23.7 cores (range, 11–44) were obtained, with an overall prostate cancer detection rate of 37.6 % (114 of 303). Moran investigated 180 patients with a median PSA of 8.1 ng/ml and 2 prior negative TRUS biopsies in which the prostates were equally divided into eight sections (four axial, two sagittal) [27]. TPMB yielded positive biopsies identifying adenocarcinoma in 68 of 180 (38 %). Novara re-biopsied 143 men using a 24-core scheme [28]. The inclusion criteria were a previous negative biopsy and a PSA ≥ 10.0 ng/ml (median 9.0), free/total ratio of <20 % or an abnormal digital rectal examination or previous high-grade prostatic intraepithelial neoplasia (HGPIN) or atypical small acinar proliferation (ASAP). The number of previous biopsies was one in 59 % of patients, two in 26 % and three or more in 15 %. Prostate cancer was detected in 26 %, ASAP in 5.6 % and HGPIN in 2.1 %. Pal investigated 40 patients with a mean PSA 21.9 ng/ml (range 4.7–87) and two previous sets of negative TRUS biopsies who underwent 36 core template-assisted transperineal prostate biopsies (6 zones) [29]. In total, 27 of 40 (68 %) patients were found to have adenocarcinoma. Of the 210 men who were re-biopsied by Pinkstaff 170 (81 %) had undergone two or more TRUS biopsies [30]. The mean number of prostate cores obtained before the template biopsy was 17.4. A mean of 21.2 cores (range 12–41) were obtained at the template biopsy, depending on prostate size. The study inclusion criteria included PSA of 10 ng/ml or greater, prostate-specific antigen velocity of 0.75 ng/mL per year or greater, or the presence of prostatic intraepithelial neoplasia and/or atypical small cell acinar proliferation on the previous biopsy. Prostate cancer was detected in 78 men (37 %) and was in the transition zone in 60 (77 %). Taira performed TPMB in

Table 5.2 Results of TPMB in men with low risk prostate cancer being considered for active surveillance (AS)

Study	Patients	Technique	Number cores	Bilateral disease or increased tumor volume (%)	Upgrading Gleason score 7 or higher (%)	Not AS candidates after TPMB (%)
Onik [32]	180	5 mm	50	61.1	22.7	44.4
Ayers [33]	101	5 mm	47	34	29	33.7
Barqawi [34]	180	5 mm	56	45.6	27.2	75.6
Vyas [35]	307	Zone	24–38	NS	29	29

373 men of whom 294 had prior negative biopsy and 79 men as the initial biopsy [31]. The biopsies were taken from 24 zones. Cancer detection rate for the initial biopsy was 75.9 %. For men with 1, 2, and 3 prior negative biopsies detection rates were 55.5, 41.7, and 34.4 % (Table 5.2).

The use of TPMB to improve intra-prostatic staging and better identify candidates for AS is becoming more common. Onik performed TPMB on 180 patients with unilateral cancer on TRUS biopsy, who were considering conservative management [32]. Biopsies were taken every 5 mm throughout the volume of the prostate, and labeling of the specimen coordinates allowed accurate reconstruction of the location and extent of a patient's cancer. A median of 50 cores were taken and 110 patients (61.1 %) were positive bilaterally, and 41 patients (22.7 %) had Gleason scores increased to 7 or higher. Of the initial 180 patients, 100 (55.6 %) were still considered AS candidates after TPMB. Ayers restaged 101 men on active surveillance using TPMB. Criteria for active surveillance were $\leq$75 years, Gleason $\leq 3+3$, PSA $\leq$ 15 ng/mL, clinical stage T1-2a, and $\leq$50 % ultrasound-guided transrectal biopsy cores positive for cancer with $\leq$10 mm of disease in a single core [33]. More significant prostate cancer was found in 34, and 44 % had disease predominantly in the anterior part of the gland. Barqawi prospectively performed 3-dimensional mapping biopsy on 180 men early stage, organ confined prostate cancer based on transrectal ultrasound guided 10–12-core biopsy [34]. Gleason score was upgraded in 49 of 180 cases (27.2 %) and up-stage in 82 (45.6 %). After TPMB 38 men elected radical prostatectomy, 11 received radiation therapy, 45 underwent whole gland cryotherapy, 60 were enrolled in a targeted focal cryotherapy clinical study and 44 elected AS. Vyas reviewed 634 patients who underwent TPMB for prior negative transrectal biopsy (174), primary biopsy in men at risk of sepsis (153); further evaluation after low-risk disease diagnosed based on a 12-core TRUS biopsy (307) [35]. Prostate cancer was found in 36 % of men after a negative TRUS with 17 % of these had disease solely in anterior sectors. As a primary diagnostic strategy, prostate cancer was diagnosed in 54 % of men (median PSA 7.4 ng/ml). Of men with Gleason $3+3$ disease on TRUS biopsy, 29 % were upgraded and went on to have radical treatment.

Taking more biopsies (by TRUS or TPMB) potentially increases the risk of diagnosing more low risk disease resulting in more definitive treatments. In this scenario, over-detection leads to over-treatment. This has been one of the criticisms of widespread use of PSA for screening. Too many men with minimally elevated PSA undergo TRUS biopsy and, despite low risk features, a large percent opt for surgery or radiation. However, the goal of TPMB is not to diagnose more cancers, but rather to improve the intra-prostatic staging so a more educated decision can be made about treatment choice. Valerio investigated 391 men who underwent TPMB (20 zones). The goal of this study was to define the index lesions [36]. Deploying a median of 1.2 (IQR = 0.9–1.7) cores/ml, cancer was diagnosed in 82.9 % (324/391) with a median of 6 (IQR = 2–9) positive cores, median maximum cancer core length at 5 mm (IQR = 3–8) and total cancer core length per zone at 7 mm (IQR = 3–13). 26.3–42.9 % had insignificant disease. When a stringent spatial relationship was used to define individual lesions, 44.4–54.6 % had one index lesion and 12.7–19.1 % had more than one area with clinically significant disease.

Precise localization of index lesions using TPMB offers the opportunity to consider focal ablation. Onik re-biopsied 110 men who were candidates for focal therapy because of low volume unilateral disease [37]. Biopsies were performed at 5 mm intervals and a median of 46 cores were taken. Bilateral cancers were demonstrated in 55 % and Gleason score was increased in 23 %. 84 patients (76 %) had at least one factor that would have potentially changed their management.

Morbidity Associated with TPMB

While the data suggests that TPMB improves cancer detection, accuracy of Gleason score, and disease volume and multifocality over TRUS biopsy, morbidity associated with the procedure has the potential to be greater than the standard TRUS biopsy. More cores are obtained, the access is transcutaneous (perineum), and patients require general or spinal anesthesia. Each of these factors could have their own complications. Complications include infection, bleeding, and urinary retention.

An increase in incidence in fluoroquinolone-resistant infections following TRUS biopsy has generated an interest in alternative biopsy and imaging modalities. Loeb performed a review of the SEER database and identified 17,472 men who underwent prostate biopsy to 134,977 matched controls [38]. Initial and repeat biopsies were associated with a significantly increased risk of hospitalization within a 30-day period compared to randomly selected controls ($p < 0.0001$). In the repeat biopsy group the mean number of biopsy procedures was 2.5. Compared to no biopsy, for every biopsy there was a 1.7-fold increase in overall hospitalizations, a 1.7-fold increase in serious infectious complications and a 2.2-fold increased risk of noninfectious urological complications. Thus, the more TRUS biopsies that a man undergoes, the greater his cumulative risk of experiencing a serious complication [38]. Minamida analyzed the prospective data from 100 patients who underwent TRUS-guided prostate biopsy from April to December 2010. A stool culture was obtained

1 month before biopsy. Patients received 500 mg levofloxacin orally once daily for 3 days, beginning 2 h before biopsy [39]. Of the 100 patients, 13 (13 %) had a stool culture positive for fluoroquinolone-resistant *E. coli*. In 4 (31 %) of these 13 patients, acute bacterial prostatitis was detected after TRUS-guided prostate biopsy. Batura started adding Amikacin to the prophylaxis of TRUS biopsy because he noted a 3.9 % infection rate (seven urinary tract infections [UTIs] and seven bacteremias). However, this approach did not eliminate all infections as 1.4 % of the subsequent 540 biopsies still developed 6 UTIs and 2 bacteremias [40]. Mosharafa evaluated the frequency and potential risk factors for infection-related complications after transrectal prostate biopsy [41]. Of the 107 patients, acute prostatitis developed in 10 (9.3 %). The most significant risk factor was prior use of a fluoroquinolone anti-microbial, with acute prostatitis developing in 7 (17.1 %) of 41 patients who had used a fluoroquinolone compared with 3 (4.5 %) of 66 patients who had not ($p=0.042$). Patients who received an enema before the procedure were slightly less likely to develop prostatitis ($p=0.061$). Of eight positive specimens, the organisms isolated were *Escherichia coli* in six, *Klebsiella pneumoniae* in one, and *Staphylococcus epidermidis* in one. Isolated gram-negative organisms were fluoroquinolone-resistant in 85.7 % of samples.

In contrast to the high infection rate associated with TRUS biopsy, especially for subsequent "confirmatory" biopsies done in the setting of AS, the TPMB, which is done as a sterile procedure, should have a very low rate of this complication. Grummet reviewed 245 TPMB biopsies that were performed at seven institutions in Australia and noted no hospital readmission for infections [42]. He also performed a literature review of 6609 TPMBs and found an infection readmission rate of 0.076 %.

While infectious complications with TPMB appear to be low, the increase number of samples taken does increase the risk of bleeding and prostate swelling leading to urinary retention. Losa reviewed 87 patients with low-risk prostate cancer who were candidates for focal therapy who underwent re-biopsy by TPMB [43]. He observed 37 cases of grade 1 complications, including 5 (6.1 %) cases of macrohematuria, 13 (16 %) of hemospermia, 11 (13.5 %) of perineal hematoma, 3 (3.7 %) of perineal hematoma and hemospermia, and 5 (6.1 %) of macrohematuria and hemospermia. Three patients (3.7 %) developed acute urinary retention. In 10 studies reporting on 2113 patients, the average urinary retention rate was 4.7 % (Table 5.3). An increase number of cores and advanced patient age were associated with higher retention rates. Of 1956 men from 9 studies, 19 (1 %) required catheter placement for clot retention or hospitalization.

Conclusions

Transperineal prostate mapping biopsy offers several advantages over TRUS biopsy including improved intra-prostatic staging, improved identification of men who are candidates for active surveillance, and better stratification of treatment selection for

Table 5.3 Complications associated with TPMB. The average retention and hospitalization rates were 4.7 and 1 %

Study	Number	Urinary retention [%]	Gross hematuria [catheter or hospitalization required (%)]
Onik [32]	180	14 [7.7]	2 [1.1]
Symons [25]	409	17 [4.2]	0 [0]
Losa [43]	87	3 [3.7]	0 [0]
Onik [37]	110	9 [8]	1 [0.9]
Vyas [35]	634	11 [1.7]	2 [0.3]
Barqawi [24]	180	9 [4.2]	9 [4.2]
Novara [28]	143	4 [3]	3 [2]
Merrick [44]	129	9 [7.1]	1 [0.8]
Buskirk [45]	157	18 [11.5]	NR
Tsivian [46]	84	5 [6]	1 [1.2]

definitive and focal therapy. There is a higher urinary retention rate with this modality compared to TRUS biopsy, but this should be weighed against the substantial reduction in UTIs and sepsis. TPMB costs more than TRUS biopsy, but is competitive with mpMRI guided biopsy. Which modality may eventually be superior will need to be determined by clinical trials.

References

1. Lee F. Transrectal ultrasound in the diagnosis, staging, guided needle biopsy, and screening for prostate cancer. Prog Clin Biol Res. 1987;237:73–109.
2. Stein BS, Vangore S, Petersen RO, Kendall AR. Immunoperoxidase localization of prostate-specific antigen. Am J Surg Pathol. 1982;6(6):553–7.
3. Horoszewicz JS, Kawinski E, Murphy GP. Monoclonal antibodies to a new antigenic marker in epithelial prostatic cells and serum of prostatic cancer patients. Anticancer Res. 1987; 7(5B):927–35.
4. Stamey TA, Yang N, Hay AR, McNeal JE, Freiha FS, Redwine E. Prostate-specific antigen as a serum marker for adenocarcinoma of the prostate. N Engl J Med. 1987;317(15):909–16.
5. Brawer MK, Lange PH. Prostate-specific antigen and premalignant change: implications for early detection. CA Cancer J Clin. 1989;39(6):361–75.
6. Catalona WJ, Smith DS, Ratliff TL, Dodds KM, Coplen DE, Yuan JJ, Petros JA, Andriole GL. Measurement of prostate-specific antigen in serum as a screening test for prostate cancer. N Engl J Med. 1991;324(17):1156–61.
7. Silverberg E, Lubera J. CA Cancer J Clin. 1987;37(1):2–19.
8. Garfinkel L. CA Cancer J Clin. 1993;43(1):5–6.
9. Garfinkel L. CA Cancer J Clin. 1995;45(1):5–7.
10. Cunningham MP. CA Cancer J Clin. 1997;47(1):3–4.
11. Siegel R, Ma J, Zou Z, Jemal A. CA Cancer J Clin. 2014;64(1):9–29.
12. Stone NN, Crawford ED, DeAntoni EP, Prostate Cancer Education Council. Screening for prostate cancer by digital rectal exam and prostate specific antigen: results of prostate cancer awareness week, 1989–1992. Urology. 1994;44(6):18–25.
13. Vallancien G, Leo JP, Brisset JM. Transperineal prostatic biopsy guided by transrectal ultrasonography. Prog Clin Biol Res. 1987;243B:25–7.

14. United States biopsy procedures outlook to 2020, Global Data, July 2014.
15. Klotz L, Vesprini D, Sethukavalan P, Jethava V, Zhang L, Jain S, Yamamoto T, Mamedov A, Loblaw A. Long-term follow-up of a large active surveillance cohort of patients with prostate cancer. J Clin Oncol. 2015;33:272–7.
16. Meiers I, Waters DJ, Bostwick DG. Preoperative prediction of multifocal prostate cancer and application of focal therapy: review 2007. Urology. 2007;70(6 Suppl):3–8.
17. Ploussard G, Salomon L, Xylinas E, Allory Y, Vordos D, Hoznek A, Abbou CC, de la Taille A. Pathological findings and prostate specific antigen outcomes after radical prostatectomy in men eligible for active surveillance--does the risk of misclassification vary according to biopsy criteria? J Urol. 2010;183(2):539–44.
18. Shapiro RH, Johnstone PA. Risk of Gleason grade inaccuracies in prostate cancer patients eligible for active surveillance. Urology. 2012;80(3):661–6.
19. Beauval JB, Ploussard G, Soulié M, Pfister C, Van Agt S, Vincendeau S, Larue S, Rigaud J, Gaschignard N, Rouprêt M, Drouin S, Peyromaure M, Long JA, Iborra F, Vallancien G, Rozet F, Salomon L, Members of Committee of Cancerology of the French Association of Urology [CCAFU]. Pathologic findings in radical prostatectomy specimens from patients eligible for active surveillance with highly selective criteria: a multicenter study. Urology. 2012;80(3):656–60.
20. Giannarini G, Autorino R, di Lorenzo G. Saturation biopsy of the prostate: why saturation does not saturate. Eur Urol. 2009;56(4):619–21.
21. Brede CM, Douville NJ, Jones S. Variable correlation of grid coordinates to core location in template prostate biopsy. Curr Urol. 2013;6(4):194–8.
22. Huo AS, Hossack T, Symons JL, PeBenito R, Delprado WJ, Brenner P, Stricker PD. Accuracy of primary systematic template guided transperineal biopsy of the prostate for locating prostate cancer: a comparison with radical prostatectomy specimens. J Urol. 2012;187(6):2044–9.
23. Katz DJ, Pinochet R, Richards KA, Godoy G, Udo K, Nogueira L, Cronin AM, Fine SW, Scardino PT, Coleman JA. Comparison of transperineal mapping biopsy results with whole-mount radical prostatectomy pathology in patients with localized prostate cancer. Prostate Cancer. 2014;2014:781438.
24. Crawford ED, Rove KO, Barqawi AB, Maroni PD, Werahera PN, Baer CA, Koul HK, Rove CA, Lucia MS, La Rosa FG. Clinical-pathologic correlation between transperineal mapping biopsies of the prostate and three-dimensional reconstruction of prostatectomy specimens. Prostate. 2013;73(7):778–87.
25. Symons JL, Huo A, Yuen CL, Haynes AM, Matthews J, Sutherland RL, Brenner P, Stricker PD. Outcomes of transperineal template-guided prostate biopsy in 409 patients. BJU Int. 2013;112(5):585–93.
26. Li H, Yan W, Zhou Y, Ji Z, Chen J. Transperineal ultrasound-guided saturation biopsies using 11-region template of prostate: report of 303 cases. Urology. 2007;70(6):1157–61.
27. Moran BJ, Braccioforte MH, Conterato DJ. Re-biopsy of the prostate using a stereotactic transperineal technique. J Urol. 2006;176(4 Pt 1):1376–81.
28. Novara G, Boscolo-Berto R, Lamon C, Fracalanza S, Gardiman M, Artibani W, Ficarra V. Detection rate and factors predictive the presence of prostate cancer in patients undergoing ultrasonography-guided transperineal saturation biopsies of the prostate. BJU Int. 2010;105(9):1242–6.
29. Pal RP, Elmussareh M, Chanawani M, Khan MA. The role of a standardized 36 core template-assisted transperineal prostate biopsy technique in patients with previously negative transrectal ultrasonography-guided prostate biopsies. BJU Int. 2012;1099(3):367–71.
30. Pinkstaff DM, Igel TC, Petrou SP, Broderick GA, Wehle MJ, Young PR. Systematic transperineal ultrasound-guided template biopsy of the prostate: three-year experience. Urology. 2005;65(4):735–9.
31. Taira AV, Merrick GS, Galbreath RW, Andreini H, Taubenslag W, Curtis R, Butler WM, Adamovich E, Wallner KE. Performance of transperineal template-guided mapping biopsy in detecting prostate cancer in the initial and repeat biopsy setting. Prostate Cancer Prostatic Dis. 2010;13(1):71–7.

32. Onik G, Miessau M, Bostwick DG. Three-dimensional prostate mapping biopsy has a potentially significant impact on prostate cancer management. J Clin Oncol. 2009;27(26):4321–6.
33. Ayres BE, Montgomery BS, Barber NJ, Pereira N, Langley SE, Denham P, Bott SR. The role of transperineal template prostate biopsies in restaging men with prostate cancer managed by active surveillance. BJU Int. 2012;109(8):1170–6.
34. Barqawi AB, Rove KO, Gholizadeh S, O'Donnell CI, Koul H, Crawford ED. The role of 3-dimensional mapping biopsy in decision making for treatment of apparent early stage prostate cancer. J Urol. 2011;186(1):80–5.
35. Vyas L, Acher P, Kinsella J, Challacombe B, Chang RT, Sturch P, Cahill D, Chandra A, Popert R. Indications, results and safety profile of transperineal sector biopsies [TPSB] of the prostate: a single centre experience of 634 cases. BJU Int. 2014;114(1):32–7.
36. Valerio M, Anele C, Freeman A, Jameson C, Singh PB, Hu Y, Emberton M, Ahmed HU. Identifying the index lesion with template prostate mapping biopsies. J Urol. 2015;193:1185. pii: S0022-5347[14]04859-9.
37. Onik G, Barzell W. Transperineal 3D mapping biopsy of the prostate: an essential tool in selecting patients for focal prostate cancer therapy. Urol Oncol. 2008;26(5):506–10.
38. Loeb S, Carter HB, Berndt SI, Ricker W, Schaeffer EM. Complications after prostate biopsy: data from SEER-Medicare. J Urol. 2011;186(5):1830–4.
39. Minamida S, Satoh T, Tabata K, Kimura M, Tsumura H, Kurosaka S, Matsumoto K, Fujita T, Iwamura M, Baba S. Prevalence of fluoroquinolone-resistant Escherichia coli before and incidence of acute bacterial prostatitis after prostate biopsy. Urology. 2011;78(6):1235–9.
40. Batura D, Rao GG, Bo Nielsen P, Charlett A. Adding amikacin to fluoroquinolone-based antimicrobial prophylaxis reduces prostate biopsy infection rates. BJU Int. 2011;107(5):760–4.
41. Mosharafa AA, Torky MH, El Said WM, Meshref A. Rising incidence of acute prostatitis following prostate biopsy: fluoroquinolone resistance and exposure is a significant risk factor. Urology. 2011;78(3):511–4.
42. Grummet JP, Weerakoon M, Huang S, Lawrentschuk N, Frydenberg M, Moon DA, O'Reilly M, Murphy D. Sepsis and 'superbugs': should we favour the transperineal over the transrectal approach for prostate biopsy? BJU Int. 2014;114(3):384–8.
43. Losa A, Gadda GM, Lazzeri M, Lughezzani G, Cardone G, Freschi M, Lista G, Larcher A, Nava LD, Guazzoni G. Complications and quality of life after template-assisted transperineal prostate biopsy in patients eligible for focal therapy. Urology. 2013;81(6):1291–6.
44. Merrick GS, Taubenslag W, Andreini H, Brammer S, Butler WM, Adamovich E, Allen Z, Anderson R, Wallner KE. The morbidity of transperineal template-guided prostate mapping biopsy. BJU Int. 2008;101(12):1524–9.
45. Buskirk SJ, Pinkstaff DM, Petrou SP, Wehle MJ, Broderick GA, Young PR, Weigand SD, O'Brien PC, Igel TC. Acute urinary retention after transperineal template-guided prostate biopsy. Int J Radiat Oncol Biol Phys. 2004;59(5):1360–6.
46. Tsivian M, Abern MR, Qi P, Polascik TJ. Short-term functional outcomes and complications associated with transperineal template prostate mapping biopsy. Urology. 2013;82(1):166–70.

Chapter 6
3D Biopsy: A New Method to Diagnose Prostate Cancer

Kevin Krughoff, Nelson N. Stone, Jesse Elliott, Craig Baer, Paul Arangua, and E. David Crawford

Introduction

Both transrectal ultrasound guided biopsy (TRUS) and transperineal mapping biopsy (TPMB) provide valuable information on the presence and grade of prostate cancer. However, both have limitations that make educated recommendations difficult for patients. TRUS biopsy identifies the correct grade and number of lesions between 30 and 50 % of the time. TPMB, in its current form, while a substantial improvement over TRUS in accurate grading and lesion identification is not optimal because of lack of standardization and antiquated technology. Additionally, TPMB usually requires anesthesia and an outpatient OR. An ideal mapping program should incorporate user friendly software to direct and record the biopsy sites, a biopsy needle and gun to sample the prostate along its length as a single specimen and a pathology component that preserve's the integrity of the core and facilitates processing.

Electronic supplementary material: The online version of this chapter (doi:10.1007/978-3-319-21485-6_6) contains supplementary material, which is available to authorized users. Videos can also be accessed at http://link.springer.com/chapter/10.1007/978-3-319-21485-6_6.

K. Krughoff, B.A.
Division of Urology, Department of Surgery, University of Colorado Denver School of Medicine, 12631 East 17th Ave., Room L15-5602, Aurora, CO 80045, USA
e-mail: kevin.krughoff@ucdenver.edu

N.N. Stone, M.D.
Professor of Urology and Radiation Oncology, Department of Urology, The Icahn School of Medicine at Mount Sinai, 1 Gustave L. Levy Place, New York, NY 10029, USA
e-mail: drnelsonstone@gmail.com

J. Elliott, B.A.
Software Development, BSCi, Inc.,
721 N. Tejon St., #200, Colorado Springers, CO 80903, USA
e-mail: jesse@bcsisims.com

© Springer International Publishing Switzerland 2016
N.N. Stone, E.D. Crawford (eds.), *The Prostate Cancer Dilemma*,
DOI 10.1007/978-3-319-21485-6_6

3D Mapping Software

An ideal mapping software program should provide a biopsy plan that directs sampling of the gland to provide a high degree of probability of encountering a lesion of a specific size. Kepner and Kepner performed an analysis of uniform core sampling to yield data on tumor volume limits on negative biopsies [1]. Based on their calculations it is possible to construct a probability graph utilizing sequential spacing and core diameter size. The requirements needed to achieve the depicted probabilities include even spacing between successive biopsy sites and one full length sample from base to apex (Fig. 6.1). For example, using a 15 gauge biopsy needle to take full core samples (base to apex) using 5 mm grid spacing would yield a probability of detecting a lesion with a radius of 2.5 mm at 90–95 %.

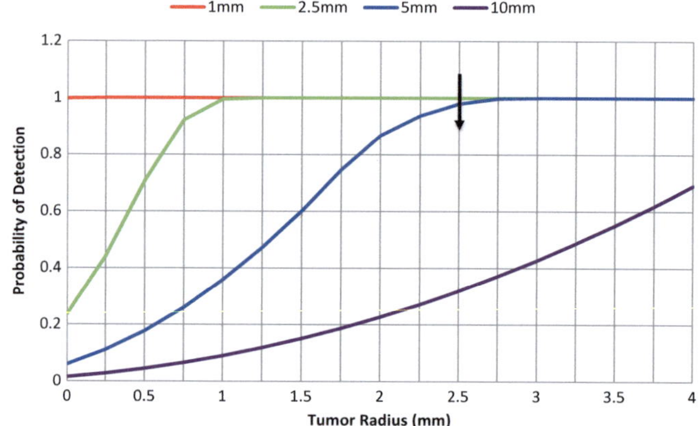

Fig. 6.1 Probability of detecting a negative biopsy based on grid spacing and needle size. In this example a 15 gauge biopsy needle is used to take full core samples (base to apex) using 5 mm grid spacing (*blue line*). The probability of detecting a lesion as indicated by the *black arrow* assumes perfectly spaced biopsies, no loss due to urethra intercept and perfect handling of capsule borders

C. Baer, Ph.D.
BCSi Inc., Colorado Springs, CO, USA
e-mail: Craig.Baer@bcsisims.com

P. Arangua, B.S., M.P.H.
Urologic Oncology, University of Colorado Denver,
1665 Aurora Court, Room 1004, Aurora, CO 80045, USA
e-mail: Paul.Arangua@ucdenver.edu

E.D. Crawford, M.D. (✉)
Professor of Urology/Surgery, Radiation Oncology, University of Colorado,
Mail Stop # F 710, PO Box # 6510, Aurora, CO 80045, USA
e-mail: edc@edavidcrawford.com

There are several constraints to using this approach with the current methodology of TPMB. When the biopsy needles are inserted in the outer template through the skin their entrance into the prostate will depend on the perineal anatomy, needle deflection, and gland movement from the needle and respiration. Stone has previously shown that brachytherapy needles, similarly placed through a perineal template can deform and deflect the prostate gland [2]. He found the median change in the base position of the prostate was 1.5 cm (range of 0–3.0 cm; $p = 0.0034$). The mean X and Y deformation was 6.8 mm (median, 7.9 mm; range, 4.3–8.1 mm) and 3.6 mm (median, 3.3 mm; range, 1.0–5.5 mm), respectively. Given the variable and significant movement of the gland when brachytherapy needles were placed, which were 17 gauge in that study, the likelihood more movement will be experienced if 15 gauge biopsy needles are used needs to be accounted for if the biopsy sites are to be uniformly distributed throughout the prostate.

A software program was developed to create a real-time 3D model of the prostate generated from intraoperative axial (transverse) image capture. Once the 3D representation is obtained a biopsy plan is generated. During the biopsy phase, the image position and the virtual biopsy sites (in axial and longitudinal) can be adjusted to match the US contours of the prostate, urethra and rectum as well the virtual biopsy sites are matched to the biopsy needle in the gland. The steps in the software program are described below in a patient undergoing TPMB.

Three-dimensional mapping biopsy (3DMB) is performed under general anesthesia with the patient in the dorsal lithotomy position. The ultrasound (US) probe is connected to a laptop running the software (3D Biopsy LLC) using a video capture card and S-video cable. After attaching the probe to a stepping device and brachytherapy grid, the probe is advanced into the rectum in 5 mm increments to visualize the prostate.

Selecting "Live Feed" broadcasts the US image in real-time to the laptop running the program (Fig. 6.2).

Once the base of the prostate is identified, the software is calibrated to the position of the US probe and dimensions of the prostate using the "Machine Calibration" function. This generates a biopsy template superimposed onto the US image with demarcations for the center of the US probe and the US field-of-view which are toggled to match the real-time US image. While the default spacing between biopsy probe positions is set to match that of a 5 mm brachytherapy template, the software-generated template can be moved, expanded, or collapsed to fit the needs of the case at hand (Fig. 6.3) .

Following calibration, the user is ready to begin outlining the prostatic capsule into the software. Using the touchscreen or mouse, the center of the prostate is demarcated and the user traces the outline of the prostatic capsule onto each axial image, moving through the prostate in axial view at 5 mm intervals from base to apex. Various options with the contouring tool allow smooth or nodal contouring (Fig. 6.4).

After outlining the capsule and position of the urethra and rectum on each axial image, the user is ready to begin planning biopsy coordinates using the "Generate Biopsy Plan" feature. In this window the biopsy needle length, spacing between needles, minimum distance from the urethra, and option for multiple biopsies at the same location are indicated. Given that the current prostate biopsy needle only takes

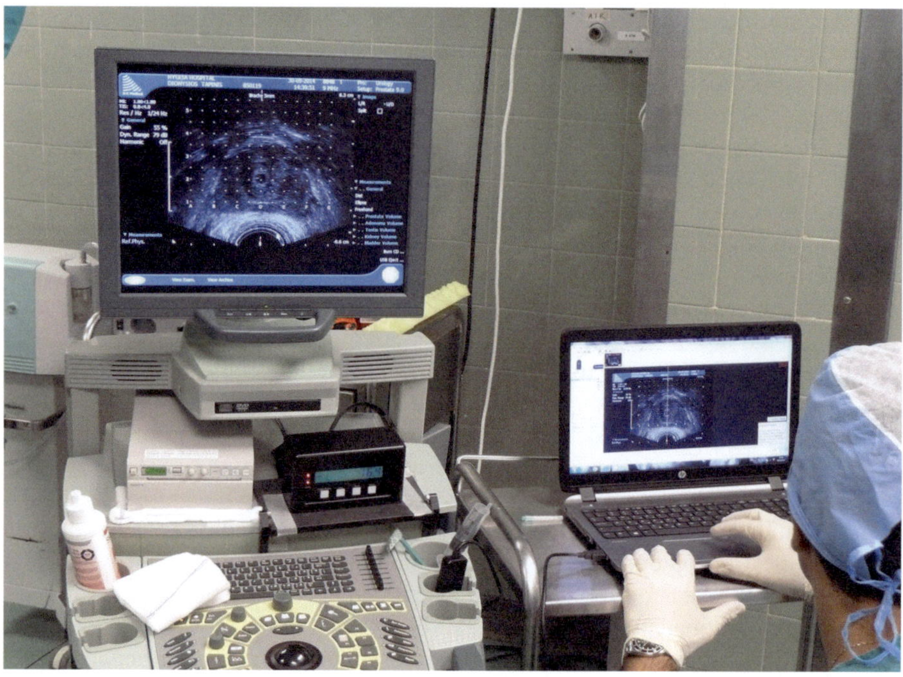

Fig. 6.2 Urologist views US image fed live into the 3D mapping program

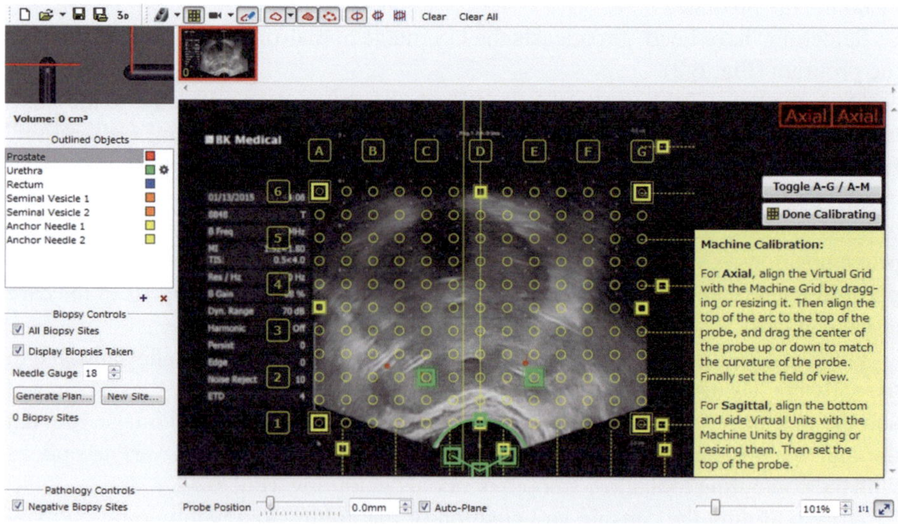

Fig. 6.3 Alignment calibration of ultrasound probe center, field of view, and grid adjustment

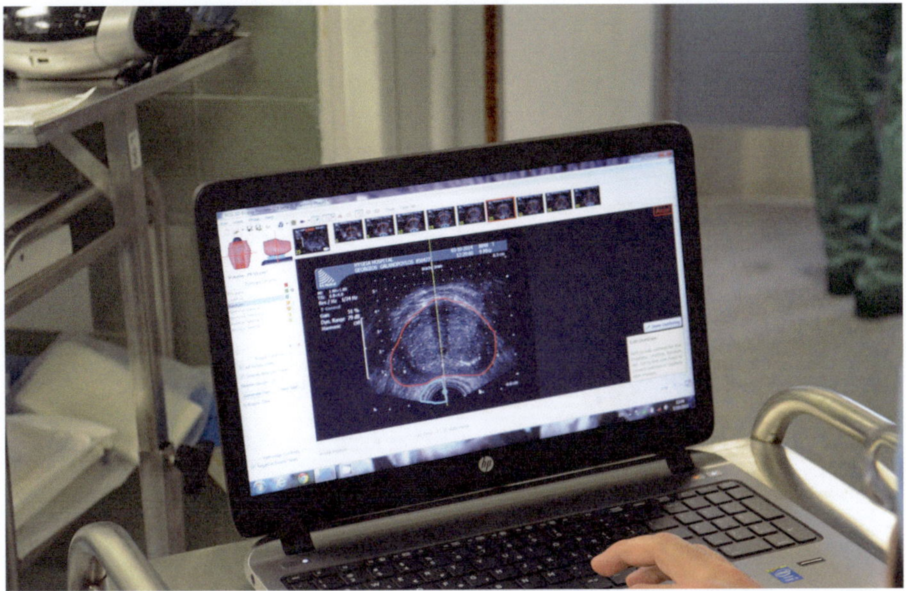

Fig. 6.4 Contouring of prostatic capsule in 5 mm slices

a 17–20 mm specimen length, this information needs to be entered into the program so the biopsy plan will generate enough in-line needles to cover the entire length of the prostate at each biopsy site. The software generates a biopsy plan covering the volume of the prostate with the user's predetermined settings, after which the user can modify specified biopsy locations as needed (Fig. 6.5).

With the biopsy plan set, the urologist is ready to begin taking needle biopsies. On axial view, the urologist approximates each biopsy location generally starting at the top left-most position on the grid corresponding to biopsy site 1. When clicking on biopsy site 1 the coordinates are displayed. The screen also displays how many in-line needles are required or in the case of a variable biopsy needle (discussed below) how long the length of the prostate is at that site. If the inserted needle is not on the grid point (it may be a 1 or 2 mm away), rather than removing the needle and reinserting it the urologist can move the virtual needle to overlap the inserted needle. When the probe switches to sagittal view the auto-plane feature of the software automatically resets to sagittal. The biopsy needle tip will be in the middle of the gland. The virtual image of this needle will also be displayed and just like in axial, the needle image needs to be matched to the inserted biopsy needle (Fig. 6.6).

The position of each biopsy is recorded and the specimen is inked at its proximal end. In general it will take approximately 1.5–2 biopsy cores per gram of prostate for adequate coverage using the brachytherapy template. Once all biopsies have been taken the user can view the overall biopsy coverage of the prostate in each

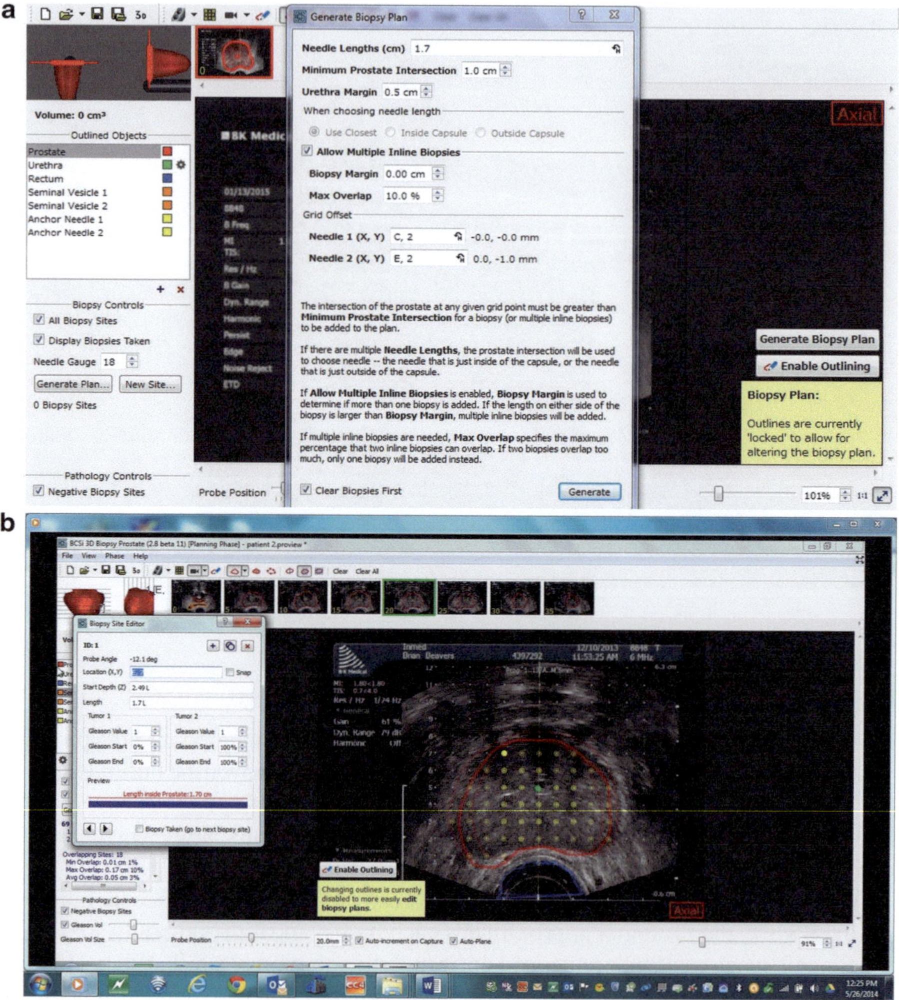

Fig. 6.5 (**a**) Dialogue box where specifications are entered before plan is generated. (**b**) Biopsy plan is generated. Biopsy site 1 is indicated in the dialogue box and by the *bright point* in the plan

axial slice or in full three-dimensional imaging to determine if any areas appear to be under-sampled. The urologist can add a new biopsy location if needed (Fig. 6.7).

The pathology is read for each core and the depth of each cancer from the inked end is recorded, giving each cancer foci a specific location along the specimen. This information for each positive biopsy, including its Gleason score and linear location is entered into the patient's 3D file creating a three-dimensional model of the cancerous lesion locations (Fig. 6.8).

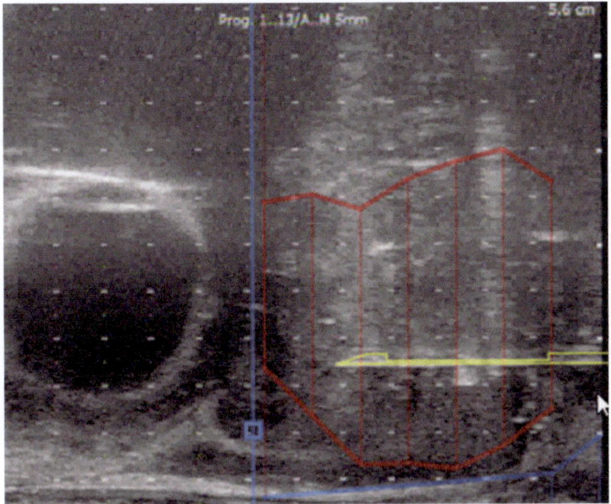

Fig. 6.6 Sagittal view of virtual needle with biopsy needle behind it

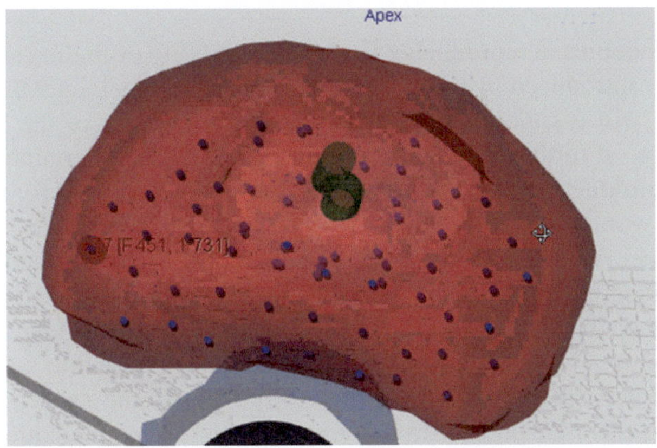

Fig. 6.7 Three-dimensional image of the prostate with biopsy core locations generated to help determine overall biopsy coverage

The 3DMB procedure allows accurate intra-prostate staging of the cancer. Of the 200–220,000 men diagnosed with prostate cancer with Gleason 6/7 disease this procedure will find that approximately one-third would be ideal AS candidates, one-third would need definitive therapy and the rest could be considered for focal therapy. If a patient is found to have cancer amenable to targeted focal therapy, the 3D map can be utilized in the OR to locate the sites to be ablated. For example, cryo-therapy probes can be inserted in the proper needle tracts and advanced to the appropriate depth utilizing the 3D map in a real-time mode. Video 6.1 demonstrates a short video of the procedure.

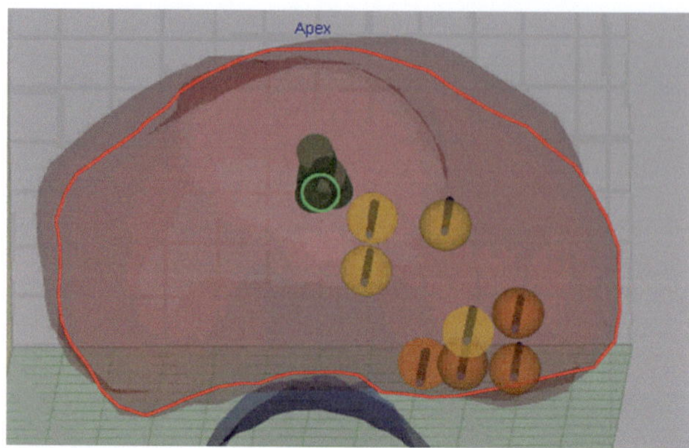

Fig. 6.8 3D model of prostate gland with biopsy results entered into patient's file. This patient who had 1/12 core positive for Gleason score 7 had 4 Gleason 6 and 3 Gleason 7 (darker lesions) on final pathology after 3DMB

Other Considerations

One of the difficulties in reproducing the high probability of finding small lesions is the uncertainty introduced by multiple in-line sticks in rows longer than the current biopsy needle will permit. Brede et al. found that deviation of the biopsy needle course increases at further depths of sampling [3–6]. This uncertainty can be overcome by the introduction of a biopsy needle specifically designed for this approach. Such a needle would require a variable length core bed and gun to fire the needle the correct distance. For example if the urologist were to click on needle #5 and the distance specified at that point was 3.2 cm, the gun would be "dialed" to that distance and fired so the core taken is 3.2 cm. This technology is under development.

Lastly, placing a long tissue specimen on telfa or directly into a formalin filled vial will not permit the pathologist to precisely identify the cancer site along the core. Handling and transport to the lab results in tissue fragmentation. To prevent this, a 6 cm fenestrated cassette which snaps closed and secures the specimen until it arrives at the lab has been developed. Upon arrival in the lab, the pathologist opens the cassette and removes the core intact on a specially developed medium.

Conclusions

The 3DMB software can identify lesions as small as 2.5 mm radius with high probability. Combined with the new needle and tissue cassette, the procedure can be performed quickly and accurately. The concern for over-diagnosis of low grade lesions should not be an issue because a patient with a few low grade lesions can elect active surveillance and not worry about repeat biopsies or risk of progression because of missed high volume or high grade disease. In this scenario, active surveillance becomes "accurate surveillance." The apparent "low risk" patient who undergoes a 3BMB and is found with high grade lesions is no longer "under diagnosed" and is referred for definitive therapy. Finally, a large number of men, who don't qualify for AS or RP, can be offered focal ablation, where a hemi-ablation or hockey-stick ablation is replaced by precise focused ablation of the individual lesions.

References

1. Kepner GR, Kepner JV. Transperineal prostate biopsy: analysis of a uniform core sampling pattern that yields data on tumor volume limits in negative biopsies. Theor Biol Med Model. 2010;17(7):23.
2. Stone NN, Roy J, Hong S, Lo YC, Stock RG. Prostate gland motion and deformation caused by needle placement during brachytherapy. Brachytherapy. 2002;1:154–60.
3. Brede CM, Douville NJ, Jones S. Variable correlation of grid coordinates to core location in template prostate biopsy. Curr Urol. 2013;6(4):194–8. doi:10.1159/000343538.
4. Huo ASY, Hossack T, Symons JLP, et al. Accuracy of primary systematic template guided transperineal biopsy of the prostate for locating prostate cancer: a comparison with radical prostatectomy specimens. J Urol. 2012;187(6):2044–9. doi:10.1016/j.juro.2012.01.066.
5. Brawer MK. The influence of prostate volume on prostate cancer detection. Eur Urol Suppl. 2002;1(6):35–9. doi:10.1016/S1569-9056(02)00055-6.
6. Symons JL, Huo A, Yuen CL, et al. Outcomes of transperineal template-guided prostate biopsy in 409 patients. BJU Int. 2013;112(5):585–93. doi:10.1111/j.1464-410X.2012.11657.x.

Chapter 7
Elastography: Can It Improve Prostate Biopsy Results?

Vassilios M. Skouteris, Spyros D. Yarmenitis, and Georgios P. Zacharopoulos

Introduction

The optimal way to biopsy prostate gland is still evolving. The ultrasound technology has evolved by adding several tools that improve the identification of the disease at early stages and avoid unnecessary biopsies.

Since original sextant scheme introduced by Hodge et al. [1], extended protocols with laterally directed biopsies have been described that considerably increased cancer detection rates [2]. Although the positivity rate was also increased by increasing the number of cores taken, the anterior part of the gland still remained the most frequent region missed by conventional TRUS biopsy [3]. Transperineal template guided biopsy having the advantage of easy access to the anterior region of the gland revealed the importance of transitional zone sampling of which its uniquely involvement in prostate cancer can exceed 50 % [4]. Pinkstaff et al. in 2005 published a study where 210 men underwent transperineal ultrasound template guided

Electronic supplementary material: The online version of this chapter (doi:10.1007/978-3-319-21485-6_7) contains supplementary material, which is available to authorized users. Videos can also be accessed at http://link.springer.com/chapter/10.1007/978-3-319-21485-6_7.

V.M. Skouteris, M.D. (✉)
Prostate Brachytherapy Department, Hygeia Hospital, Hygeia Group,
4 Er. Stavrou Str. And Kifissias Av., Maroussi, Athens 15123, Greece
e-mail: basileskout@hotmail.com

S.D. Yarmenitis, M.D.
Radiology Department, Hygeia Hospital, Hygeia Group,
4 Er. Stavrou Str. And Kifissias Av., Maroussi, Athens 15123, Greece
e-mail: s.yarmenitis@hygeia.gr

G.P. Zacharopoulos, M.D., M.Sc., Ph.D.
Ultrasound Department, Hygeia Hospital, Hygeia Group,
4 Er. Stavrou Str. And Kifissias Av., Maroussi, Athens 15123, Greece
e-mail: g.zacharopoulos@hygeia.gr

© Springer International Publishing Switzerland 2016
N.N. Stone, E.D. Crawford (eds.), *The Prostate Cancer Dilemma*,
DOI 10.1007/978-3-319-21485-6_7

prostate biopsy. All of them had at least one negative transrectal biopsy in the past with 81 % of them having more than one. The mean number of cores obtained was 21. Prostate cancer in the transitional zone was detected in 77 % of the patients and in 46 % of them cancer was solely localized in that region [5].

Transperineal prostate biopsy guided by a template represents the most accurate and uniform way to sample the entire gland [6–8]. One of the advantages of this technique is that is a transcutaneous procedure performed through the perineum and not through the anterior rectal wall, diminishing the risk of infection to negligible levels. Grummet et al. reported almost zero percent of sepsis and hospital readmission rate after 245 transperineal prostate biopsies [9]. Another advantage is that puncture sites are guided by a template (or grid) similar to the one used for brachytherapy or cryotherapy. This allows a uniform mapping of the gland at constant 5 mm intervals increasing the cancer detection rate from 25 to 60 %. Ayres et al. reported in 2012 that 101 patients already diagnosed with prostate cancer by transrectal biopsy and were on active surveillance, they underwent restaging by transperineal template guided biopsy. The criteria used for surveillance were: age $\leq$ 75 years, PSA $\leq$ 15 ng/ml, clinical stage $\leq$T2a, $\leq$50 % cores positive on transrectal biopsy and $\leq$10 mm positive in each core. The results showed that 34 % of the patients had more significant disease than falsely originally estimated and 44 % of them had disease predominantly in the anterior part of the gland. As a result of the above, 33 % of them stopped surveillance and proceed to a radical treatment [10].

In 2009, Onik and his colleagues restaged 180 patients who were considering conservative management of their disease by transperineal mapping biopsy. All patients had unilateral, Gleason 6, prostate cancer found on TRUS biopsy. The mapping biopsy was carried out transperineally using a brachytherapy grid and biopsies were taken every 5 mm throughout the volume of the gland, under TRUS guidance. Median 50 cores were obtained. Their results showed that in 61.1 % (110 patients) the disease was bilateral and in 25 % (45 patients) Gleason score was upgraded to 7 or higher [11].

Initially puncture sites of biopsy schemes were guided solely by grey scale imaging. Afterwards the addition of Doppler ultrasound improved blood flow information to the suspicious areas. Elastography is a technique that produces images about the mechanical characteristics of the tissues. It uses ultrasound imaging modality to detect and visually record shear deformation of a tissue by the shearing forces of an ultrasonic waveform and the elastic restoring forces of the tissue against this deformation. Two types of shearing effects may be observed, simple shear that displaces a single dimension of a tissue body resulting in simple shape deformation and pure shear that displaces a whole surface of the tissue body resulting in horizontal expansion of it.

In clinical practice ultrasound (US) elastograms may be illustrated as static images of the tissue strain usually under the term "Strain or Compression Elastography" or as dynamic tissue displacement measurements. The latter method comprises various techniques that are commonly grouped under the term "Shear Wave Elastography" and offer the capability to quantitatively measure the shear wave properties. Both elastography methods can be used to detect the elastographic properties of normal prostate tissue against those of cancerous lesions.

Several publications report a significant improvement in the detection of prostatic cancer by the use of strain elastography and also a better performance in the guidance of targeted needle biopsy sampling [12–18]. However, some controversial reports exist that show inability of the method to satisfactorily distinguish prostate cancer from chronic prostatitis or to confirm improvements of biopsy guidance [19, 20].

In regard with Shear Wave elastography, a few reports at the moment with promising results, support an improved Negative Predictive Value rate by using a cut-off stiffness value of 35–37 kPa of malignant lesions [18, 20].

Major limitations of Strain Elastography are the non-uniform compression force over the prostate gland and the intra- and inter-operator dependency. Limitations of Shear Wave elastography mainly include the slower real time frame rate and the small elasticity sampling box that cannot include the whole organ.

Transrectal Ultrasound and Elastography

In our institution prostate transrectal US elastography is obtained with a Hitachi Hi-Vision Preirus machine (Hitachi Hi Vision Preirus, Hitachi Medical Corporation, Tokyo, Japan) with an EUP-U531 intracavity probe, performing at 8.0–4.0 MHz with Tissue Harmonics and Compound Imaging in b-mode and the fourth generation Hitachi Real-Time Elastography (HI-RTE) technique.

In a period of 10 months, 153 consecutive male patients were evaluated (mean age: 63.6 years, range: 37–84). In all patients a standard b-mode TRUS scan was followed by a color Doppler scan and Real-Time Compression Elastography (RTCE). The b-mode TRUS findings were categorized as type 1: no focal lesions, type 2: ill-defined focal lesions and type 3: definite focal lesion(s) (Fig. 7.1).

Using the Hitachi elasticity color code mapping that encodes stiff tissues as blue and soft as red (Fig. 7.2), elastic properties of the peripheral zone were classified as type 1: normal stiffness (evenly mixed red, orange, yellow, and green hues), type 2: inhomogeneous/inconclusive stiffness, and type 3: definite focal lesions of increased stiffness (blue). Intact prostate fibrofatty margin (capsule) was illustrated as an Orange/Red rim in the RTCE images (Figs. 7.3 and 7.4).

An US guided needle biopsy was then performed. In 122/153 patients 12 core biopsies were taken. The rest 31 patients had 6–8 core biopsies. In both B-mode and RTCE scans, type 1 images were interpreted as negative, type 3 images as positive and type 2 images as inconclusive. Ultrasound findings were compared to the results of the core biopsies. Inconclusive were the B-mode TRUS scans in 14/153 (9 %) patients. Three of these were among the 46 prostate cancer patients (7 %) while 11 were among the 107 non-cancer patients (10 %). Inconclusive were the RTCE scans in 8/153 (5 %) patients. Three of these were among the 46 cancer patients (7 %) while five were among the 107 non-cancer patients (5 %). Disruption of the normal prostatic capsule red rim in RTCE was found in 11 (73 %) of the 15 cancer patients that were histologi-

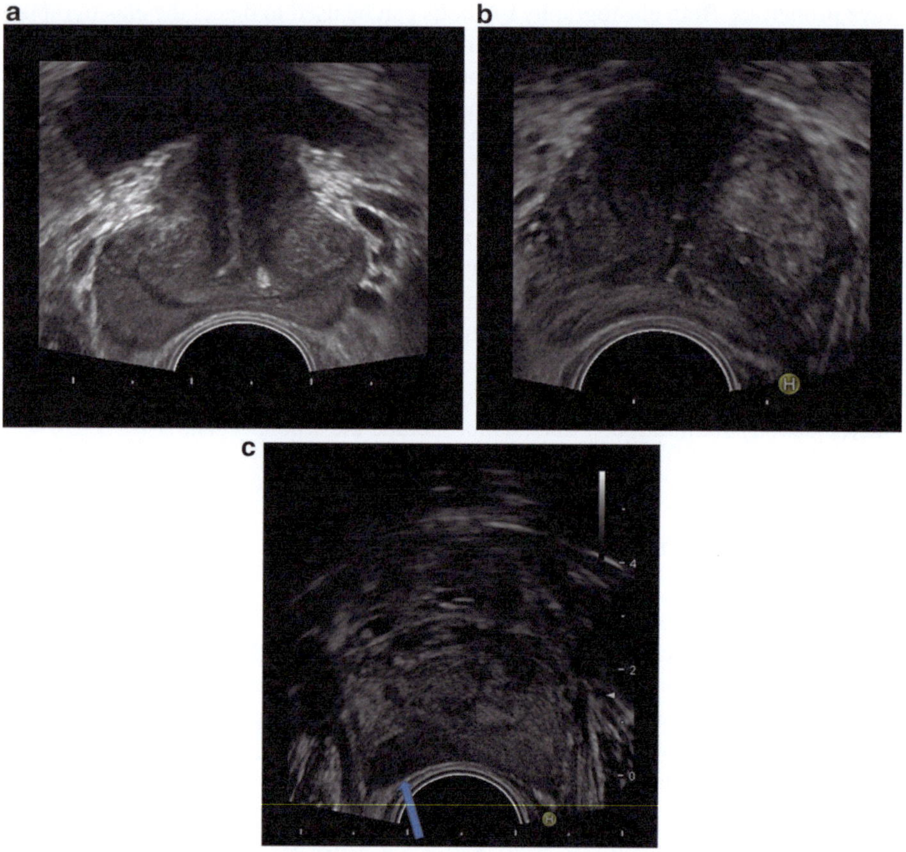

Fig. 7.1 (**a**) B mode TRUS findings classification. Type 1, no focal lesion. (**b**) B mode TRUS findings classification. Type 2, intermediate or ill-defined focal lesions. (**c**) B mode TRUS findings classification. Type 3, definite focal lesion (*blue arrow*)

Fig. 7.2 Color coding of strain or compression elastography

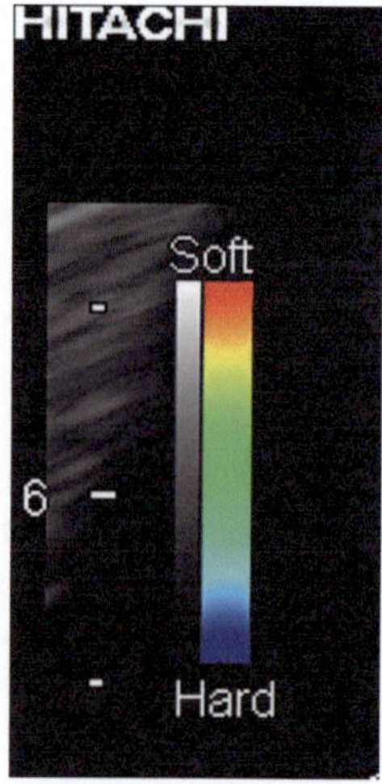

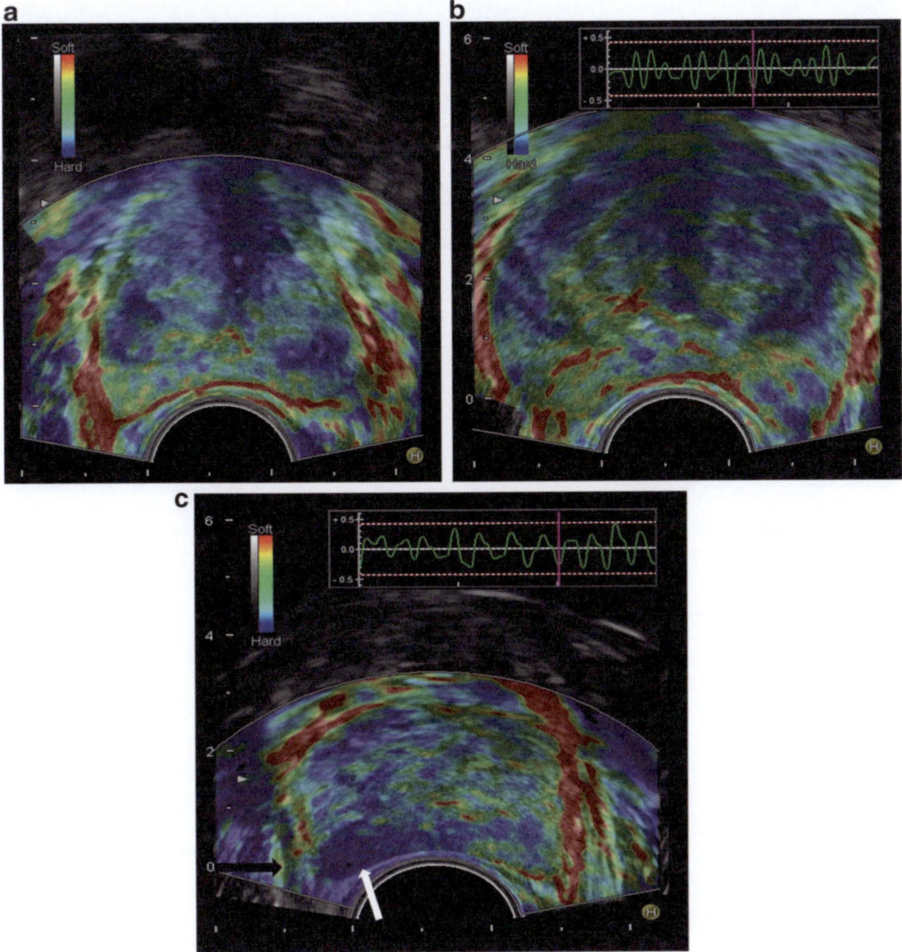

Fig. 7.3 (**a**) Prostatic peripheral zone RTCE TRUS findings classification. Normal stiffness. (**b**) Prostatic peripheral zone RTCE TRUS findings classification. Inhomogeneous/inconclusive stiffness. (**c**) Prostatic peripheral zone RTCE TRUS findings classification. Definite focal lesion of increased stiffness (*white arrow*), capsule disruption (*black arrow*)

cally proven to have neoplasia extended beyond the prostatic capsule. Sensitivity, specificity, positive and negative predictive values are summarized in Table 7.1.

These data suggest that RTCE improves the diagnostic rate of TRUS in detecting peripheral zone prostatic cancer and yields more robust information in the presence of cancer lesions. It can discriminate the inconclusive results of baseline B-mode images. Thus the number of needle core samples may be reduced. It also may enhance the role of TRUS in prostatic cancer local staging (Video 7.1). Even our data show that addition of elastography to TRUS increases accuracy it' s efficacy has never been compared to the pathologic result obtained through transperineal tem-

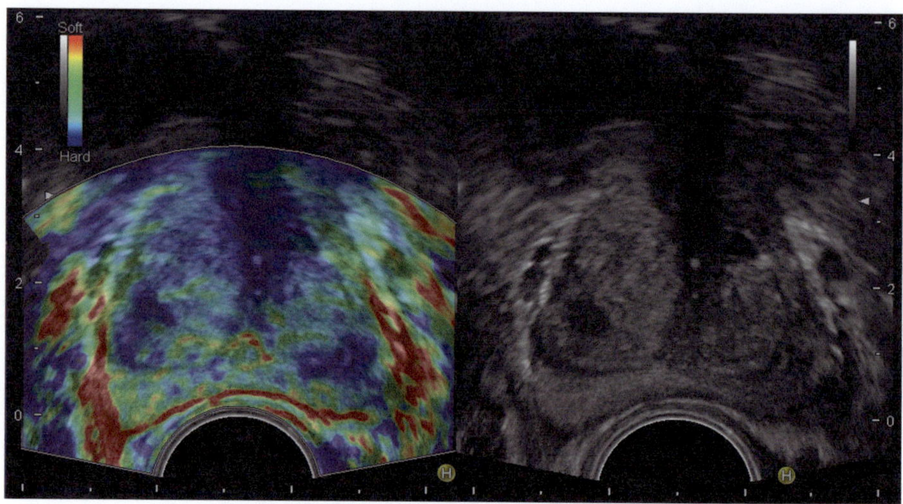

Fig. 7.4 An important characteristic or advantage of strain elastography is the ability of assessing the integrity of prostatic capsule. In this figure we can see that the capsule looks normal, intact on both sides. Peripheral zone has normal elastographic appearance and we can see few hard lesions in the transitional zone, bilaterally, which proved to be non cancerous

Table 7.1 Results of TRUS biopsy with elastography

	Needle biopsy positive	Needle biopsy negative	
TRUS positive	39	21	PPV 65 %
TRUS negative or inconclusive	8	85	NPV 91 %
	(Sensitivity 83 %)	(Specificity 80 %)	
RTCE positive	43	9	PPV 83 %
RTCE negative or inconclusive	4	97	NPV 96 %
	(Sensitivity 91 %)	(Specificity 92 %)	

plate guided prostate biopsy. As previously mentioned, this biopsy technique provides the most reliable and uniform access to all regions of the prostate and for this reason we believe it represents a highly accurate method for assessing the effectiveness of elastography and its capability in distinguishing cancerous foci from normal prostate parenchyma. Our institution started offering transperineal mapping biopsy to patients in 2008 and elastography was added to the procedure in 2011, a year after ultrasound department was equipped with the ultrasound elastography machine.

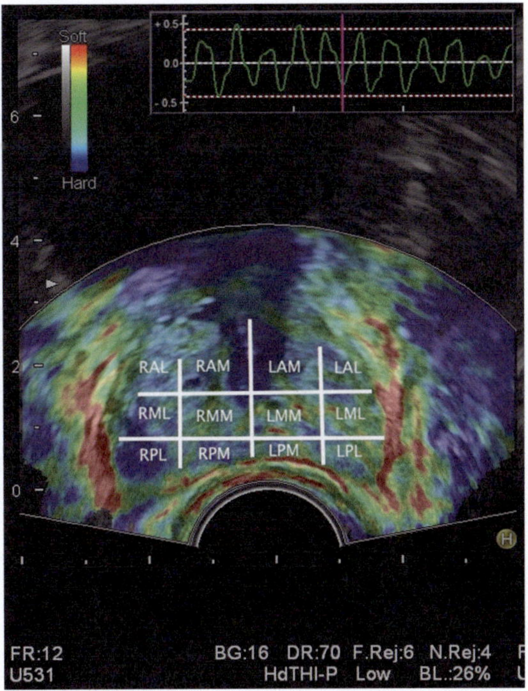

Fig. 7.5 Radiologist marks hard-suspicious area on elastography (e.g., RPL). He will then reassure that this area is sampled during mapping biopsy and the samples marked accordingly

Technique of Transperineal Biopsy and Elastography

Patients at risk for prostate cancer were referred for transrectal ultrasound elastography followed by a transperineal biopsy. The patient is placed at a right lateral decubitus position with the knees elevated towards the chest and a local anesthetic gel is introduced in the rectum. Prostate is divided in six quadrants in each lobe, anterior-lateral (AL), anterior/medial (AM), middle/lateral (ML), middle/medial (MM), posterior/lateral (PL) and posterior/medial (PM). The radiologist performing the ultrasound locates suspicious-hard lesions on elastography areas and carefully maps the quadrant in which they are present in order after to note which sample taken during the transperineal biopsy corresponds to that area (Fig. 7.5). After completion of elastography, the patient is brought in the operating room where the team is present consisting of an urologist and the radiologist who previously performed the elastographic evaluation. The patient is now placed in the dorsal lithotomy position and a Foley catheter is placed, draining in the bladder. The purpose of the urethral catheter is to clearly identify the anatomic relations and to prevent any urethral injury during the procedure. The stepping device is attached to the table and ultrasound probe fixed to it (B&K Leopard, model 8558 probe, B&K Medical, Winthrop, Mass) and inserted to the rectum. Prostate image is adjusted to fit template's coordinates on the ultrasound screen. That is a crucial adjustment since the holes of the

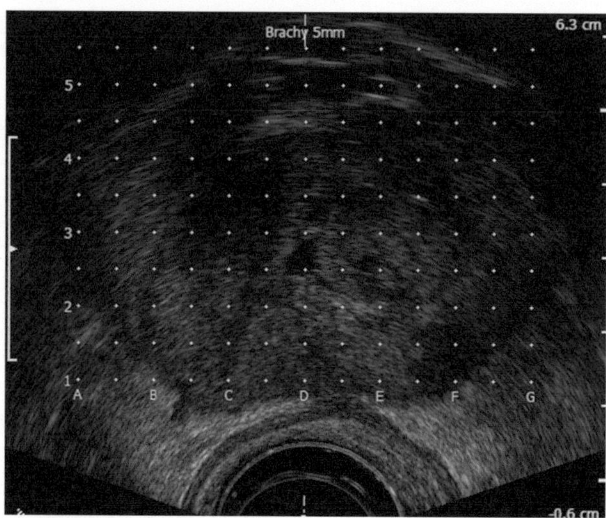

Fig. 7.6 Superimposed template on transverse ultrasound image of prostate. Samples were obtained at 5 mm intervals throughout whole prostate volume. Sampling starts from right lobe and anterior lateral part (e.g., C capital 4) working our way down till the most medial/posterior part (e.g., D capital 1)

grid have to have access to all parts of the prostate. Sampling then starts under general anesthesia, in transverse plane beginning from the right lobe and most anterior/lateral part, working our way down till the most medial/posterior part (Fig. 7.6). Once the needle is visible, image is switched to sagittal and the needle is pulled back until the tip reaches the apex of the gland. The biopsy device is then fired and the sample taken. In cases where prostate length exceeds sample length (1.8 cm), e.g., in a gland with 4 cm length, two cores are taken one from the base till middle of the gland and one from the middle till the base. If length extends beyond 4 cm, a third core at the same level can be taken to cover the entire sagittal distance of the gland. The biopsy instrument used ("gun") was the disposable 18G "Max-Core", with 25 cm long needle (CR Bard, Covington, GA, USA). When right lobe is finished, we switch and biopsy the left side. Samples are carefully put to the corresponding labeled vials according to their region and the radiologist is reassuring that positive-hard areas on elastography are mapped correctly, sampled and marked (Figs. 7.5 and 7.7). Once the procedure is finished, patient is brought to the recovery room and Foley catheter is removed. If the patient is unable to urinate catheter is reinserted the same day. When the pathology report is available urologist and radiologist check if cancerous areas correspond to the positive elastographic quadrants (Figs. 7.8, 7.9, 7.10, and 7.11).

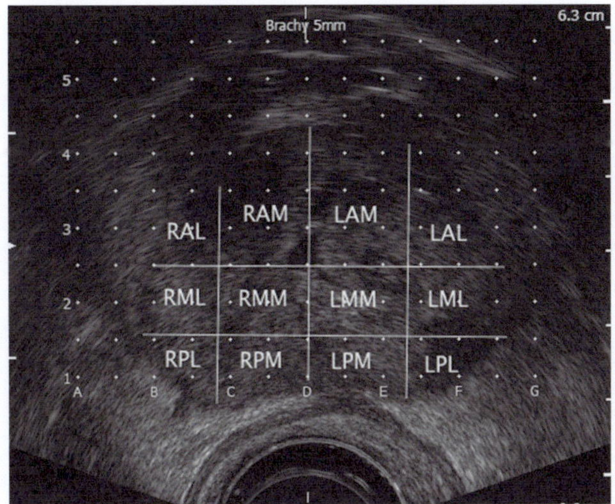

Fig. 7.7 Radiologist reassures during mapping biopsy that area RPL is sampled and marks down names of cores (e.g., B capital 1, B small 1, B capital 1½, B small 1½)

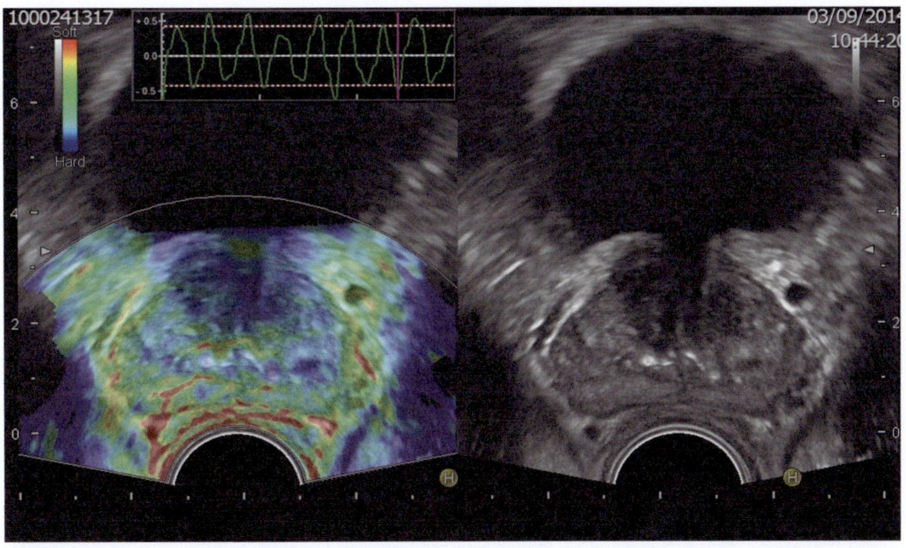

Fig. 7.8 Normal elastographic appearance of peripheral zone, few hard areas present in the transitional zone. Mapping biopsy revealed 3/15 positive cores from the right lobe (RAL, RML, RMM) and 5/19 positive from the left lobe (LAL, LAM, LML, LPL, LMM), Gleason 7 (4+3)

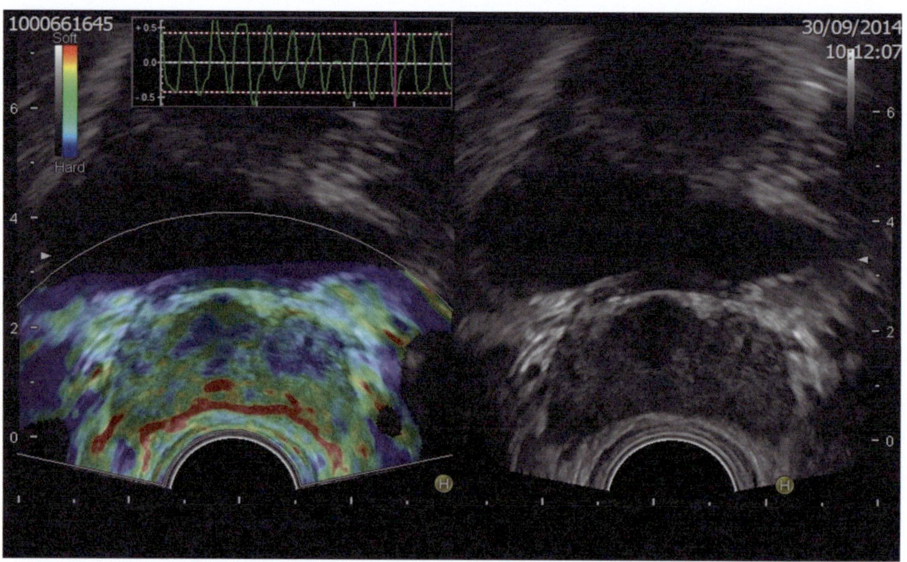

Fig. 7.9 Normal elastographic appearance of peripheral zone, few hard areas present in the transitional zone. Mapping biopsy revealed a Gleason 7 (3 + 4) prostate cancer, with 4/25 cores positive from the right lobe (4xRAM) and 8/31 positive from the left lobe (2xLAM, LAL, 4xLMM, LML)

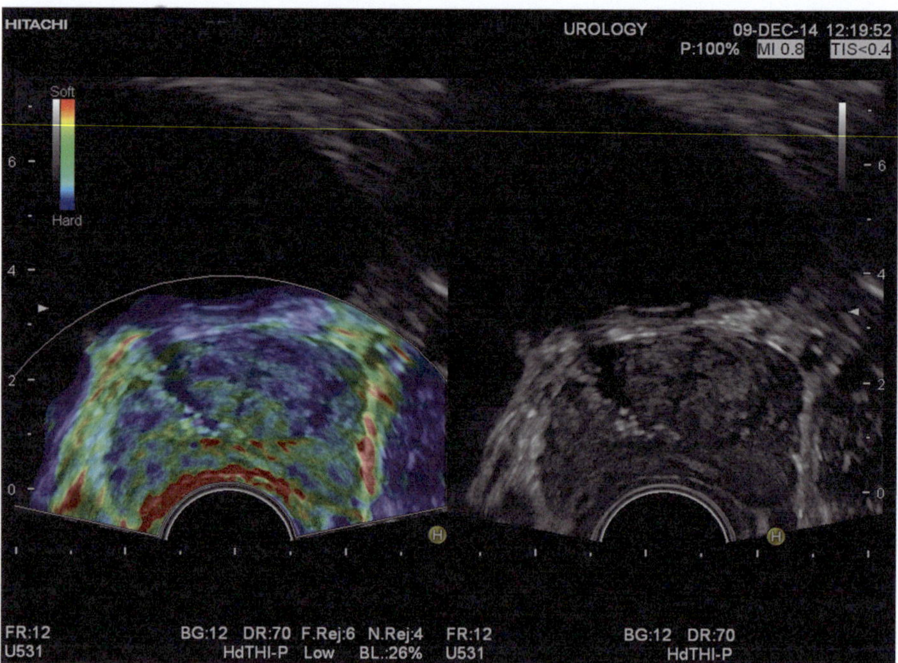

Fig. 7.10 Normal elastographic appearance of peripheral zone, few hard areas present in the transitional zone not pathologic. Mapping biopsy revealed one core positive for adenocarcinoma out of 20 (total 44) in the right lobe (RPL quadrant), Gleason 6 (3 + 3)

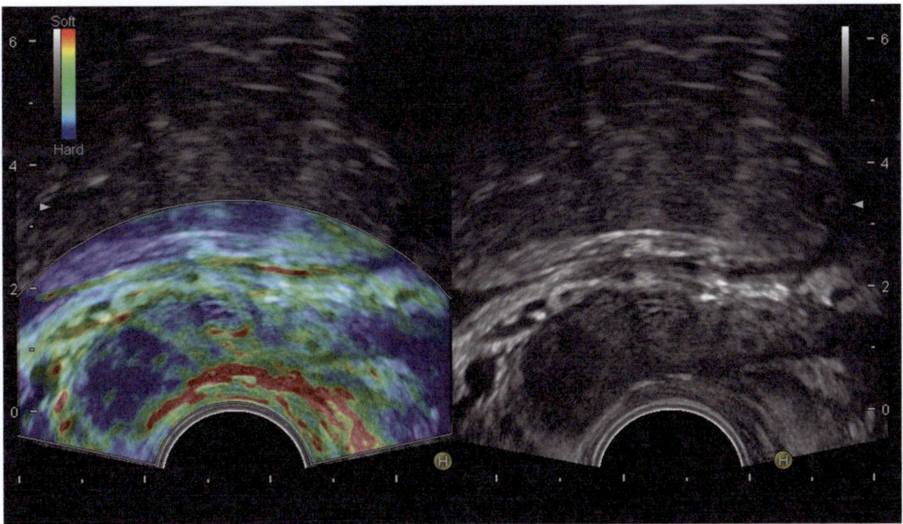

Fig. 7.11 Extensive hard lesion occupying the right peripheral zone with signs of capsular disruption on both sides. Few hard areas also present on the transitional zone bilaterally. Mapping biopsy revealed 9/17 positive cores on the right lobe (2xRML, 5xRPL, 1xRMM, 1xRPM) and 9/23 positive from the left lobe (1xLAL, 7xLPL, 1xLPM), Gleason 9 (5+4)

Results of Transperineal Template-Guided Biopsy with Elastography

From July 2008 till December 2014, 149 consecutive patients underwent transperineal mapping biopsy. In the last 15 of them "3D biopsy" software (see Chap. 6) was used to guide and record the biopsy procedure. 73 patients (49 %) had abnormal findings on digital rectal examination (DRE) and 52 of them previously underwent negative transrectal biopsies in 1–3 occasions (one: 33 patients, two: 16 patients, three: 3 patients). 83 (55.7 %) of the patients were submitted to TRUS compression elastography before the mapping biopsy and the pathology results were used to make comparisons between elastography and transperineal biopsy findings. Median patient age was 66 years (range 48–86), mean PSA 8 ng/dl (range 1–118), mean prostate volume (PV) 46 cm^3 (range 18–137) and mean PSA density (PSAD) 0.2037 (range 0.02–4.21) (Table 7.2).

Preparation the night before the biopsy included a fleet enema around 19:00 and light, low in fiber supper was suggested. Patients were prescribed an a-blocker and oral fluoroquinolone for 10 days total (five pre and five post-procedure). PV, residual urine, international prostate symptom score (IPSS) and quality of life measurements were determined prior and 1 week after procedure (Table 7.3). Associations were tested by ANOVA and two-tail T test and correlations/odds ratios estimated by chi-square (Pearson).

Table 7.2 Patient characteristics of 149 men undergoing transperineal mapping biopsy

Variable	Mean	Median	Range
Age (years)	66	66	48–86
PSA (ng/ml)	8.1	6.3	1–118
PSAD	0.193	0.129	0.02–4.21
Prostate Volume (cm^3)	46	45.5	18–147

Table 7.3 Factors comparison before and after (1 week) transperineal biopsy

Variable	IPSS	Residual volume	Prostate volume
Before TPMB	4.6	14.1	49.1
After TPMB	6.6	18.9	57.2
p value	<0.001	<0.001	<0.001

A median 46 cores (range 18–84) were obtained, 23 from each lobe. 67 men (44.96 %) were diagnosed with prostate cancer and of the 52 with prior negative transrectal biopsy, 25 (48.1 %) were proved positive for prostate adenocarcinoma through the transperineal route. 20 (80 %) of them, were characterized as clinical significant cancers according to Epstein criteria (2005). Mean number of positive cores was 6.7 (range 1–26), Gleason score was 6 in 25 (37.3 %), 7 in 36 (53.7 %) and 8–10 in 6 (9 %). Positive biopsy was associated only with a positive DRE (61.5 % vs. 26.5 %, $p<0.001$, OR 4.5), and a positive family history (88.9 % vs. 36.5 %, $p=0.002$, OR 13.9). PSA level, prior negative biopsy and number of cores taken were not significant predictors of a positive biopsy. Mean PSAD for negative biopsy was 0.1359 and for positive biopsy 0.2885 ($p=0.057$). Of the Gleason scores 6, 10/24 (41.6 %) had PSAD ≤ 0.15 and ≤ 2 positive cores ($p=0.004$) but 16/35 (45.7 %) with Gleason score 7 also had PSAD ≤ 0.15.

Compression elastography was positive in 33/46 (71.7 %) of the positive biopsies in the peripheral zone ($p=0.007$, OR 5.1, 95 % CI 1.5–17.1) and had an ROC area of 0.690. But efficacy of elastography in the other zones of prostate as well as in determining bilateral disease was lower than in the periphery. Mapping biopsy found cancer located in the remaining zones of prostate where elastography was negative in 18/40 (45 %) of patients. Elastography also incorrectly evaluated that disease existed only in one lobe in 19/36 (52.7 %) patients where transperineal route proved that bilateral localization was present. When results in the peripheral zone where stratified according to prostate volume we found out that in patients with PV < 40 cm^3 ($n=28$) elastography could identify cancer in 85.7 % of the cases (24 patients) compared to 44.4 % (8/18 patients) in glands with PV ≥ 40 cm^3.

Conclusions

Prostate elastography gives valuable information in the peripheral zone of the prostate where the majority of prostate cancers arise but efficacy in prediction of bilateral disease and cancer involvement in other zones of the gland is limited. It improves the detection rate over b-mode TRUS guided biopsy.

Gland size significantly affects elastography results, as in smaller glands predicting of cancerous areas is more accurate. When prostate volume is increasing efficacy of elastography is diminished.

References

1. Hodge KK, McNeal JE, Stamey TA. Ultrasound guided transrectal core biopsies of the palpably abnormal prostate. J Urol. 1989;142(1):66–70.
2. Chon CH, Lai FC, McNeal JE, Presti Jr JC. Use of extended systematic sampling in patients with a prior negative prostate needle biopsy. J Urol. 2002;167(6):2457–60.
3. Meng MV, Franks JH, Presti Jr JC, Shinohara K. The utility of apical anterior horn biopsies in prostate cancer detection. Urol Oncol. 2003;21(5):361–5.
4. Merrick GS, Gutman S, Andreini H, Taubenlag W, et al. Prostate cancer distribution in patients diagnosed by transperineal template-guided saturation biopsy. Eur Urol. 2007;52(3):723–4.
5. Pinkstaff DM, Igel TC, Petrou SP, Broderick GA, Wehle MJ, Young PR. Systematic transperineal ultrasound-guided template biopsy of the prostate: three-year experience. Urology. 2005;65(4):735–9.
6. Dimmen M, Vlatkovic L, Hole KH, Nesland JM, Brennhovd B, et al. Transperineal prostate biopsy detects significant cancer in patients with elevated prostate-specific antigen (PSA) levels and previous negative transrectal biopsies. BJU Int. 2012;110:E69.
7. Epstein JI, Sanderson H, Carter HB, Scharfstein DO. Utility of saturation biopsy to predict insignificant cancer at radical prostatectomy. Urology. 2005;66(2):356–60.
8. Nafie S, Mellon JK, Dormer JP, Khan MA. The role of transperineal template prostate biopsies in prostate cancer diagnosis in biopsy naïve men with PSA less than 20ng/ml. Prostate Cancer Prostatic Dis. 2014;17(2):170–3.
9. Grummet JP, Weerakoon M, Huang S, Lawrentschuk N, Frydenberg M, Moon DA, O'Reilly M, Murphy D. Sepsis and 'superbugs': should we favour the transperineal over the transrectal approach for prostate biopsy? BJU Int. 2014;114(3):384–8.
10. Ayres BE, Montgomery BS, Barber NJ, Pereira N, Langley SE, Denham P, Bott SR. The role of transperineal template prostate biopsies in restaging men with prostate cancer managed by active surveillance. BJU Int. 2012;109(8):1170–6.
11. Onik G, Miessau M, Bostwick DG. Three-dimensional prostate mapping biopsy has a potentially significant impact on prostate cancer management. J Clin Oncol. 2009;27(26):4321–6.
12. Salomon G, Kollerman J, Thederan I, et al. Evaluation of prostate cancer detection with ultrasound real-time elastography: a comparison with step section pathological analysis after radical prostatectomy. Eur Urol. 2008;54:1354–62.
13. Pallwein L, Mitterberger M, Struve P, et al. Real-time elastography for detecting prostate cancer: preliminary experience. BJU Int. 2007;100:42–6.
14. Brock M, von Bodman C, Sommerer F, et al. Comparison of real-time elastography with greyscale ultrasonography for detection of organ-confined prostate cancer and extra capsular extension: a prospective analysis using whole mount sections after radical prostatectomy. BJU Int. 2011;108:E217–22.
15. Brock M, von Bodman C, Palisaar RJ, et al. The impact of real-time elastography guiding a systematic prostate biopsy to improve cancer detection rate: a prospective study of 353 patients. J Urol. 2012;187:2039–43.
16. Walz J, Marcy M, Pianna JT, et al. Identification of the prostate cancer index lesion by real-time elastography: considerations for focal therapy of prostate cancer. World J Urol. 2011;29: 589–94.
17. Aigner F, Pallwein L, Junker D, et al. Value of real-time elastography targeted biopsy for prostate cancer detection in men with prostate specific antigen 1.25 ng/ml or greater and 4.00 ng/ml or less. J Urol. 2010;184:913–7.

18. Aboumarzouk OM, Ogston S, Huang Z, et al. Diagnostic accuracy of transrectal elastosonography (TRES) imaging for the diagnosis of prostate cancer: a systematic review and meta-analysis. BJU Int. 2012;110:1414–23.
19. Kapoor A, Mahajan G, Sidhu BS. Real-time elastography in the detection of prostate cancer in patients with raised PSA level. Ultrasound Med Biol. 2011;37:1374–81.
20. Kamoi K, Okihara K, Ochiai A, et al. The utility of transrectal real-time elastography in the diagnosis of prostate cancer. Ultrasound Med Biol. 2008;34:1025–32.

Chapter 8
Multiparametric MRI of the Prostate as a Tool for Prostate Cancer Detection, Localization, and Risk Assessment

Marc A. Bjurlin, Neil Mendhiratta, and Samir S. Taneja

Introduction

Advances in multiparametric magnetic resonance imaging (mpMRI) hold promise for the improved detection and characterization of prostate cancer [1]. MpMRI combines diffusion-weighted imaging, dynamic contrast-enhanced sequences, or spectroscopy with conventional T2-weighted sequences. With a combination of anatomic and functional imaging sequences to identify suspicious regions in the prostate, pre-biopsy mpMRI has the potential to improve prostate cancer detection and risk stratification through MRI-targeted biopsy [2]. In this chapter we review the role of mpMRI in prostate cancer detection, the outcomes of MRI-targeted biopsy, and the critical concepts currently under evaluation in validation of an MRI-based prostate cancer risk stratification strategy.

Limitations of Contemporary Systematic Biopsy Technique and Methods for Prostate Cancer Detection

The contemporary random 12-core systematic biopsy strategy relies on sampling efficiency for cancer detection and is consequently subject to sampling error. Cancers are often small, intermingled with benign stroma, and not uniformly distributed

M.A. Bjurlin, D.O. • S.S. Taneja, M.D. (✉)
Division of Urologic Oncology, Department of Urology, NYU Langone
Medical Center, 150 E 32nd Street, 2nd Floor, New York, NY 10016, USA
e-mail: marc.bjurlin@gmail.com; samir.taneja@nyumc.org

N. Mendhiratta, B.A.
School of Medicine, NYU Langone Medical Center,
550 1st Avenue, New York, NY 10016, USA
e-mail: Neil.Mendhiratta@nyumc.org

© Springer International Publishing Switzerland 2016
N.N. Stone, E.D. Crawford (eds.), *The Prostate Cancer Dilemma*,
DOI 10.1007/978-3-319-21485-6_8

within the gland. As a result, clinically significant cancers frequently go undetected. Under-sampling of the prostate during ultrasound-guided biopsy also leads to incorrect risk stratification in a subset of men with a potential for categorization of clinically significant tumors as low volume or low grade. Random non-targeted prostate biopsies risk inadequate sampling of a cancer lesion often at its periphery. This may reveal a small length of tumor in a core with a low Gleason score, when in fact a clinically significant lesion may exist adjacent to the biopsy site. Approximately 30–50 % of men over age 50 years harbor clinically insignificant PCa at autopsy. These clinically insignificant cancers are often identified by chance during a systematic biopsy approach, contributing, in part, to the problem of over-detection and over-treatment of indolent PCa. Repeat biopsy increases detection of clinically insignificant PCa. The recent trend of overcoming sampling error through increasing core number, or repeating biopsies, further escalates the risk of identifying small, indolent cancers which may have little to do with the patient's PSA elevation [3].

Introducing pre-biopsy mpMRI and MRI-targeted biopsy in the evaluation of men at risk for prostate cancer has the potential to address many of the shortcomings of contemporary clinical approaches to prostate cancer diagnosis using systematic biopsy. Potential advantages of pre-biopsy mpMRI and MRI-targeted biopsy include increased detection of high-risk prostate cancer, reduced detection of low risk, indolent disease, utilization of fewer biopsy cores, reduction of the number of men needing biopsy, and better sampling of cancer leading to more accurate risk stratification [4, 5].

Multiparametric MRI: Image Sequences

T2-Weighted Imaging

T2-weighted MR images, reflecting tissue water content, have high spatial resolution and clearly define the prostate's zonal anatomy, distinguishing the peripheral zone (high signal intensity) from the central zone (surrounding the ejaculatory ducts in the posterior prostate base and exhibiting decreased T2 signal intensity) and transition zones (surrounding the urethra, extending anteriorly and superiorly from the level of the verumontanum, and exhibiting heterogeneous, often swirled, signal intensity) (Fig. 8.1) [6]. In the peripheral zone, PCa can appear as an area of low signal intensity. The degree of intensity decrease differs with the Gleason score, with higher Gleason score components showing lower signal intensities [7]. T2-weighted imaging results in false-positive findings, as low signal intensity can also be the consequence of benign abnormalities including acute and chronic prostatitis, atrophy, scars, post-irradiation or hormonal treatment effects, hyperplasia, and post-biopsy hemorrhage. Partly related to the heterogeneous appearance of BPH with areas of both increased and decreased signal intensity, cancer in transition zone may be more difficult to discern than in the peripheral zone, particularly for the less experienced radiologist. However, morphological features such as homogeneously low signal

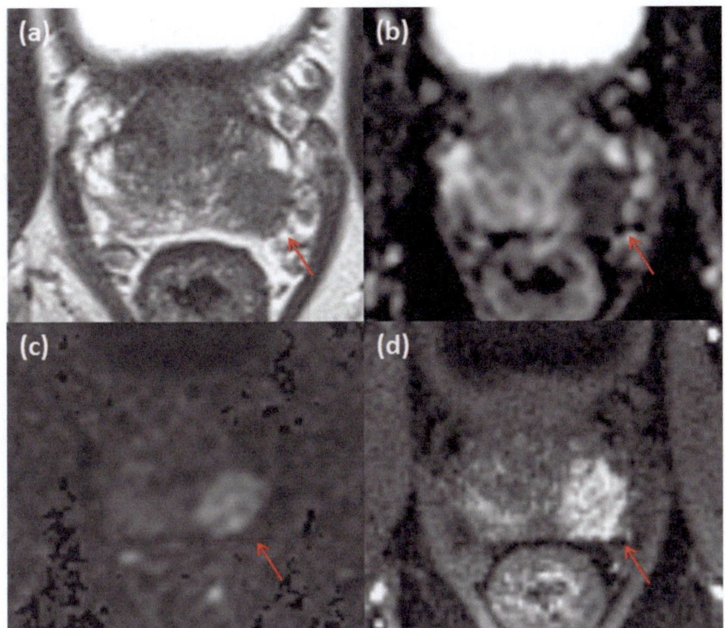

Fig. 8.1 Sixty-six year-old biopsy naïve male with a PSA of 6.2 underwent mpMRI demonstrating a Likert scale suspicion score of 5/5 in the left posterolateral base to mid peripheral zone lesion: T2WI (**a**), ADC (**b**), DWI (*b*-value 1500) (**c**), and DCE (single time-point (**d**)). Systematic biopsy demonstrated Gleason score 6 (3+3) prostate cancer while MRI-targeted biopsy demonstrated Gleason score 8 (4+4) cancer in 4/4 cores. *Red arrow* points to lesion

intensity, ill-defined irregular edges of the suspicious lesion, invasion into the urethra or the anterior fibromuscular stroma, and lenticular shape are helpful for detection of transition zone tumor [8].

Diffusion-Weighted Imaging

Diffusion-weighted (DW) MRI measures random motion of water molecules. The strength of the gradient that determines the degree of diffusion-weighting is reflected by the sequence's *b*-value. By performing DWI with multiple *b*-values, it is possible to compute the apparent diffusion coefficient (ADC) based on the signal intensity measured at each *b*-value image to quantify the restriction of water diffusion (Fig. 8.1). Traditionally, a maximal *b*-value of around 1000 s/mm^2 has been used. More recent data show that use of higher *b*-values up to 2000 s/mm^2 helps eliminate background signal from normal prostate and may increase the accuracy of PCa detection [9], within both the peripheral zone and transition zone [10]. However, modern MRI hardware and careful attention to sequence optimization is required to maintain image quality when using these very high *b*-values. On ADC maps, PCa frequently shows low ADC [11], and an inverse correlation exists between quantitative ADC values and the Gleason score [12]. While ADC does correlate with final Gleason score, the confidence intervals are widely overlapping, limiting the ability to use ADC as a surrogate of Gleason score. This is an area of ongoing investigation and technical optimization aimed to improve ADC's predictive ability in the future. Limitations of DWI include low signal-to-noise ratio and image distortion, both of which become more problematic at higher *b*-values. Nonetheless, DWI is a widely available technique with relatively straightforward acquisition and post-processing. Moreover, given its strong association with tumor aggressiveness, it may prove to be the primary sequence for tumor detection and characterization [13].

Perfusion Imaging

Dynamic contrast-enhanced (DCE) MRI consists of a series of fast T1-weighted sequences covering the prostate before and after rapid injection (2–4 mL/s) of a bolus of a gadolinium chelate. Given the serial rapid imaging of the prostate, DCE-MRI allows assessment of contrast kinetics within focal lesions (Fig. 8.1). PCa typically enhances faster and to a greater extent than surrounding prostate, and will also show more rapid washout of contrast in a fraction of cases. Even though prostatitis-related enhancement is usually diffuse and non-focal in nature, and BPH-related enhancement is often well-encapsulated and spherical, the non-specific nature of these patterns limits the utility of DCE findings in isolation, resulting in DCE often being applied largely as an adjunct to interpretations based primarily on findings on T2WI and DWI. A simple approach to evaluating DCE-MRI is through a subjective visual assessment of the raw dynamic images. Alternatively, semi-quantitative parameters, such as the time-to-peak, wash-in rate, and washout rate, may be computed to allow pixel-wide construction of parametric perfusion maps. A compartment-based model may also be performed to generate truly quantitative metrics. This has largely been performed using a Tofts model, which provides the parameter k^{trans} (transfer constant), reflecting the forward transfer rate constant between the plasma and extravascular extracellular space and is elevated in PCa [14].

One limitation of DCE-MR imaging relates to overlap of cancer with prostatitis in the peripheral zone and marked overlap with vascularized BPH nodules in the transition zone. Another limitation is the reduced spatial resolution due to fast imaging.

Accuracy in Detection/Performance Characteristics

While these individual sequences all have utility in PCa detection, results are optimized by multiparametric (mp) MRI, combining all of the sequences in an integrated fashion (Fig. 8.1). MpMRI offers superior diagnostic power for PCa detection and can assist risk stratification based on lesion size, extent, and ADC value [15]. In one study, mpMRI sensitivity exceeded 80 % for detecting 0.2 cm³ of Gleason 4 + 3 or above and 0.5 cm³ of ≥Gleason 3 + 4 [16]. In another study using a 3 T magnet, addition of DCE and/or DW imaging to T2-weighted MRI significantly improved sensitivity from 63 % to 79–81 % in the peripheral zone, while maintaining a stable specificity [17]. Yoshizako et al. demonstrated the combined use of DW, DCE, and T2-weighted MRI to increase accuracy in detection of transition zone cancer compared to T2WI alone, from 64 to 79 % [18]. Nevertheless, given moderate specificity, mpMRI findings require biopsy to confirm the presence of tumor and assess Gleason score [15]. PCa MRI suspicion scores have been developed for improved standardization of MRI interpretation and reporting [19, 20].

MRI Suspicion Score

Prostatic abnormalities, often termed regions of suspicion, identified on mpMRI have the potential to localize high-risk prostate cancer. Lesions are commonly scored on a Likert scale as 2 (low probability), 3 (equivocal), 4 (high probability), or 5 (very high probability), or the standard-based Prostate Imaging-Reporting and Data System (PI-RADS) as I (very low), II (low), III (indeterminate), IV (high), V (very high), as previously described [21–23]. The performance characteristics of MRI suspicion score in predicting the likelihood of cancer are highly interpreter-dependent. Individual institutional variation in reporting of Likert scales of suspicion results in variability in cancer detection rates observed on biopsy. This serves as a primary impetus for the implementation of a standardized reporting scheme such as PI-RADS. Most recently in version 2 of PI-RADS (Tables 8.1 and 8.2), the standardized scheme has been greatly simplified [23].

MRI suspicion score strongly predicts the likelihood of cancer on MRI-targeted biopsy. In a study of 105 subjects with prior negative biopsy and elevated PSA values who underwent mpMRI targeted biopsy, a highly suspicious MRI abnormality was the most significant predictor of significant cancer on multivariate analysis [24]. Yerram et al. evaluated 125 patients with only low suspicion prostatic lesions on mpMRI and determined these lesions are associated with either negative biopsies or low-grade tumors suitable for active surveillance [25]. Our institution has also reported a positive trend between increasing suspicion score on mpMRI and detection of high-grade (GS ≥ 7 PCa) disease, but not with detection of Gleason score 6 cancer [5].

Negative Predictive Value of MRI

One potential benefit of the utilization of pre-biopsy MRI in clinical practice would be the opportunity to reduce biopsy utilization among men at risk. A growing body of literature has begun to address the negative predictive value (NPV) of MRI in

Table 8.1 PI-RADS 2.0 mpMRI interpretation

Score	T2W (PZ)	T2W (TZ)	DWI (PZ and TZ)	Score	DCE (PZ and TZ)
1	Uniform hyperintense signal intensity	Homogenous intermediate signal intensity	No abnormality on ADC and high b-value DWI	(−)	No early enhancement, or Diffuse enhancement not corresponding to a focal finding on T2 and/or DWI or Focal enhancement corresponding to a lesion demonstrating features of BPH on T2WI
2	Linear/wedge-shaped hypointensity or diffuse mild hypointensity	Circumscribed hypointense or heterogenous encapsulated nodules	Indistinct hypointense on ADC		
3	Heterogenous signal intensity or non-circumscribed, rounded, moderate hypointensity	Heterogenous signal intensity with obscured margins	Focal mildly/moderately hypointense on ADC and isointense/mildly hyperintense on high b-value DWI		
4	Circumscribed, homogenous moderate hypointense focus/ mass confined to prostate and <1.5 cm in greatest dimension	Lenticular or non-circumscribed, homogenous, moderately hypointense, and <1.5 cm in greatest dimension	Focal markedly hypointense on ADC and markedly hyperintense on high b-value DWI; <1.5 cm in greatest dimension	(+)	Focal, and; Earlier than or contemporaneously with enhancement of adjacent normal prostatic tissues, and; Corresponds to suspicious finding on T2W and/or DWI
5	Same as 4 but ≥1.5 cm in greatest dimension or definite extraprostatic extension/ invasive behavior	Same as 4 but ≥1.5 cm in greatest dimension or definite extraprostatic extension/invasive behavior	Same as 4 but ≥1.5 cm in greatest dimension or definite extraprostatic extension/ invasive behavior		

Adapted from Radiology ACo. MR Prostate Imaging Reporting and Data System version 2.0. 2015; http://www.acr.org/Quality-Safety/Resources/PIRADS/, (2015). Creative Commons Attribution-NonCommercial-NoDerivatives 4.0 International License

Table 8.2 PI-RADS 2.0 scoring rubric

Score	Peripheral zone			Transition zone		
	DWI	T2W	DCE	DWI	T2W	DCE
1	1	Any	Any	Any	1	Any
2	2	Any	Any	Any	2	Any
3	3	Any	(−)	≤4	3	Any
4	3	Any	(+)	5	3	Any
	4	Any	Any	Any	4	Any
5	5	Any	Any	Any	5	Any

Adapted from Radiology ACo. MR Prostate Imaging Reporting and Data System version 2.0. 2015; http://www.acr.org/Quality-Safety/Resources/PIRADS/, (2015). Creative Commons Attribution-NonCommercial-NoDerivatives 4.0 International License

ruling out cancer in men for whom there is clinical suspicion. A normal or low suspicion MRI has the potential to allow men to avoid an unnecessary prostate biopsy, and secondarily to reduce the over-detection of indolent disease.

Kumar et al. evaluated 36 men who had a PSA between 4 and 10 ng/mL and a magnetic resonance spectroscopic image (MRSI) that did not show any malignant voxels [26]. Of the 26 men who met follow-up criteria, an initial MRSI negative for a lesion suspicious for malignancy maintained a high negative predictive value (96.2 %), even after an average period of more than 2 years. The authors concluded that a prostate biopsy can be deferred in patients with an increased serum PSA of 4–10 ng/mL and a negative MRSI. Squillaci et al. reported on suspicious lesion on transrectal ultrasound that was further evaluated by mpMRI with proton MR spectroscopy (MRSI). This study reported a NPV for overall cancer detection of T2W-MRI alone, MRSI alone, and combined MRI/MRSI as 69 %, 91 %, and 74 %, respectively [27]. Manenti et al. also showed the prostate biopsy results of 39 men undergoing mpMRI with MRSI, reporting a similar NPV of T2W-MRI, MRSI, and combined MRI/MRSI of 77 %, 74 %, and 74 %, respectively [28].

Although the NPV of mpMRI is high in terms of overall cancer detection rates (CDR), a paucity of data exists on the NPV of mpMRI for clinically significant prostate cancer. In our institutional experience we evaluated 75 men presenting for prostate biopsy who underwent pre-biopsy mpMRI that was negative for suspicious foci, defined as a MRI suspicion score of 1/5 as previously described [21]. Overall, cancer was detected in 14 (18.7 %) men [29]. One (1.3 %) was found to have Gleason 3 + 4 and the remaining 13 (17.3 %) were found to have Gleason sum 6 (GS6). No Gleason sum ≥ 7 (GS ≥ 7) were detected in men without prior biopsy or on active surveillance. Overall, the NPV for detecting any cancer on systematic 12-core biopsy for men with a negative MRI was 81.3 % and 98.7 % for detecting GS ≥ 7. These NPV were 86.2 % and 100 % for men without prior biopsy, 88.0 % and 96 % for men with a prior negative biopsy, and 61.9 % and 100 % for men on active surveillance. On multivariate analysis, no prior biopsy and a prior negative biopsy were significantly associated with decreased cancer detection on systematic prostate biopsy with a negative mpMRI.

In a recent prospective trial of 226 men who had 3 T mpMRI prior to primary biopsy, Pokorny et al. reported negative biopsies in 56/81 (69 %) men with normal mpMRI [30]. However, this group included men with both PIRADS 1 and 2 mpMRI scores. Among the 25 men with normal mpMRI and prostate cancer on biopsy, 80 % had low-risk disease (low volume Gleason score 3 + 3 or very low volume Gleason score 3 + 4), making the NPV for intermediate/high risk disease 94 %. The authors highlight that mpMRI with MRI targeted prostate biopsy reduces the detection of low-risk prostate cancer and reduces the number of men requiring biopsy while improving the overall rate of detection of intermediate/high-risk prostate cancer, a conclusion that is supported by several additional studies [31, 32].

These findings, taken together, lend further support to the utility of mpMRI in predicting negative biopsy among men with clinical suspicion for prostate cancer. The performance characteristics of mpMRI appear to have a high clinical NPV where mpMRI may ultimately be a useful tool to rule out clinically significant prostate cancer on initial evaluation, therefore avoiding unnecessarily prostate biopsies. Validation of this concept will require standardized prospective study.

Correlation of MRI with Surgical Pathology: Disease Localization

There is strong evidence that mpMRI accurately localizes prostate cancer foci larger than 0.2 mL and/or high-grade disease [30, 33]. Accurate identification of index tumor location on mpMRI, followed by fusion of the MR image with a transrectal ultrasound image, could potentially guide targeted biopsy of such index tumors with greater accuracy. Moreover, for image-guided focal therapy, imaging must be able to guide therapy and accurately define margins of the tumor to allow accurate treatment and follow-up. The findings of mpMRI have been compared with whole mount radical prostatectomy specimens and have been evaluated to address the concordance of the index tumor location and the index tumor volume.

In initial studies comparing MRI with whole mount radical prostatectomy specimens to determine tumor site and size concordance, Villers et al. assessed the value of pelvic phased array DCE MRI for predicting the intraprostatic location and volume of clinically localized prostate cancers [16]. Sensitivity, specificity, and positive and negative predictive values for cancer detection by magnetic resonance imaging were 77 %, 91 %, 86 % and 85 % for foci greater than 0.2 cc, and 90 %, 88 %, 77 % and 95 % for foci greater than 0.5 cc, respectively. Kim et al. [34] and Nakashima et al. [35] observed similar performance characteristics of MRI in determining cancer foci location and size. More recent studies which have incorporated modern multiparametric sequences have shown that mpMRI has >90 % specificity in detecting index tumors [36, 37]. In a multi-institutional study of 135 men who had pre-biopsy MRI, MR-TRUS image-fusion biopsy, and robotic radical prostatectomy, followed by whole mount step section of the specimen, MR-TRUS fusion biopsy accurately identified the location of the index tumor in

95 % of patients. In the remaining 5 % of patients, the index tumor was invisible on MRI; each of these tumors was very small (histological tumor volume ≤ 0.4 mL for radical prostatectomy specimens). These data suggest that MR-TRUS image-fusion biopsies could become a valuable tool in identifying the location of clinically important prostate cancer. However, not all prostate cancer lesions are detectable on MRI, even when using advanced technology. The MRI visibility of prostate cancer depends on cancer volume, grade, histology, and location in comparison to the histological architecture of normal adjacent prostate tissue.

Determining tumor volume concordance, rather than the index lesions site, appears to be a more challenging undertaking with varied success. In a series of 75 men, Isebaert et al. correlated mpMRI and histopathological tumor volumes after radical prostatectomy [38]. Tumor volume was found to be the most accurately assessed by means of DW MRI ($r=0.75$). In a retrospective analysis of 135 men, Baco et al. determined a coefficient for correlation between index lesion volume on MRI and histology was $r=0.663$ [39]. The authors acknowledge the absence of significant agreement between the two and additional MRI variables are necessary to improve tumor volume estimations. Turkbey et al. evaluated 135 patients who underwent multiparametric 3 T endorectal coil magnetic resonance imaging of the prostate and subsequent radical prostatectomy [37]. They observed a positive correlation between histopathology tumor volume and MRI tumor volume (Pearson coefficient 0.633). MRI accurately estimated the index tumor volume independent of Gleason score. MRI had a better accuracy than clinical variables (serum PSA, patient age) in the distinction of tumors larger than 0.5 cm^3.

In our institutional experience, Le Nobin et al. evaluated the level of agreement in volumes of prostate cancer index lesions between histopathology and MRI in 37 men [40]. The authors addressed many of the shortcoming of previous whole mount studies, such as imprecise estimates of pathological volume as the reference standard, suboptimal techniques for achieving co-registration of MRI and pathological images, and the use of correlative statistical methods (such as the Pearson correlation coefficient), by investigating the accuracy of volume estimates from 3 T multiparametric MRI using novel co-registration software. The volume estimates of prostate cancer using MRI tended to substantially underestimate histopathological volumes, with a wide variability in extent of underestimation across cases. Rud et al. similarly compared tumor volume and tumor burden between MRI and histology from radical prostatectomy specimens in 199 men and observed MRI underestimates both tumor volume and tumor burden compared with histology [36]. The rate of detection of the index tumor was 92 %, while the overall rate of detection of tumors with a histology tumor volume of >0.5 mL was 86 %. Cornud et al. studied 84 men who had a mpMRI prior to prostatectomy and analyzed mpMRI and pathological tumor volume [41]. The authors similarly observed a wide variation in overestimation and underestimation of MRI tumor volume compared to pathological volume.

In the context of potential focal ablation, Anwar et al. analyzed mpMRI of 20 men who underwent radical prostatectomy with the aim of defining the contour of treatable intraprostatic tumor foci in prostate cancer [42]. By comparing histopathological tumor maps from whole-mount step sections the authors calculated the margin of error between imaging and histopathological contours at both capsular and non-capsular surfaces and the treatment margin required to ensure at least 95 % tumor coverage if the patient was to undergo targeted therapy. They concluded mpMRI can be used to accurately contour these tumor foci; complete tumor coverage is achieved by expanding the treatment contour at the non-capsular margin by 5 mm. Our institutional experience has shown that MRI underestimates histologically determined tumor boundaries, especially for high MRI suspicion score and high Gleason score lesions [43]. A 9 mm treatment margin around an MRI-visible lesion consistently ensures treatment of the entire histological tumor volume during focal ablative therapy. In assessing tumor volume and tumor margins, mpMRI tended to underestimate lesion size for high-grade tumors while overestimating the size of low-grade tumors. The latter may relate, in part, to stromal reaction and inflammation in the surrounding tissues.

Outcomes of MRI-Targeted Biopsy in Clinical Practice

There are a number of potential benefits of MRI-targeted biopsy which are reported in the literature; however, these still need to be proven though further studies. In theory, accurate localization of significant cancer prior to biopsy may potentially correct limitations of systematic biopsy. Accurate targeting of biopsy cores should reduce false-negative biopsies and improve accuracy in risk classification through better sampling of tumor, with the intent of detecting high-risk disease and avoiding indolent cancer (Table 8.3). Secondarily, a reduction in false-negative biopsies could reduce the necessity for repeat biopsies, thereby reducing cost. Because targeted biopsy relies upon image guidance, fewer cores potentially would be required, additionally reducing cost. Finally, if metrics can be established to demonstrate the lowest risk parameters for detection of clinically significant disease, avoidance of biopsy among men falling below that threshold may reduce the number of biopsies performed and secondarily reduce over-detection. These principles remain to be fully proven, but there is a growing body of evidence to support the assertion.

Several institutions, including our own, have now accrued a mature dataset highlighting the outcomes of MRI-targeted biopsy. In our institutional experience of 601 men, we also found that MRI-US fusion-targeted biopsy detects more high-grade cancer compared to systematic biopsy while limiting over-detection of indolent disease in all men presenting for prostate biopsy [5]. The National Cancer Institute has shown an increased detection of high-risk prostate cancer and decreased detection of low-risk prostate cancer in their experience of 1003 targeted MR/ultrasound fusion biopsies [4]. Collectively, the published literature suggests that overall cancer detection is decreased by MR-targeted biopsy compared to systematic biopsy, but higher grade cancers are detected with fewer cores, and insignificant cancers are detected less often [24, 44].

Table 8.3 Summary of trials of MRI-ultrasound fusion-targeted biopsy in which the cancer detection rate (CDR) of clinically significant cancer was reported

Investigators	Study size	Biopsy history	MRI field strength and additional sequences[a]	TB technique	SB technique	Definition of clinically significant cancer	Overall CDR (TB)	Overall CDR (SB)	Clinically significant CDR (TB)	Clinically significant CDR (SB)
Mozer et al. [47]	152	100 % BN	1.5 T	Transrectal	12-core TRUS	CCL $\geq$ 4 mm or GS $\geq$ 3+4	54 %	57 %	43 %	37 %
Sonn et al. [24]	105	100 % PNB	3.0 T	Transrectal	12-core TRUS	CCL $\geq$ 4 mm or GS $\geq$ 3+4	24 %	28 %	22 %	15 %
Wysock et al. [59]	125	54 % BN 27 % PNB 19 % AS	3.0 T	Transrectal	12-core TRUS	GS $\geq$ 3+4	Cohort: 36 % BN: 40 %	Cohort: NR BN: 55 %	Cohort: 23 % BN: 33 %	Cohort: NR BN: 33 %
Kuru et al. [61]	347	51 % BN 49 % PNB	3.0 T	Transperineal	24-core Transperineal	NCCN criteria (intermediate or high risk)	51 %	50 %	41 %	38 %
Fiard et al. [64]	30	43 % BN 57 % PNB	3.0 T	Transrectal	12-core TRUS	$\geq$ 10 mm cancer or GS $\geq$ 3+4	55 %	43 %	50 %	33 %
Rastinehad et al. [65]	105	33 % BN 67 % PNB	3.0 T	Transrectal	12-core TRUS	Epstein criteria	51 %	49 %	45 %	32 %
Sonn et al. [66]	171	38 % PNB 62 % AS	3.0 T	Transrectal	12-core TRUS	GS $\geq$ 3+4	35 %	44 %	13 %	12 %
Siddiqui et al. [4]	1003	20 % BN 43 % PNB 37 % AS	3.0 T Spectroscopy	Transrectal	12-core TRUS	GS $\geq$ 4+3	46 %	47 %	17 %	12 %

TB MR-targeted biopsy, *SB* systematic biopsy, *BN* biopsy naive, *PNB* prior negative biopsy, *AS* active surveillance, *CCL* cancer-core length, *GS* Gleason score
[a]All studies used T2-weighted, diffusion-weighted, and dynamic contrast-enhanced magnetic resonance imaging sequences, with any additional sequences listed above

Among Men with No Previous Biopsy

The use of MRI among men with no previous biopsy has been studied but currently its cost-effectiveness and true benefit are yet to be determined by larger randomized studies, as such its use is currently investigational. Haffner et al. reported a seminal series of 555 consecutive patients undergoing pre-biopsy MRI followed by systematic biopsy and visual estimation biopsy of MRI abnormalities. The overall cancer detection rate (CDR) was 54 % using extended systematic biopsy and 63 % amongst the 351 cases with an abnormal MRI [2]. Although systematic biopsy detected 66 more cases of cancer, 53 were deemed clinically insignificant. The MRI-targeted approach detected more high-grade cases and better quantified the cancer through increased cancer length per biopsy core. Delongchamps et al. also examined the use of pre-biopsy mpMRI in 391 consecutive patients and reported CDR of 41 % using systematic biopsy and 43 % using cognitive or fusion-targeted biopsy [45]. Targeted biopsy was significantly better at detecting high Gleason score ($>3+3$) cancer, missing only 2/63 (3 %) high-grade cancers detected by systematic biopsy while detecting an additional 17 high-grade cancers missed by systematic biopsy and avoiding detection of 39 Gleason 6 cancers [45]. Among 1448 men with pre-biopsy DW-MRI prior to initial biopsy, Watanabe et al. reported a CDR of 70.1 % in 890 patients with MRI lesions who underwent both targeted and systematic biopsy, compared to a CDR of only 13.1 % in 558 patients with no MRI lesions who only underwent systematic biopsy [46]. CDR was 90.1 % in 141 patients with anterior cancers found on MRI, an area easily missed with standard systematic biopsy [46]. A number of additional studies have demonstrated similar results (Table 8.1) [2, 47, 48].

Among Men with Previous Negative Biopsy

In a series of 438 consecutive patients with elevated PSA and at least one prior negative biopsy who underwent mpMRI, Hoeks et al. reported a CDR of 41 % (108/265) using in-bore targeted biopsy, with 87 % (94/108) of these cancers found to be clinically significant [49]. Vourganti et al. report on 195 patients with previous negative biopsy and suspicious mpMRI, finding a CDR of 37 % (73/195) using a combination of MRI-US fusion biopsy and systematic biopsy [50]. In addition to detecting nine additional high-grade cancers missed by systematic biopsy, fusion biopsy leads to pathological upgrading in 28/73 (38.4 %) patients [50]. Sonn et al. found a CDR of 34 % (36/105) in men with previous negative biopsy with 72 % (26/36) being clinically significant [24]. MRI-US fusion biopsy detected clinically significant cancer in 21/23 (91 %) men compared to only 15/28 (54 %) men with systematic biopsy. A highly suspicious MRI lesion was the most significant predictor of significant cancer on multivariate analysis [24]. Even in patients with up to four prior negative biopsies, Labanaris et al. found that among 170/260 (65 %) of patients with a suspicious MRI, PCa was detected on 96/170 (56 %) targeted biopsies compared to only 30/170 (18 %) systematic biopsies [51]. A subgroup analysis of our institutional cohort demonstrated that among 172 men with prior negative biopsies and suspicious lesions on MRI, targeted biopsies missed no high-grade cancers, while detecting 15/31 (48 %) additional high-grade cancers missed by systematic biopsy. Additionally, the majority of cancers detected by systematic biopsy and missed or mischaracterized by targeted biopsy was found to be low volume and met clinical criteria for insignificant disease [52].

Among Men with Low-Risk Cancer

The performance of mpMRI and MRI-US fusion biopsy for monitoring patients with prostate cancer on active surveillance has yielded positive results which may improve risk stratification in these men [53, 54]. In a study of 388 consecutive patients with low-risk disease who underwent mpMRI and confirmatory visual estimation co-registration biopsy, Vargas et al. reported that 20 % (79/388) of patients were upgraded on confirmatory biopsy [55]. A 5-point MRI suspicion scale demonstrated excellent risk stratification, with a high sensitivity for upgrading on confirmatory biopsy (0.87–0.98) for a score of 5/5 [55]. In a study of 281 men, Ouzzane et al. showed mpMRI-targeted biopsy reclassified 10 % of patients who were eligible for active surveillance based on systematic biopsy [54]. In a recent study of 152 men meeting active surveillance criteria who underwent MRI-US fusions biopsy, Walton Diaz et al. determined that stable findings on mpMRI are associated with Gleason score stability and mpMRI appears promising as a useful aid for reducing the number of biopsies in the management of patients on active surveillance [56]. Additionally, Kim et al. demonstrated that among 287 men on active surveillance, high ADC values on DWI were strongly predictive of clinically insignificant, organ-confined disease [57]. MpMRI-based nomograms may further confirm eligibility for active surveillance and may decrease the number of repeat biopsies in patients on active surveillance by as much as 68 % [58].

Limitations of MRI-Targeted Biopsy

While MRI-targeted biopsy has the potential to overcome the limitations of standard TRUS-guided biopsy, it is not without several potential limitations itself. MRI-targeted biopsy incurs additional cost which remains to be justified through larger cohort studies. Imaging quality and quality of image-interpretation serves as a major barrier to widespread implementation in the community. Targeting methods are not purely defined and may still miss cancer. This targeting strategy may result in additional biopsies due to a false-positive MRI. Lastly, MRI-targeted biopsy may overestimate cancer risk, where further studies are needed to define the significance of pathology findings within the targeted biopsy.

Technique of MRI-Targeted Biopsy

Visual Estimation MR-Targeted TRUS Biopsy

Visual estimation allows adaptation of MRI-targeted biopsy in clinical practice without significant upfront cost, but carries a significant learning curve and lacks real-time feedback regarding accuracy. The effectiveness of visual estimation-targeted biopsy in detecting PCa varies between studies, likely reflecting inconsistencies in targeting precision, but generally visual estimation appears inferior to software co-registration [59, 60]. In a series of 351/555 (63 %) patients with a positive MRI, Haffner et al. detected clinically significant PCa in 45 % (248/555) of patients by systematic biopsy compared to 43 % (236/555) by visual estimation biopsy, but 53/66 cancers missed by targeted biopsy were clinically insignificant [2]. In contrast, Labanaris et al. reported CDR of 56 % by targeted visual estimation MRI-targeted biopsy alone but only 18 % by systematic biopsy alone in 170/260 (65 %) patients with a positive MRI [51]. Collectively, the currently published studies suggest improved accuracy and efficiency compared to systematic biopsy but also demonstrate that experience with visual estimation biopsy varies by investigator experience and likely, in part, due to variable practices in imaging approach.

Software Co-registered MRI-Targeted TRUS Biopsy

Software co-registration potentially overcomes the limitation of cognitive fusion through reproducible methods for identification of MRI lesions on ultrasound. A number of commercial platforms have become available [56]. These applications vary by method of co-registration (mechanical, electromagnetic, or real-time) and utilize different hardware platform for aligning the biopsy with the co-registered image. MRI/US fusion biopsy potentially has greater reproducibility due to less operator dependence and by providing real-time feedback of actual biopsied locations. Disadvantages include a high upfront cost for the software/device, dependence on the software for accuracy, and associated learning curve and operator training.

Table 8.3 summarizes reported outcomes of systematic biopsy vs. targeted biopsy using MRI/US fusion platforms evaluating clinically significant PCa. Siddiqui et al. recently reported that the combination of extended systematic and targeted biopsy using the Philips/PercuNav device resulted in diagnosing 30 % more high-risk cancers vs. standard biopsy (173 vs. 122 cases, $P<0.001$) and 17 % fewer low-risk cancers (213 vs. 258 cases, $P<0.001$) [4]. Sonn et al. report similar positive results using the Eigen/Artemis device, reporting a CDR of 53 % (90/171) with a higher percentage of positive cores (21 % vs. 7 %) and higher detection of Gleason ≥ 7 (38 % vs. 31 %) cancers using targeted biopsy [24]. Our institution experience with the Eigen/Artemis device has yielded similar results (Fig. 8.2) [5]. Patients with highly suspicious MRI lesions (5/5 grade) had a 94 % rate of cancer diagnosis compared to only 43 % in patients with low suspicious lesions (2/5 grade) [24]. High

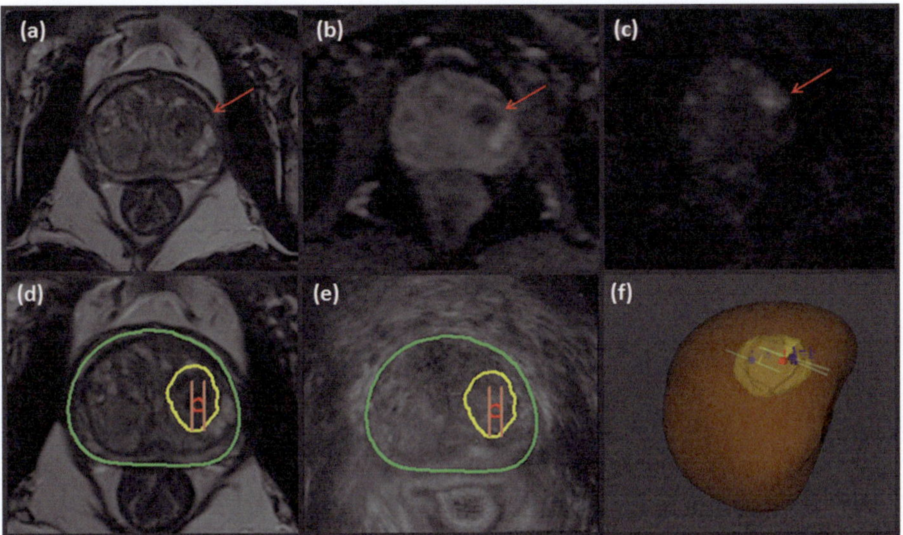

Fig. 8.2 Suspicious lesion visualized as (**a**) hypointense area on T2W image, (**b**) restricted diffusion with low ADC, and (**c**) high signal on diffusion-weighted image. Targeted biopsy workflow showing segmented prostate and lesion on (**d**) T2-weighted MRI, (**e**) transrectal ultrasound, and (**f**) 3D reconstruction of prostate and suspicious region

detection rates have also been demonstrated with transperineal MRI/US fusion biopsy. Kuru et al. reported a CDR of 58 % (200/347) (58 %) using the MedCom/ BiopSee device, with a CDR of 82.6 % (86/104) in patients with highly suspicious lesions compared to only 15 % (14/94) in patients with a normal mpMRI [61].

In Bore MRI-Guided Biopsy

Hoeks et al. reported on 265 patients with suspicious lesions on mpMRI with prior negative TRUS biopsies that underwent transrectal in-bore MRGB, resulting in CDR of 41 % with 87 % of these detected cancers found to be clinically significant [49]. Multiple studies have corroborated this result, demonstrating that in-bore MRGB is a feasible diagnostic technique in patients with prior negative biopsy with a median detection rate of 42 %, significantly higher than reported detection rates for repeat systematic biopsy [62]. This in-bore biopsy strategy has the advantages of real-time feedback of needle placement, fewer sampled cores, and a low likelihood of missed target. It has the disadvantage of increased cost, use of scanner time (opportunity cost), and an inability to routinely sample the remaining gland. Additionally, in applying in bore MRI-guided biopsy, urologists are largely removed from the diagnostic pathway with concerning implications for the ultimate management of the disease.

Comparative Studies

While many studies compare targeted to systematic biopsy, only a few studies have compared the CDR between different targeted techniques. Recently, Cool and colleagues analyzed 225 simulated targeted biopsies by both visual estimation and MRI–ultrasound fusion and found MRI-targeted TRUS-guided prostate biopsy using cognitive registration appears to be inferior to MRI-TRUS fusion, with fewer than 50 % of clinically significant PCA lesions successfully sampled [60]. Wysock et al. prospectively compared MRI/US fusion biopsy using the Eigen/Artemis system vs. visual estimation targeting for 125 consecutive men with suspicious regions on pre-biopsy mpMRI and found that fusion targeting had improved accuracy for smaller MRI lesions and trended toward increased detection compared to visual targeting for all cancer (32.0 % vs. 26.7 %) as well as Gleason sum ≥ 7 cancers (20.3 % vs. 15.1 %) [59]. Delongchamps et al. reported that cognitive fusion was not significantly better than systematic random biopsies, while both software co-registration devices tested (Esaote/MyLabTMTwice and Koelis/Urostation) significantly increased CDR compared to systematic biopsies using conditional logistic regression analysis in a cohort of 391 patients [45]. Yet to be explored are the relationship of clinical factors such as prostate size, PSA, and location of MRI lesion on the accuracy of targeting by cognitive or co-registered approach. While more comparative studies examining the efficacy of different techniques are needed, it is possible that the decision for an institution or practice to utilize a particular type of MRI-targeted biopsy will be largely influenced by local factors such as cost, space, and operator experience with MRI interpretation. Recently through a consensus meeting, guidelines were published regarding conduct and standards in reporting MRI-targeted biopsy studies [63].

Conclusions

MpMRI represents a potential tool for addressing many of the limitations of contemporary systematic biopsy as MRI suspicion score correlated with significant disease. MpMRI appears to have a high negative predictive value, potentially reducing the need for a prostate biopsy in men with a normal MRI. However, there appears to be substantial variation in estimation of MRI tumor volume compared to pathological volume. Among men with no previous biopsy, targeted prostate biopsy using MRI guidance has the potential to reduce false negatives, improve risk classification, and contribute to reduction of repeat biopsies and over-detection. Among men with previous negative biopsy, but persistent suspicion, it has the potential to increase cancer detection and reduce further repeat biopsy. Among men with cancer contemplating surveillance, MR-targeted biopsy potentially improves risk stratification and reduces the need for repetitive biopsy. The optimal method for MR-targeted biopsy is not yet established, but emerging methods of co-registration may offer wider accessibility to the approach. Further comparative studies to standard of practice and evaluation of cost-effectiveness are warranted prior to consideration of wide adoption.

Acknowledgement   Neil Mendhiratta and Samir S. Taneja are supported by the Joseph and Diane Steinberg Charitable Trust.

References

1. Bjurlin MA, Meng X, Le Nobin J, et al. Optimization of prostate biopsy: the role of magnetic resonance imaging targeted biopsy in detection, localization and risk assessment. J Urol. 2014;192(3):648–58.
2. Haffner J, Lemaitre L, Puech P, et al. Role of magnetic resonance imaging before initial biopsy: comparison of magnetic resonance imaging-targeted and systematic biopsy for significant prostate cancer detection. BJU Int. 2011;108(8 Pt 2):E171–8.
3. Bjurlin MA, Carter HB, Schellhammer P, et al. Optimization of initial prostate biopsy in clinical practice: sampling, labeling and specimen processing. J Urol. 2013;189(6):2039–46.
4. Siddiqui MM, Rais-Bahrami S, Turkbey B, et al. Comparison of MR/ultrasound fusion-guided biopsy with ultrasound-guided biopsy for the diagnosis of prostate cancer. JAMA. 2015;313(4):390–7.
5. Meng X, Rosenkrantz AB, Mendhiratta N et al. Relationship of pre-biopsy multiparametric MRI and biopsy indication with MRI-US fusion-targeted prostate biopsy outcomes. Paper presented at: American Urological Association Annual Meeting, New Orleans, LA, 17 May 2015.
6. Hricak H, Dooms GC, McNeal JE, et al. MR imaging of the prostate gland: normal anatomy. AJR Am J Roentgenol. 1987;148(1):51–8.
7. Wang L, Mazaheri Y, Zhang J, Ishill NM, Kuroiwa K, Hricak H. Assessment of biologic aggressiveness of prostate cancer: correlation of MR signal intensity with Gleason grade after radical prostatectomy. Radiology. 2008;246(1):168–76.
8. Akin O, Sala E, Moskowitz CS, et al. Transition zone prostate cancers: features, detection, localization, and staging at endorectal MR imaging. Radiology. 2006;239(3):784–92.
9. Kim CK, Park BK, Kim B. High-b-value diffusion-weighted imaging at 3 T to detect prostate cancer: comparisons between b values of 1,000 and 2,000 s/mm². AJR Am J Roentgenol. 2010;194(1):W33–7.
10. Katahira K, Takahara T, Kwee TC, et al. Ultra-high-b-value diffusion-weighted MR imaging for the detection of prostate cancer: evaluation in 201 cases with histopathological correlation. Eur Radiol. 2011;21(1):188–96.
11. Mazaheri Y, Vargas HA, Akin O, Goldman DA, Hricak H. Reducing the influence of b-value selection on diffusion-weighted imaging of the prostate: evaluation of a revised monoexponential model within a clinical setting. J Magn Reson Imaging. 2012;35(3):660–8.
12. Hambrock T, Hoeks C, Hulsbergen-van de Kaa C, et al. Prospective assessment of prostate cancer aggressiveness using 3-T diffusion-weighted magnetic resonance imaging-guided biopsies versus a systematic 10-core transrectal ultrasound prostate biopsy cohort. Eur Urol. 2012;61(1):177–84.
13. Turkbey B, Shah VP, Pang Y, et al. Is apparent diffusion coefficient associated with clinical risk scores for prostate cancers that are visible on 3-T MR images? Radiology. 2011;258(2):488–95.
14. Parker GJ, Tofts PS. Pharmacokinetic analysis of neoplasms using contrast-enhanced dynamic magnetic resonance imaging. Top Magn Reson Imaging. 1999;10(2):130–42.
15. Turkbey B, Choyke PL. Multiparametric MRI and prostate cancer diagnosis and risk stratification. Curr Opin Urol. 2012;22(4):310–5.
16. Villers A, Puech P, Mouton D, Leroy X, Ballereau C, Lemaitre L. Dynamic contrast enhanced, pelvic phased array magnetic resonance imaging of localized prostate cancer for predicting

tumor volume: correlation with radical prostatectomy findings. J Urol. 2006;176(6 Pt 1): 2432–7.

17. Delongchamps NB, Rouanne M, Flam T, et al. Multiparametric magnetic resonance imaging for the detection and localization of prostate cancer: combination of T2-weighted, dynamic contrast-enhanced and diffusion-weighted imaging. BJU Int. 2011;107(9):1411–8.

18. Yoshizako T, Wada A, Hayashi T, et al. Usefulness of diffusion-weighted imaging and dynamic contrast-enhanced magnetic resonance imaging in the diagnosis of prostate transition-zone cancer. Acta Radiol. 2008;49(10):1207–13.

19. Jung JA, Coakley FV, Vigneron DB, et al. Prostate depiction at endorectal MR spectroscopic imaging: investigation of a standardized evaluation system. Radiology. 2004;233(3):701–8.

20. Barentsz JO, Richenberg J, Clements R, et al. ESUR prostate MR guidelines 2012. Eur Radiol. 2012;22(4):746–57.

21. Rosenkrantz AB, Kim S, Lim RP, et al. Prostate cancer localization using multiparametric MR imaging: comparison of Prostate Imaging Reporting and Data System (PI-RADS) and Likert scales. Radiology. 2013;269(2):482–92.

22. Rosenkrantz AB, Lim RP, Haghighi M, Somberg MB, Babb JS, Taneja SS. Comparison of inter-reader reproducibility of the prostate imaging reporting and data system and likert scales for evaluation of multiparametric prostate MRI. AJR Am J Roentgenol. 2013;201(4):W612–8.

23. Radiology ACo. MR Prostate Imaging Reporting and Data System version 2.0. 2015. http://www.acr.org/Quality-Safety/Resources/PIRADS/

24. Sonn GA, Natarajan S, Margolis DJA, et al. Targeted biopsy in the detection of prostate cancer using an office based magnetic resonance ultrasound fusion device. J Urol. 2013;189(1):86–91.

25. Yerram NK, Volkin D, Turkbey B, et al. Low suspicion lesions on multiparametric magnetic resonance imaging predict for the absence of high-risk prostate cancer. BJU Int. 2012;110(11 Pt B):E783–8.

26. Kumar R, Nayyar R, Kumar V, et al. Potential of magnetic resonance spectroscopic imaging in predicting absence of prostate cancer in men with serum prostate-specific antigen between 4 and 10 ng/ml: a follow-up study. Urology. 2008;72(4):859–63.

27. Squillaci E, Manenti G, Mancino S, et al. MR spectroscopy of prostate cancer. Initial clinical experience. J Exp Clin Cancer Res. 2005;24(4):523–30.

28. Manenti G, Squillaci E, Carlani M, Mancino S, Di Roma M, Simonetti G. Magnetic resonance imaging of the prostate with spectroscopic imaging using a surface coil. Initial clinical experience. Radiol Med. 2006;111(1):22–32.

29. Wysock JS, Zattoni F, Meng X et al. Predictive value of negative 3T multiparametric prostate MRI on 12 core biopsy results. Submitted.

30. Pokorny MR, de Rooij M, Duncan E, et al. Prospective study of diagnostic accuracy comparing prostate cancer detection by transrectal ultrasound-guided biopsy versus magnetic resonance (MR) imaging with subsequent MR-guided biopsy in men without previous prostate biopsies. Eur Urol. 2014;66(1):22–9.

31. Itatani R, Namimoto T, Atsuji S, et al. Negative predictive value of multiparametric MRI for prostate cancer detection: outcome of 5-year follow-up in men with negative findings on initial MRI studies. Eur J Radiol. 2014;83(10):1740–5.

32. Villeirs GM, De Meerleer GO, De Visschere PJ, Fonteyne VH, Verbaeys AC, Oosterlinck W. Combined magnetic resonance imaging and spectroscopy in the assessment of high grade prostate carcinoma in patients with elevated PSA: a single-institution experience of 356 patients. Eur J Radiol. 2011;77(2):340–5.

33. Hoeks CM, Barentsz JO, Hambrock T, et al. Prostate cancer: multiparametric MR imaging for detection, localization, and staging. Radiology. 2011;261(1):46–66.

34. Kim CK, Park BK, Kim B. Localization of prostate cancer using 3T MRI: comparison of T2-weighted and dynamic contrast-enhanced imaging. J Comput Assist Tomogr. 2006;30(1): 7–11.

35. Nakashima J, Tanimoto A, Imai Y, et al. Endorectal MRI for prediction of tumor site, tumor size, and local extension of prostate cancer. Urology. 2004;64(1):101–5.

36. Rud E, Klotz D, Rennesund K, et al. Detection of the index tumour and tumour volume in prostate cancer using T2-weighted and diffusion-weighted magnetic resonance imaging (MRI) alone. BJU Int. 2014;114(6b):E32–42.
37. Turkbey B, Mani H, Aras O, et al. Correlation of magnetic resonance imaging tumor volume with histopathology. J Urol. 2012;188(4):1157–63.
38. Isebaert S, Van den Bergh L, Haustermans K, et al. Multiparametric MRI for prostate cancer localization in correlation to whole-mount histopathology. J Magn Reson Imaging. 2013;37(6): 1392–401.
39. Baco E, Ukimura O, Rud E, et al. Magnetic resonance imaging-transectal ultrasound image-fusion biopsies accurately characterize the index tumor: correlation with step-sectioned radical prostatectomy specimens in 135 patients. Eur Urol. 2015;67:787–94.
40. Le Nobin J, Orczyk C, Deng FM, et al. Prostate tumour volumes: evaluation of the agreement between magnetic resonance imaging and histology using novel co-registration software. BJU Int. 2014;114(6b):E105–12.
41. Cornud F, Khoury G, Bouazza N, et al. Tumor target volume for focal therapy of prostate cancer-does multiparametric magnetic resonance imaging allow for a reliable estimation? J Urol. 2014;191(5):1272–9.
42. Anwar M, Westphalen AC, Jung AJ, et al. Role of endorectal MR imaging and MR spectro-scopic imaging in defining treatable intraprostatic tumor foci in prostate cancer: quantitative analysis of imaging contour compared to whole-mount histopathology. Radiother Oncol. 2014;110(2):303–8.
43. Le Nobin J, Rosenkrantz AB, Villers A et al. Image guided focal therapy of MRI-visible pros-tate cancer: defining a 3D treatment margin based on MRI-histology co-registration analysis. J Urol. 2015. doi: 10.1016/j.juro.2015.02.080.
44. Puech P, Rouviere O, Renard-Penna R, et al. Prostate cancer diagnosis: multiparametric MR-targeted biopsy with cognitive and transrectal US-MR fusion guidance versus systematic biopsy—prospective multicenter study. Radiology. 2013;268:461–9.
45. Delongchamps NB, Peyromaure M, Schull A, et al. Prebiopsy magnetic resonance imaging and prostate cancer detection: comparison of random and targeted biopsies. J Urol. 2013;189(2):493–9.
46. Watanabe Y, Terai A, Araki T, et al. Detection and localization of prostate cancer with the targeted biopsy strategy based on ADC map: a prospective large-scale cohort study. J Magn Reson Imaging. 2012;35(6):1414–21.
47. Mozer P, Rouprêt M, Le Cossec C, et al. First round of targeted biopsies using magnetic reso-nance imaging/ultrasonography fusion compared with conventional transrectal ultrasonography-guided biopsies for the diagnosis of localised prostate cancer. BJU Int. 2015;115(1):50–7.
48. Numao N, Yoshida S, Komai Y, et al. Usefulness of pre-biopsy multiparametric magnetic reso-nance imaging and clinical variables to reduce initial prostate biopsy in men with suspected clinically localized prostate cancer. J Urol. 2013;190(2):502–8.
49. Hoeks CM, Schouten MG, Bomers JG, et al. Three-Tesla magnetic resonance-guided prostate biopsy in men with increased prostate-specific antigen and repeated, negative, random, sys-tematic, transrectal ultrasound biopsies: detection of clinically significant prostate cancers. Eur Urol. 2012;62(5):902–9.
50. Vourganti S, Rastinehad A, Yerram NK, et al. Multiparametric magnetic resonance imaging and ultrasound fusion biopsy detect prostate cancer in patients with prior negative transrectal ultrasound biopsies. J Urol. 2012;188(6):2152–7.
51. Labanaris AP, Engelhard K, Zugor V, Nutzel R, Kuhn R. Prostate cancer detection using an extended prostate biopsy schema in combination with additional targeted cores from suspi-cious images in conventional and functional endorectal magnetic resonance imaging of the prostate. Prostate Cancer Prostatic Dis. 2010;13(1):65–70.
52. Mendhiratta N, Meng X, Rosenkrantz AB, et al. Pre-biopsy MRI and MRI-ultrasound fusion-targeted prostate biopsy in men with previous negative biopsies: improved cancer detection and risk stratification. Paper presented at American Urological Association Annual Meeting, New Orleans, LA, 17 May 2015.

53. Turkbey B, Mani H, Aras O, et al. Prostate cancer: can multiparametric MR imaging help identify patients who are candidates for active surveillance? Radiology. 2013;268(1):144–52.
54. Ouzzane A, Renard-Penna R, Marliere F, et al. MRI-targeted biopsy improves selection of patients considered for active surveillance for clinically low-risk prostate cancer based on systematic biopsies. J Urol. 2015. doi: 10.1016/j.juro.2015.02.2938.
55. Vargas HA, Akin O, Afaq A, et al. Magnetic resonance imaging for predicting prostate biopsy findings in patients considered for active surveillance of clinically low risk prostate cancer. J Urol. 2012;188(5):1732–8.
56. Logan JK, Rais-Bahrami S, Turkbey B, et al. Current status of magnetic resonance imaging (MRI) and ultrasonography fusion software platforms for guidance of prostate biopsies. BJU Int. 2014;114(5):641–52.
57. Kim TH, Jeong JY, Lee SW, et al. Diffusion-weighted magnetic resonance imaging for prediction of insignificant prostate cancer in potential candidates for active surveillance. Eur Radiol. 2015;25:1786–92.
58. Siddiqui MM, Truong H, Rais-Bahrami S, et al. Clinical implications of a multiparametric MRI based nomogram applied to prostate cancer active surveillance. J Urol. 2015;193:1943–9.
59. Wysock JS, Rosenkrantz AB, Huang WC, et al. A prospective, blinded comparison of magnetic resonance (MR) imaging-ultrasound fusion and visual estimation in the performance of MR-targeted prostate biopsy: the PROFUS Trial. Eur Urol. 2014;66(2):343–51.
60. Cool DW, Zhang X, Romagnoli C, Izawa JI, Romano WM, Fenster A. Evaluation of MRI-TRUS fusion versus cognitive registration accuracy for MRI-targeted, TRUS-guided prostate biopsy. AJR Am J Roentgenol. 2015;204(1):83–91.
61. Kuru TH, Roethke MC, Seidenader J, et al. Critical evaluation of MRI-targeted TRUS-guided transperineal fusion biopsy for detection of prostate cancer. J Urol. 2013;190(4):1380–6.
62. Overduin CG, Futterer JJ, Barentsz JO. MRI-guided biopsy for prostate cancer detection: a systematic review of current clinical results. Curr Urol Rep. 2013;14(3):209–13.
63. Moore CM, Kasivisvanathan V, Eggener S, et al. Standards of reporting for MRI-targeted biopsy studies (START) of the prostate: recommendations from an International Working Group. Eur Urol. 2013;64(4):544–52.
64. Fiard G, Hohn N, Descotes JL, Rambeaud JJ, Troccaz J, Long JA. Targeted MRI-guided prostate biopsies for the detection of prostate cancer: initial clinical experience with real-time 3-dimensional transrectal ultrasound guidance and magnetic resonance/transrectal ultrasound image fusion. Urology. 2013;81(6):1372–8.
65. Rastinehad AR, Turkbey B, Salami SS, et al. Improving detection of clinically significant prostate cancer: magnetic resonance imaging/transrectal ultrasound fusion guided prostate biopsy. J Urol. 2014;191(6):1749–54.
66. Sonn GA, Chang E, Natarajan S, et al. Value of targeted prostate biopsy using magnetic resonance-ultrasound fusion in men with prior negative biopsy and elevated prostate-specific antigen. Eur Urol. 2014;65(4):809–15.

Chapter 9
Genomic Markers

Neal D. Shore and Karen Ventii

Introduction

Patients being evaluated for the detection of prostate cancer often face critical interventional decisions, such as whether or not to do an initial biopsy or perform a repeat biopsy after an initial negative one. Furthermore, if diagnosed with prostate cancer, a decision to choose an interventional treatment vs. an active surveillance strategy has now become an appropriate discussion.

Use of genomic and proteomic markers/assays may improve the precision of risk assessment and shared educational patient–physician review, thus enhancing decision-making for physicians and patients, especially when the traditional clinical parameters (PSA, DRE, pathology) may not provide the most accurate assessment of indication for biopsy nor indication for treatment option. Certainly, a patient with low-risk, newly diagnosed prostate cancer may benefit from a more precise, personalized assessment of their individual tumor biology.

The currently commercially available array of biomarkers aims to improve risk assessment, guide diagnostic strategies and ultimately enhance treatment outcomes through more targeted screening, more accurate diagnosis, and improved risk stratification, which should lead to improved treatment recommendations and subsequent selection of therapy [1].

N.D. Shore, M.D., F.A.C.S. (✉)
Carolina Urologic Research Center,
823 82nd Parkway, 4 Nelson Court, Myrtle Beach, SC 29572, USA
e-mail: nshore@gsuro.com

K. Ventii, Ph.D.
Emory University, 1510 Clifton Rd., Atlanta, GA 30322, USA
e-mail: kventii@gmail.com

© Springer International Publishing Switzerland 2016
N.N. Stone, E.D. Crawford (eds.), *The Prostate Cancer Dilemma*,
DOI 10.1007/978-3-319-21485-6_9

Who Is Best Suited for an Initial Biopsy?

- PSA testing became the cornerstone of early prostate cancer detection after its approval approximately 30 years ago. However, due to the low disease mortality rate, controversies have emerged with early detection strategies, and concerns regarding subsequent overdiagnosis with the attendant concern of overtreatment with the associated morbidities for the patient and additional cost to the healthcare system.
- Biomarker assays have been developed to help reduce unnecessary initial biopsies, unnecessary repeat biopsies, and enhanced information for ultimate treatment strategies when prostate cancer is newly diagnosed.

PSA

After its approval by the Food and Drug Administration (FDA) in 1986, the availability of PSA dramatically influenced prostate cancer early diagnosis [2, 3]. In the United States, approximately 19 million men receive annual PSA testing, which resulted in more than 1.3 million biopsy procedures and a resultant 240,890 new prostate cancer diagnoses [4].

Nonetheless, reliance on PSA testing alone for the detection of prostate cancer has inherent limitations. First, the test is prostate-specific but not prostate cancer, and it often gives false-positive or false-negative results. Most men with an elevated PSA level (above 4.0 ng/mL) [5] are not found to have prostate cancer; only approximately 25 % of men undergoing biopsy for an elevated PSA level actually have the disease. Conversely, a negative result may give false assurances that the tumor is not detected, when, in fact, a cancer may still exist. Secondly, the test does not always differentiate indolent from aggressive cancers and thus its early detection may not impact eventual mortality from the disease [5] and can lead to overtreatment. This limitation of PSA testing was largely responsible for the recent recommendation of the USPTF against continued routine screening [6].

The Prostate, Lung, Colorectal and Ovarian (PLCO) Cancer Screening trial was a large, population-based randomized trial designed and sponsored by the National Cancer Institute to determine the effects of screening on cancer-related mortality and secondary endpoints in men and women aged 55–74. Regarding the prostate cancer arm of the trial, after 13 years of follow-up, there was no evidence of a survival benefit for planned annual screening compared with mandated screening. Additionally, there was no clinical impact with benefit for scheduled vs. unplanned screening related to age, baseline comorbidity, or pretrial PSA testing [7]. PLCO had a high rate of previous screening (~50 %) in the control arm, thus limiting its conclusions. However, Crawford and colleagues have reported a survival benefit for screening in men without significant comorbidities [8].

Eleven-year follow-up results from the European Randomized Study of Screening for Prostate Cancer study demonstrated that screening does significantly reduce death from prostate cancer [9]. A potential reason for these differing results is that in the US-based PLCO Cancer Screening trial, at least 44 % of participants in the control arm were already PSA-tested prior to being randomized into the study [7], confounding the interpretation of the results.

Roobol and colleagues [10] stated that there was "poor compliance with biopsy recommendations" in PLCO, as the trial did not mandate biopsies. Screening test results were sent to the participant and his physician, and together they decided upon subsequent biopsy.

In order to improve the sensitivity and specificity of serum PSA, several PSA derivatives and isoforms (e.g., PSA isoforms, PSA density, etc.) have been used. The National Comprehensive Cancer Network (NCCN) recommends PSA density when assessing for very low-risk prostate cancer patients [11].

Of note, the Goteborg trial, a prospective randomized trial of 20,000 men born between 1930 and 1944, showed that the benefit of prostate cancer screening compared favorably to other cancer screening programs. Prostate cancer mortality was reduced by almost half, over 14 years of follow-up [12].

Prostate Health Index (Phi)

Efforts have been made to reduce PSA-associated over-biopsying, which may lead to overtreatment in very-low- and low-risk patients. Phi was approved by the FDA for use in 2012 in those with serum PSA values between 4 and 10 ng/mL in an effort to reduce the burden of biopsies in men with a low probability of prostate cancer. NCCN guidelines describe Phi as markers of specificity (along with PCA3 and percent-free PSA) to be used in those considered for additional biopsy [13].

The Phi (Phi = [−2] proPSA/fPSA×PSA1/2); proPSA is a PSA subtype and fPSA is free PSA initially developed as an additional diagnostic biomarker in men with a serum PSA level of 2–10 ng/mL in European trials; an elevated proPSA/fPSA ratio is associated with prostate cancer [14].

Phi score trials have reported a high diagnostic accuracy rate and can be used in prostate cancer diagnosis. Phi score may be useful as a tumor marker in predicting patients harboring more aggressive disease and guiding biopsy decisions [15].

Phi also predicts the likelihood of progression during active surveillance. Tosoian and colleagues showed that both baseline and longitudinal values of Phi predicted which men would be reclassified to higher-risk disease on repeat biopsy during a median follow-up of 4.3 years after diagnosis. Baseline and longitudinal measurements of Phi had confidence indices of 0.788 and 0.820 for upgrading on repeat surveillance biopsy, respectively. In contrast, an earlier study in the Johns Hopkins active surveillance program, PCA3 did not reliably predict short-term biopsy progression during active surveillance [16].

In patients with persistent suspicion of prostate cancer and a negative biopsy, testing with PCA3 and Phi has been proposed as a way to reduce the number of unnecessary repeat biopsies [17].

4KScore

4KScore is a newly available commercial assay panel that is designed to help predict which men with an elevated PSA will have high-grade disease upon tumor biopsy. By combining measures of total, free, and intact PSA with human kallikrein 2 (hK2) and other clinical parameters, the 4KScore was shown to be better than PCPT (Prostate Cancer Prevention Trial) at predicting the occurrence of high-grade disease on biopsy [18]. The 4Kscore Test results have recently been validated in a prospective, blinded clinical study conducted at 26 urology centers across the United States on 1012 patients [19]. The test has been shown to identify the risk of aggressive prostate cancer for the individual patient, including high-grade prostate cancer pathology and poor prostate cancer clinical outcomes within 20 years, with both high sensitivity and negative predictive value for aggressive prostate cancer [20]. Ongoing clinical utility trials are still pending.

Who Can Safely Avoid a Repeat Biopsy?

- For patients with an initial negative prostate biopsy, who are still believed to be at risk for prostate cancer, biomarker tests (PCA3 and ConfirmMDx) may be considered to clarify avoiding proceeding to a repeat (second) biopsy.
- In the presence of persistent risk factors (e.g., elevated PSA), repeat prostate biopsies are frequently used to detect occult cancer in men with previous negative findings, leading to unnecessary morbidity and increased healthcare costs [21].
- Some studies on repeated biopsy procedures have shown that initial prostate biopsy histopathology has a 20–30 % false-negative rate [21].

PCA3

PCA3 is a noncoding messenger RNA that has been demonstrated to be elevated in >90 % of men with known prostate cancer, but not significantly elevated in normal prostatic glands or in benign prostatic hypertrophy. The PCA3 test is a urine-based assay approved by the FDA as a diagnostic test in the setting of a previous negative prostate biopsy. It may be helpful in deciding when to proceed or not re-biopsy, and thus avoid the attendant potential morbidity and associated healthcare costs, while supplementing the diagnostic information obtained from monitoring a patient's PSA kinetics [22]. The higher the PCA3 score, the higher the probability of prostate cancer, whereas a lower score suggests a lower likelihood. The mean PCA3 score was statistically significantly higher in men with a positive prostate cancer biopsy, or those with atypical small acinar proliferation and/or high-grade prostatic intraepithelial neoplasia (HGPIN), compared with men who had a negative biopsy in a large cohort of prospectively evaluated men [23]. PCA3 testing may fail to identify transition zone cancers because the DRE may not elude cells for the assay evaluation into the urine.

ConfirmMDx

ConfirmMDx is a tissue-based epigenetic assay designed to improve decision-making for a repeat prostate biopsy after an initial negative biopsy when there remains concern that a cancer may still be present. It is performed on the paraffin-embedded blocked biopsy samples, and has had assay validation extending back to 24 months from the prior biopsy. The assay detects an epigenetic field effect resulting from increased hypermethylation of three distinct prostate cancer-specific genes. The field effect, or halo effect of cancerization, purports to detect significant genetic abnormalities within/around the cancerous lesion, and thus may be detected despite the normal histologic appearance of the epithelium, hence, effectively extending the interpretative coverage of the biopsy core. This test may help in the identification of men who should proceed to a repeat biopsy while also assist in the avoidance of many unnecessary repeat biopsies [24, 25]. Use of this assay on initial biopsies has been reported to enhance the negative predictive value over histopathologic review [26]. A prospective clinical utility trial (Prostate Assay Specific Clinical Utility at Launch; PASCUAL) is underway to assess the role of this assay in lowering the repeat biopsy rate. With favorable trial findings, it is expected that unrestricted Medicare coverage will be granted (with the Registry requirement removed) [27].

PCMT

PCMT is a tissue-based test that identifies a deletion in mitochondrial DNA that indicates cellular change associated with prostate cancer. It detects the presence of malignant cells in normal-appearing tissue across an extended area. Recent clinical data indicate that this test may be useful for identifying men who do not require a repeat biopsy [28]. A nested case-controlled study demonstrates that the deletion has clinical utility in identifying those patients who may have had cancer missed by sampling error on a prior biopsy procedure. The sensitivity of the assay is 85 % and importantly it has a negative predictive value of 92 % [28, 29]. Additional trials are still pending.

PTEN

Dysregulation of PTEN, a tumor suppressor gene, which is remarkably common deletion for many solid tumor malignancies, has been associated with poor prognosis in prostate cancer. Evidence suggests that loss (homozygous/heterozygous) of

PTEN is associated with higher Gleason grade, risk of progression, and recurrence after therapy [30]. Additionally, it has been reported to be associated with increased risk with advanced localized and metastatic disease [31]. The PTEN assay is a prognostic fluorescence in situ hybridization test, typically ordered in conjunction with prostate biopsy tests which will indicate partial or complete deletions of the gene. Understanding the deletion presence with regard to homozygosity and heterozygosity requires further clinical validation and clinical utility trials.

Who Should Undergo Interventional Therapy or Consider Active Surveillance?

- Physicians and patients can evaluate disease monitoring (active surveillance) as an alternative to interventional treatment after careful consideration of the patient's prostate cancer risk, general health, and age. Biomarkers should assist with this shared decision-making.

Oncotype DX®

The Onco*type* DX® is a multi-gene RT-PCR expression assay that has been prospectively validated in several contemporary cohorts as an accurate predictor of adverse pathology in men with NCCN very-low-, low- and low-intermediate-risk prostate cancer [32]. Using very small biopsy tumor volumes, the assay measures expression of 17 cancer-related genes from four relevant biological pathways, employing five reference genes as threshold validation. These are combined to calculate a Genomic Prostate Score (GPS), which adds independent predictive information beyond standard clinical and pathologic parameters. The report that generates a score between 0 and 100 reveals the patient's underlying tumor, which may help guide initial treatment decision at the time of biopsy. The assay has been clinically validated in two separate independent cohorts confirming Onco*type* DX® as a predictor of adverse pathology from the prostate needle biopsy and demonstrating the test's ability to predict the risk of biochemical recurrence after surgery [33, 34]. There is an ongoing clinical utility trial designed to demonstrate the assay's usefulness with physician–patient shared decision making regarding a decision to proceed with interventional therapy vs. active surveillance.

Prolaris®

Prolaris® is a tissue-based cell cycle progression signature test that assesses 31 cell cycle progression genes to provide a risk assessment of prostate cancer-specific progression and 10-year disease-specific mortality when combined with standard pathologic parameters [35]. It is designed as a risk stratification tool to help refine treatment/monitoring strategy for patients with prostate cancer. Prolaris has been validated in both the biopsy and post-prostatectomy settings. The prognostic value of the Prolaris score has been validated in nine cohorts and over 6000 patients. Data from these studies demonstrate that Prolaris is more predictive of mortality than Gleason score, PSA, age, clinical stage or extent of disease individually and almost doubles the total predictive information when they are combined [36–41]. PROCEDE 500 is a prospective registry study that was designed to evaluate the impact of the Prolaris test on physician treatment recommendations for patients with prostate cancer. It demonstrated that 65 % of physicians changed their original treatment plans for men with prostate cancer based on results from the Prolaris test [42]. A larger prospective clinical utility trial, PROCEDE 1000, has been completed and the final analysis has been accepted for presentation at the AUA Annual Meeting 2015.

Decipher®

The Decipher® RNA assay directly measures the biological risk for metastatic prostate cancer after radical prostatectomy. The test assesses the activity of 22 RNA markers associated with metastatic disease and has been demonstrated to be independently prognostic of prostate cancer death in a high-risk surgical cohort. It generates a genomic risk score to predict the probability of the patient developing metastasis within 5 years of surgery or 3 years of biochemical recurrence. Patients are identified as high, average or low risk based on their predicted probability of developing metastasis. In a validation study, over 70 % of high-risk patients had low genomic classifier (GC) scores and good prognosis, whereas patients with high GC scores had a cumulative incidence of metastasis over 25 % [43, 44]. The test has also demonstrated clinical utility. In a recent study, an average of 39 % of physicians changed patient treatment planning with the benefit of Decipher results [45]. The assay has recently received an LCD (Local Coverage Determination) approval for its indications in assessing post-prostatectomy risk for adjuvant therapy.

ProMark

ProMark is a prognostic biopsy-based prostate cancer test. It uses immunofluorescent imaging analysis to quantify protein biomarker expression and classify patients' tumors. A clinical validation study demonstrated that ProMark can differentiate indolent from aggressive disease, based on data from standard formalin-fixed, paraffin-embedded tissue. The ability to monitor treatment effects and to identify therapeutic targets at the time of treatment consideration is a major unmet need in prostate cancer. Additional assay validation and clinical utility trials are underway [46].

Markers to Assist Post-prostatectomy Evaluation

Both Prolaris® and Decipher® are approved in the post-prostatectomy space, to help enable application of directed, multimodal or adjuvant therapy for patients following radical prostatectomy (RP). Prolaris® testing is particularly well-suited for post-prostatectomy patients with higher risk features to better estimate the risk of biochemical recurrence (BCR) [36, 47]. For Decipher®, 60 % of clinically high-risk men post prostatectomy were reclassified as low risk by Decipher and 98.5 % of men classified as low risk by Decipher did not develop metastasis within 5 years of radical prostatectomy [48].

Clinical Utility and Value of Biomarkers

A biomarker must be measurable, reproducible, linked to relevant clinical outcomes, and demonstrate clinical utility. Clinical utility demonstrates how much additional information the biomarker provides relative to what is currently available; both cost and clinical utility affect reimbursement. Although the FDA does not formally request clinical utility in the biomarker development process, it is a vital consideration that will impact on how widely the marker is used and ultimately reimbursed by private and public payers. For example, clinical utility would be a deciding factor when comparing the value of a costly molecular analysis of a tumor compared to inexpensive clinical parameters routinely available in practice to assess prognosis [49].

Molecular diagnostic researchers should ensure that the analytic validity of a biomarker test has been established prior to the evaluation of clinical utility. In planning clinical utility studies for biomarkers, protocols should specify the patient population intended to benefit from the decision guided by the test result. For validation studies of all types, prior evidence from early studies must be obtained from cohorts relevant to the intended use population.

Ideally, clinical validation studies should use metrics that are clinically useful to physicians in order to assess the strength of association between the biomarker assay and prostate cancer. Ideally, such studies should include outcome measures that assess the potential benefits and challenges from the patient perspective, recognizing that these outcomes may occur at different time points and are the result of clinical management decisions guided by test results.

Biomarker platforms that enable healthcare professionals to accurately interpret and communicate the results of biomarker diagnostic and predictive testing for patients and their caregivers must be prospectively validated before their contemporaneous use should be promoted.

Conclusion

Prostate cancer biomarkers have the potential to assist clinicians in improving decisions regarding whom to biopsy, whom to avoid a repeat biopsy, whom to enhance risk assessment, and thereby reduce unnecessary biopsy strategies as well as over overtreatment, thus achieving more selective therapy for patients with high-risk disease. In effect, clinicians can strive for better outcomes and hopefully remain cost neutral or better yet, achieve cost savings to the healthcare system. In the last few years, there has been rapid development of many new and novel biomarkers. These biomarkers should offer and assist clinicians with improved decision-making on when to biopsy, whom to re-biopsy and how to assist patients with treatment decisions.

References

1. Crawford ED, Ventii K, Shore ND. New biomarkers in prostate cancer. Oncology. 2014;28:135–42.
2. Catalona WJ, Smith DS, Ratliff TL, et al. Measurement of prostate-specific antigen in serum as a screening test for prostate cancer. N Engl J Med. 1991;324(17):1156–61.
3. Chou R, Croswell JM, Dana T, et al. Screening for prostate cancer: a review of the evidence for the U.S. Preventive Services Task Force. Ann Intern Med. 2011;155(11):762–71.
4. Siegel R, Ma J, Zou Z, Jemal A. Cancer statistics, 2014. CA Cancer J Clin. 2014;64:9–29.
5. Institute NC: Prostate-specific antigen (PSA) test.
6. Moyer VA, U.S. Preventive Services Task Force. Screening for prostate cancer: U.S. Preventive Services Task Force recommendation statement. Ann Intern Med. 2012;157(2):120–34.
7. Andriole GL, Crawford ED, Grubb III RL, et al. Prostate cancer screening in the randomized Prostate, Lung, Colorectal, and Ovarian Cancer Screening Trial: mortality results after 13 years of follow-up. J Natl Cancer Inst. 2012;104(2):125–32.
8. Crawford ED, Grubb III R, Black A, et al. Comorbidity and mortality results from a randomized prostate cancer screening trial. J Clin Oncol. 2011;29(4):355–61.
9. Schroder FH, Hugosson J, Roobol MJ, et al. Prostate-cancer mortality at 11 years of follow-up. N Engl J Med. 2012;366(11):981–90.
10. Roobol MJ, Bangma CH, Loeb S. Prostate-specific antigen screening can be beneficial to younger and at-risk men. CMAJ. 2013;185(1):47–51.
11. Oncology NCPGI: Prostate Cancer. Version 2.2014. 2014.
12. Hugosson J, Carlsson S, Aus G, et al. Mortality results from the Goteborg randomised population-based prostate-cancer screening trial. Lancet Oncol. 2010;11(8):725–32.
13. NCCI: Updates Prostate Cancer Early Detection. Version 1.2014. 2014.
14. Le BV, Griffin CR, Loeb S, et al. [-2]Proenzyme prostate specific antigen is more accurate than total and free prostate specific antigen in differentiating prostate cancer from benign disease in a prospective prostate cancer screening study. J Urol. 2010;183(4):1355–9.
15. Wenying Wang MW, Wang L, Adams TS, Tian Y, Xu J. Diagnostic ability of %p2PSA and prostate health index for aggressive prostate cancer: a meta-analysis. Sci Rep. 2014;4:5012.
16. Tosoian JJ, Loeb S, Feng Z, et al. Association of [-2]proPSA with biopsy reclassification during active surveillance for prostate cancer. J Urol. 2012;188(4):1131–6.
17. Porpiglia F, Russo F, Manfredi M, et al. The roles of multiparametric magnetic resonance imaging, PROSTATE CANCER3 and prostate health index-which is the best predictor of prostate cancer after a negative biopsy? J Urol. 2014;192:60–6.

18. Daniel WL. The 4KscoreTM test as a predictor of high-grade prostate cancer on biopsy. American Urological Association Annual Meeting; 2014.
19. Lin DW. The 4Kscore test as a predictor of high-grade prostate cancer on biopsy. AUA; 2014.
20. Lilja HJ, Vickers AJ, Sjoberg D, et al. Improving the specificity of prostate cancer screening for early detection of lethal disease. J Clin Oncol. 2014;32:5s. suppl; abstr 5081.
21. Wojno KJ, Costa FJ, Cornell RJ, et al. Reduced rate of repeated prostate biopsies observed in ConfirmMDx clinical utility field study. Am Health Drug Benefits. 2014;7(3):129–34.
22. De La Taille A, Irani J, Graefen M, et al. Clinical evaluation of the PROSTATE CANCER3 assay in guiding initial biopsy decisions. J Urol. 2011;185(6):2119–25.
23. Crawford ED, Rove KO, Trabulsi EJ, et al. Diagnostic performance of PROSTATE CANCER3 to detect prostate cancer in men with increased prostate specific antigen: a prospective study of 1,962 cases. J Urol. 2012;188(5):1726–31.
24. Stewart G, et al. Clinical utility of a multiplexed epigenetic gene assay to detect cancer in histopathologically negative prostate biopsies: results of the multicenter MATLOC study. American Urological Association (AUA) 2012 Annual Scientific Meeting, 211; 2012.
25. Trock BJ, Brotzman MJ, Mangold LA, et al. Evaluation of GSTP1 and APC methylation as indicators for repeat biopsy in a high-risk cohort of men with negative initial prostate biopsies. BJU Int. 2012;110(1):56–62.
26. Stewart GD, Van Neste L, Delvenne P, et al. Clinical utility of an epigenetic assay to detect occult prostate cancer in histopathologically negative biopsies: results of the MATLOC study. J Urol. 2013;189(3):1110–6.
27. Clinicaltrials.Gov., Nct02250313.: PASCUAL (Prostate Assay Specific Clinical Utility at Launch) Study.
28. Robinson K, Creed J, Reguly B, et al. Accurate prediction of repeat prostate biopsy outcomes by a mitochondrial DNA deletion assay. Prostate Cancer Prostatic Dis. 2010;13(2):126–31.
29. Parr RL, Mills J, Harbottle A, et al. Mitochondria, prostate cancer, and biopsy sampling error. Discov Med. 2013;15(83):213–20.
30. Lotan TL, Carvalho FL, Peskoe SB, et al. PTEN loss is associated with upgrading of prostate cancer from biopsy to radical prostatectomy. Mod Pathol. 2015;28:128–37.
31. Chaux A, Peskoe SB, Gonzalez-Roibon N, et al. Loss of PTEN expression is associated with increased risk of recurrence after prostatectomy for clinically localized prostate cancer. Mod Pathol. 2012;25(11):1543–9.
32. Knezevic D, Goddard AD, Natraj N, et al. Analytical validation of the Oncotype DX prostate cancer assay—a clinical RT-PCR assay optimized for prostate needle biopsies. BMC Genomics. 2013;14:690.
33. Cullen J, Rosner IL, Brand TC, et al. A biopsy-based 17-gene genomic prostate score predicts recurrence after radical prostatectomy and adverse surgical pathology in a racially diverse population of men with clinically low- and intermediate-risk prostate cancer. Eur Urol. 2015;68(1):123–31.
34. Klein EA, Cooperberg MR, Magi-Galluzzi C, et al. A 17-gene assay to predict prostate cancer aggressiveness in the context of Gleason grade heterogeneity, tumor multifocality, and biopsy undersampling. Eur Urol. 2014;66:550–60.
35. Kar AJ, Scholz MC, Fegan JE, David Crawford E, Scardino PT, Kaldate RR, Brawer MK. The effect of cell cycle progression (CCP) score on treatment decisions in prostate cancer: results of an ongoing registry trial. J Clin Oncol 32, 2014 (suppl 4; abstr 277).
36. Cuzick J, Swanson GP, Fisher G, et al. Prognostic value of an RNA expression signature derived from cell cycle proliferation genes in patients with prostate cancer: a retrospective study. Lancet Oncol. 2011;12(3):245–55.
37. Cuzick J, Stone S, Yang ZH, et al. Validation of a 46-gene cell cycle progression RNA signature for predicting prostate cancer death in a conservatively managed watchful waiting needle biopsy cohort. American Urological Association; 2014.
38. Bishoff JT, Freedland SJ, Gerber L, et al. Prognostic utility of the cell cycle progression score generated from biopsy in men treated with prostatectomy. J Urol. 2014;192(2):409–14.

39. Freedland SJ, Gerber L, Reid J, et al. Prognostic utility of cell cycle progression score in men with prostate cancer after primary external beam radiation therapy. Int J Radiat Oncol Biol Phys. 2013;86(5):848–53.
40. Cooperberg MR, et al. Development and validation of the biopsy-based genomic prostate score (GPS) as a predictor of high grade or extracapsular prostate cancer to improve patient selection for active surveillance. AUA; 2013.
41. Cuzick J, Berney DM, Fisher G, et al. Prognostic value of a cell cycle progression signature for prostate cancer death in a conservatively managed needle biopsy cohort. Br J Cancer. 2012;106(6):1095–9.
42. Crawford ED, Scholz MC, Kar AJ, et al. Cell cycle progression score and treatment decisions in prostate cancer: results from an ongoing registry. Curr Med Res Opin. 2014;30(6):1025–31.
43. Badani K, Thompson DJ, Buerki C, et al. Impact of a genomic classifier of metastatic risk on postoperative treatment recommendations for prostate cancer patients: a report from the DECIDE study group. Oncotarget. 2013;4(4):600–9.
44. Karnes RJ, Bergstralh EJ, Davicioni E, et al. Validation of a genomic classifier that predicts metastasis following radical prostatectomy in an at risk patient population. J Urol. 2013;190(6):2047–53.
45. Lobo JM, Dicker AP, Buerki C, et al. Evaluating the clinical impact of a genomic classifier in prostate cancer using individualized decisionanalysis. PLoS One. 2015;10(3):e0116866.
46. Fred Saad MS, Choudhury S, Capela T, Ernst C, Hurley A, Small C, Kaprelyants A, Hussain S, Chang H, Giladi E, Dunyak J, Coupal L, Nifong T, Latour M, Berman D, Blume-Jensen P. Distinguishing aggressive versus nonaggressive prostate cancer using a novel prognostic proteomics biopsy test, ProMark. 2014 ASCO Annual Meeting J Clin Oncol 2014;32:5s. (suppl; abstr 5090).
47. Cooperberg MR, Simko JP, Cowan JE, et al. Validation of a cell-cycle progression gene panel to improve risk stratification in a contemporary prostatectomy cohort. J Clin Oncol. 2013;31(11):1428–34.
48. Ross AE, Feng FY, Ghadessi M, et al. A genomic classifier predicting metastatic disease progression in men with biochemical recurrence after prostatectomy. Prostate Cancer Prostatic Dis. 2014;17(1):64–9.
49. Scher HI, Morris MJ, Larson S, Heller G. Validation and clinical utility of prostate cancer biomarkers. Nat Rev Clin Oncol. 2013;10(4):225–34.

Part II
Treatment

Chapter 10
Current Status of Clinical Trials in Active Surveillance

Laurence Klotz

Background

The identification of men with indolent, clinically insignificant prostate cancer began in the 1950s, when TURP became widely adopted for BPH. Ten percent of men having this operation were found to have clinically unsuspected prostate cancer; in most cases this was small volume, low-grade disease (stage T1a). Remarkably, there was a widespread and uncontroversial consensus that this cancer did not warrant treatment [1]. The incidence of micro-focal low grade disease increased dramatically with the advent of PSA testing in North America and Europe in the late 1980s. This continued unabated until 2012, when the US Preventive Services Task Force announced a level D recommendation against PSA screening [2], followed by equivocal recommendations regarding PSA screening by several other respected national health policy organizations [3]. Screening remains a topic of intense controversy and disagreement. (Most experts believe that PSA screening provides a mortality benefit at the cost of significant overdiagnosis; if overtreatment is avoided, the mortality benefit is compelling.) However, the consequences of the USPSTF recommendation (and that of other groups) have been a steady drop in the rate of PSA testing and referral for biopsy over the last few years.

The USPSTF recommendation against PSA screening was driven in large part by concerns about overdiagnosis and overtreatment of clinically insignificant disease [3]. Despite the historical consensus about conservative management of T1a disease post TURP, from the beginning of the PSA era around 1988 until the task force recommendation in 2012, more than 90 % of patients diagnosed with low-risk prostate cancer by PSA and biopsy in the US were treated with definitive therapy.

L. Klotz, M.D. (✉)
Sunnybrook Health Sciences Centre,
2075 Bayview Ave., MG408, Toronto, ON, Canada, M4N 3M5
e-mail: Laurence.Klotz@sunnybrook.ca

© Springer International Publishing Switzerland 2016
N.N. Stone, E.D. Crawford (eds.), *The Prostate Cancer Dilemma*,
DOI 10.1007/978-3-319-21485-6_10

However, following the task force recommendation, and bolstered by substantial evidence regarding the indolent nature of low-grade disease and the favorable outcome with expectant management, an increasing consensus about the value and benefit of active surveillance has emerged. The most recent available data are that the proportion of patients with low-risk disease managed conservatively increased from about 10 % in 2000 to 35 % in 2010 [4, 5].

Metastatic Potential of Low-Risk Prostate Cancer

Prostate cancers have heterogeneous biology and behavior. Some cancers are aggressive, and others have little or no metastatic potential. Some small cancers, due to lack of telomerase, VEGF, or other biological machinery conferring cellular immortality, may even undergo spontaneous involution and disappear [6]. Several large clinical series have reported a rate of metastasis for surgically confirmed Gleason 6 (where there is no possibility of occult higher grade cancer lurking in the prostate) that is virtually zero [7]. Occult higher grade cancer is present in about 25–40 % of men initially diagnosed with Gleason 6 on biopsy [8, 9].

A natural limitation of assessing the outcome of conservative (no treatment) series is that, since the diagnosis is based on needle biopsy, it is possible, indeed probable, that occult higher grade cancer present at the time of diagnosis was responsible for disease progression in the subset of patients who proceed to develop metastases. The long-term mortality reported for biopsy Gleason 6 managed with no intervention is remarkably similar, about 25 % [10]. The occult high-grade cancers thus are likely responsible for most of the prostate cancer deaths reported in conservative management series.

One way to address the under-grading problem in assessing the true natural history of Gleason 6 is to examine the outcome when the entire prostate has been evaluated, i.e., by surgical pathological grading after radical prostatectomy. One multicenter study of 24,000 men with long-term follow up after surgery included 12,000 with surgically confirmed Gleason 6 cancer [7]. The 20-year prostate cancer mortality was 0.2 %. About 4000 of these were treated at MSKCC; of these, 1 died of prostate cancer; a pathological review of this patient revealed Gleason 4 + 3 disease in the primary; in other words, it was misclassified as Gleason 6 [11]. A second study of 14,000 men with surgically confirmed Gleason 6 disease found only 22 with lymph node metastases; review of these cases showed that all 22 were misclassified, and had higher grade cancer in the primary tumor. The rate of node-positive disease in the 14,000 patients with no Gleason 4 or 5 disease in their prostates was therefore zero. (A limitation of this study was that patients had, in most cases, a limited node dissection; but given the large cohort size, the message is still clear) [12].

Of course, an alternative explanation for the very low rate of metastasis following surgery for Gleason 6 cancer is the treatment effect, i.e., that the intervention is completely successful, and commonly alters the natural history of the disease. This is analogous to the surgical management of basal cell carcinomas of the skin, which may become lethal due to the effects of local invasion if neglected, but in early cases are almost always cured by surgical resection. An important distinction is that basal cell carcinomas do not metastasize, even when locally advanced. Higher grade prostate cancer clearly does metastasize. Thus, one would expect, if Gleason 6 had metastatic potential occasional Gleason 6 cancers would have micro-metastasized prior to surgery or recur locally with subsequent metastasis. This has rarely if ever been observed. Further, if resection of a small basal cell carcinoma of the skin had the same effects on quality of life as a radical prostatectomy, dermatologists would also be considering conservative management in the "low-risk" cases! Notwithstanding that absence of a metastatic potential does not preclude categorizing a lesion as cancer, it has been proposed to change the designation "cancer" for micro-focal Gleason 6 to "Indolent Lesions of Epithelial Origin" (IDLE tumors) [13].

An interesting case report with longitudinal genetic sequencing described a patient who was managed stably on surveillance for Gleason 6 disease for 15 years, including 12 sets of biopsies showing Gleason 6 only or normal tissue. Fifteen years after diagnosis he was re-biopsied for a sharp rise in PSA and found to have Gleason 9 and 10 cancer with metastases. The expression of PTEN, ERG, P53, and Ki-67 switched from uniformly normal in the first 12 biopsies to abnormal in the last one. This case confirms that the activation of genetic switches resulting in histological grade progression can occur in low-grade cancer (or in normal prostate epithelium). Fortunately, these kinds of cases are rare in clinical practice [14].

The published literature on surveillance includes 23 prospective studies. The largest and most mature 14 studies encompassing about 5000 men are summarized in Table 10.1 [15–29]. The conclusions to be drawn from these studies and the areas of continued uncertainty are summarized as below:

The studies use a range of eligibility criteria, from inclusive to stringent. This heterogeneity with respect to eligibility reflects a difference in risk tolerance by the investigators. Inclusion criteria include all low-risk patients (Gleason 6 and PSA < 10 ng/mL, regardless of cancer volume), and selected intermediate risk (Gleason 7 with small amounts of pattern 4, or PSA between 10 and 20 ng/mL). For those groups with more inclusive criteria, particularly the Toronto, Rotterdam, and UCSF series, the potential advantages of surveillance outweigh what is hoped to be a small increased risk of metastasis occurring during the period of surveillance. In contrast, the centers adopting a more stringent inclusion approach restrict surveillance to very low-risk patients by NCCN guidelines (1–2 cores positive, <50 % of core involvement, and PSA density <0.15). For these groups, the increased risk of metastatic disease outweighs the benefits of surveillance for the low- and intermediate-risk groups. Several decision analyses suggest that a very substantial increase in prostate cancer mortality with surveillance compared to radical intervention for all would be required before surveillance would not have a net benefit for the low- and intermediate-risk groups [30]. However, this remains an area of debate.

The rate of radical intervention in men on active surveillance is consistently around 30 % at 5–10 years. This is remarkably similar to the rate of occult higher grade cancer known to be present in men found to have Gleason 6 on systematic biopsy.

Table 10.1 Outcomes of AS in large prospective series

References	n	Median follow-up (months)	% treated overall; % treatment free	Overall/disease specific survival (%)	% BCR post deferred treatment
Klotz et al. [15, 16], University of Toronto	993	92	30 %; 72 % at 5 years	79/97 at 10 years	25 % (6 % overall)
Bul et al. [17], Multicentre, Europe	2500	47	32 %; 43 % at 10 years	77/100 at 10 years	20 %
Dall'Era et al. [18] UCSF	328	43	24 %; 67 % at 5 years	100/100 at 5 years	NR
Kakehi et al. [19], Multicentre, Japan	118	36	51 %; 49 % at 3 years	NR	NR
Tosian et al. [20], Johns Hopkins, USA	407	NR	36 %; NR	NR	NR: 50 % "incurable" based on RP pathology
Roemeling et al. [21], Rotterdam Netherlands	273	41	29 %; 71 % at 5 years	89/100 at 5 years	NR [31 % of 13 RP positive margins]
Soloway et al. [22], Miami, USA	99	35	8 %; 85 % at 5 years	NR	NR
Patel et al. [23], Memorial Sloan Kettering, USA	88	35	35 %; 58 % at 5 years	NR	NR
Barayan [24] McGill, Canada	155	65	20 %	NR	NR
Rubio-Briones [25] Spain	232	36	27 %	93 % at 5 years/99.5 %	
Godtman [26]	439		63 %	81/99.8	14 %
Thomsen [27] Denmark	167	40	35 %/60 % 5 years		
Selvadurai [28] UK	471	67	30 %	98/99.7	12 %
Eggener [29]	262	29	15 %; 25 % at 5 years	NR	5 %

The intervention rate does vary between series, reflecting differences in eligibility criteria and triggers for intervention.

Most groups have reported a consistent rate of re-classification and radical treatment for at least 5 years after diagnosis, typically around 5 %/year. Most patients who are re-classified in the first 5 years likely harbored higher grade cancer at the time of diagnosis. This experience defines an opportunity for improvement in the surveillance algorithm. It is likely that the increasing use of MRI will identify those patients harboring higher grade, usually anterior cancers, earlier, resulting in a shift of the intervention curve to the left. This should result in improved outcome for those patients with a "wolf in sheep's clothing," i.e., an occult higher grade cancer present but not detected by the TRUS biopsy.

Death from prostate cancer is uncommon. Most of these studies have a duration of follow up that is insufficient to preclude an increased risk of prostate cancer mortality as a result of surveillance with certainty. In the most mature surveillance cohort with a median follow up of 8 years and range of 2–18 years, the actuarial prostate cancer mortality at 15 years was 5 % [16]. The commonest cause of death in AS cohorts is cardiovascular disease. In the Toronto cohort, the cumulative hazard ratio (or relative risk) of non-prostate-cancer death rate with a median follow up of 9 years was ten times that for prostate cancer.

A challenge to the surveillance concept is the pivotal Swedish study reported that the risk of prostate cancer mortality in patients managed by watchful waiting was low for many years, but tripled after 15 years of follow up [31]. ("Watchful waiting" meant no opportunity for selective delayed intervention, whereas about 30 % of patients in the surveillance series have had radical treatment.) In the Toronto experience, 70 patients have been followed for 14 years; about 1.5 % have had late disease progression (metastasis developing 8 or more years after diagnosis) but there is no evidence of a sharp increase in mortality to date. Thus a critical question in this field is what the long-term prostate cancer mortality will be beyond 15 years. It will be 5–7 years before the most mature existing cohorts have a median of 15 years of follow-up. To date, however, there is no evidence of a dramatic increase in late prostate cancer mortality.

PSA density has been identified by many groups as a biomarker for higher risk disease, including in the most recent update of the Epstein criteria [32]. A low PSA density is a proxy for low volume of disease, and vice versa; this, in turn, is correlated with the risk of higher grade cancer. A PSA density of <0.15 is an indicator of a more benign phenotype.

If Gleason 6 does not metastasize, and therefore is generally not a threat to the patient's life, what is the significance of higher volume of Gleason 6? This has become clear in several recent publications. Higher volume Gleason 6 is a predictor for an increased risk of occult higher grade cancer [33–35]. In one study, total cancer biopsy length of >8 mm predicted for a significantly increased risk of high-grade disease [36]. Thus, high volume Gleason 6 patients require close scrutiny to exclude as accurately as possible the presence of higher grade disease. With the exception of very young patients, they otherwise do not require treatment.

Race is relevant. African Americans on AS have a higher rate of risk re-classification and PSA failure after treatment than Caucasian men [37]. Black men who are surveillance candidates also have a higher rate of large anterior cancers than Caucasians. Another study suggested that AA men may be at higher risk for disease reclassification [38]. Japanese men younger than age 60 have a lower rate of histological cancer than Caucasian men [39]. Thus, the finding of low-grade prostate cancer in young Asian men is less common, and the risk of overdiagnosis may be less. However, Black and Asian patients diagnosed with low-grade prostate cancer includes men who have little or no probability of a prostate cancer-related death during their remaining lives, and active surveillance is still an appealing option for those who have been appropriately risk-stratified.

The utility of surveillance compared to surgery and radiation has been modeled by several groups. One propensity score analysis compared 452 men from the Toronto surveillance cohort to 6485 men who had RP, 2264 treated with external beam radiotherapy and 1680 with brachytherapy. There was no difference in prostate cancer mortality between the groups while there was improved overall survival in the surveillance group due to an increase in other cause mortality in the radiation patients [40]. A decision analysis of surveillance compared to initial treatment showed that surveillance had the highest QALE even if the relative risk of prostate cancer-specific death for initial treatment vs. active surveillance was as low as 0.6 [30]. (In fact, it is almost certainly 0.95 or better at 15 years.)

An attempt to carry out a prospective randomized trial comparing active surveillance to radical intervention (surgery or radiation) for men with low-risk prostate cancer was undertaken by the NCIC, the intergroup mechanism (CTEP) in the US, and the UKCCR beginning in 2004 (the START trial). The START trial was to enroll 2100 patients, with a primary outcome of prostate cancer mortality. Unfortunately, despite the widespread co-operative group support for the trial, it failed to accrue sufficiently, closing after 4 years with only 240 patients registered.

While surveillance has become more widely accepted over the last decade, the modification of the Gleason system in 2005 has resulted in a decrease in the number of newly diagnosed Gleason 6 compared to 7. Many Gleason 7 cases, who would have been graded as Gleason 6 before 2005, also have clinically insignificant disease. In particular, where the component of pattern 4 is small (<10 %), these patients are likely to have a similar natural history to those with Gleason $3+3$, reflecting stage migration [41]. A recent analysis of Gleason 7 patients having radical prostatectomy found that those who otherwise fulfilled criteria for very low-risk disease (PSA < 10, T1c, ≤positive cores, and PSA density <0.15) had only a 12 % chance of Gleason $4+3$ or higher cancer [42].

Active Surveillance Technique

Implementation of AS has evolved over the last 15 years. The published series reflect an approach which relied on serial systematic biopsies and PSA kinetics. All groups mandate a confirmatory biopsy within the first 3–12 months, targeting the areas of the prostate that have been shown to harbor significant cancer in patients initially diagnosed with Gleason 6. These are the regions that are typically undersampled on the initial diagnostic biopsy, namely the anterior prostate, prostatic apex and base. The interval of biopsy after this varied between annual (Johns Hopkins) and 4–5 years (Toronto).

A major development in the field is the increasing use of multiparametric MRI. We emphasize that none of the favorable results reported in the 14 cohorts summarized herein employed mpMRI until recently. However, the ability to identify large high-grade cancers by imaging is compelling. Some groups are now using mpMRI routinely in men who are surveillance candidates, with biopsy of a target when present. Others use MRI selectively, i.e., in those patients whose biopsy shows substantial volume increase, those who are upgraded to Gleason $3+4$ and surveillance is still desired as a management option, or whose PSA kinetics suggest more aggressive disease (usually defined as a PSADT<3 years). Multiparametric MRI, including T2-weighted image, dynamic contrast-enhanced image, and diffusion-weighted image, should be performed. Identification of an MRI target suspicious for high-grade disease should warrant a targeted biopsy; or, if the lesion is large and unequivocal, intervention.

Eighty-five to 90 % of patients who are upgraded are increased to Gleason $3+4$ [33]. Upgrading to Gleason 8 or higher occurs in 10 % or less of upgraded patients. In many of these patients, the presence of a small amount of Gleason 4 cancer does not alter the indolent course, and conservative management may still be feasible.

MRI has an emerging and potentially game-changing role in the management of AS patients. There are two potential benefits: reassurance that no higher risk disease is present in those with no visualized disease; and, in the subset harboring higher grade disease, earlier identification of this cancer. With respect to the former, the key metric is the negative predictive value. This has been reported to be 97 % for a group of about 300 surveillance candidates at MSKCC [43]. A study of the performance of MRI in the Toronto cohort showed that a non-suspicious MRI was highly correlated with a lack of clinically significant lesions. MRI-targeted biopsy was 6.3× more likely to yield a core positive for GS7 cancer compared with TRUS Bx (25 % of 141 vs. 4 % of 874, $P<0.001$). The negative predictive value of mpMRI for Gleason 7 or greater cancer was 100 % [44]. A recent report from Hopkins confirmed that a non-suspicious MRI was highly correlated with a lack of pathologically significant lesions in an AS population [45]. Another recent study showed that the performance of MRI was particularly effective in men with a PSA >5.2 (which includes most men with diagnosed untreated prostate cancer) [46].

If these results of single-centre cohorts are validated, the performance of MRI as a diagnostic test would permit a level of confidence in a negative MRI that would allow it to replace the biopsy in men with an elevated PSA. This would decrease the number of men requiring biopsies (a major unmet need) and facilitate earlier identification of clinically significant disease. A limitation is that the skill set for accurate interpretation of mpMRI is demanding and not yet widely prevalent.

PSA kinetics are now used as a guide to identify patients at higher risk, but not to drive the treatment decision. This is a shift in practice. In most centers reporting surveillance outcomes, prior to the availability of mpMRI, men with worrisome PSA kinetics (doubling time <3 years or PSA velocity >2 ng/mL/year) were treated. In the PRIAS multi-institutional AS registry, 20 % of men being treated had intervention based on a PSA doubling time <3 years [17].

A rapid rise in PSA is sensitive for aggressive disease but lacks sufficient specificity to be reliable. For example, in a report of the five men dying of metastatic prostate cancer in the Toronto cohort, all had a PSA doubling time <2 years [47]. However, the lack of specificity is a critical flaw. In a study of PSA kinetics in a large surveillance cohort, false-positive PSA triggers (doubling time <3 years, or PSA velocity >2 ng/mL/year) occurred in 50 % of stable untreated patients, none of whom went on to progress, require treatment, or died of prostate cancer [48]. An overview of all of the studies of more than 200 patients examining the predictive value of PSA kinetics in localized prostate cancer concluded that PSA kinetics had no independent predictive value beyond the absolute value of PSA [49].

Active surveillance is highly cost-effective. A recent economic analysis estimated that avoiding treatment in men with clinically insignificant prostate cancer would save \$1.32 billion per year in the US alone [50].

Ongoing Clinical Trials

The Protect trial, a randomized phase 3 study [51], recruited men between age 50 and 69 for a PSA test, and mandated biopsies for those with a $PSA \geq 3.0$ ng/mL. Those diagnosed with prostate cancer were randomized between active surveillance, radical prostatectomy, or conformal radiotherapy. Two thousand eight hundred and ninety-six men were diagnosed with prostate cancer (4 % of tested men and 39 % of those who had a biopsy), of whom 2417 (83 %) had clinically localized disease (mostly T1c, Gleason score 6). One thousand six hundred and forty-three (62 %) agreed to be randomly assigned (545 to active monitoring, 545 to radiotherapy, and 553 to radical prostatectomy). The primary end point is prostate cancer mortality at 10 years, and the data from this pivotal study are expected to be reported in 2016.

Diet may play a role in preventing progression of low-risk disease, and many epidemiological studies suggest that a vegetable based diet may be beneficial. The MEAL study is a 2-year randomized, phase 3 clinical trial in 464 patients allocated to receive either a validated telephone-based diet counseling intervention for 2 years or a published diet guideline [52]. The primary outcome is clinical progression defined by PSA value and pathological findings on follow-up prostate biopsy. Secondary outcome variables include incidence of surgical and non-surgical treatments for prostate cancer, prostate cancer-related patient anxiety and health-related quality of life.

The Study of Active Monitoring in Sweden (SAMS) is a prospective, multicentre study of active surveillance for low-risk prostate cancer, consisting of randomization between standard re-biopsy and follow-up and extensive initial re-biopsy coupled with less intensive follow-up and no further scheduled biopsies (SAMS-FU) [53]. There is also an observational arm (SAMS-ObsQoL). SAMS-FU is planned to randomize 500 patients and SAMS-ObsQoL to include at least 500 patients during 5 years. The primary endpoint is conversion to active treatment.

Conclusion

Active surveillance is an effective solution to the widely recognized problem of overtreatment of screen-detected prostate cancer. Many prospective phase 2 studies including more than 5000 patients have reported a low rate of prostate cancer metastasis and death. A randomized phase 3 trial comparing surveillance to radical intervention was launched in 2007—it failed to accrue adequately and closed unsuccessfully. Mild uncertainty remains related to the outcome after >15 years follow-up. Adoption of an active surveillance program for low-risk disease could reduce overall mortality without an increase in prostate cancer deaths and provide substantial cost savings (estimated at up to $1.32 billion/year in the US). The approach to surveillance continues to evolve, and the incorporation of improved imaging and molecular biomarkers is certain to improve individual risk characterization, and therefore long-term outcome. This should also reduce the need for periodic biopsies. A dispassionate re-assessment of PSA screening based on these improved metrics should lead to a re-consideration of the value of early detection by organizations such as the USPSTF. The minimum standard currently is a confirmatory biopsy targeting the anterolateral horn and anterior prostate within 6–12 months. PSA should be performed every 6 months and subsequent biopsies every 3–5 years until the patient is no longer a candidate for definitive therapy. The role of mpMRI in men on surveillance is currently the subject of intensive investigation, and should be clarified within the next few years. Currently it is indicated for men with a grade or volume increase, or adverse PSA kinetics. Treatment should be offered for most patients with upgraded disease.

References

1. Byar DA, The VA Cooperative Urology Research Group. Survival of patients with incidentally found microscopic cancer of the prostate: results of a clinical trial of conservative treatment. J Urol. 1972;108:908.
2. http://www.uspreventiveservicestaskforce.org/uspstf12/prostate/prostateart.htm
3. https://www.auanet.org/education/guidelines/prostate-cancer-detection.cfm
4. Cooperberg MR, Broering JM, Carroll PR. Time trends and local variation in primary treatment of localized prostate cancer. J Clin Oncol. 2010;28(7):1117–23.
5. Weiner AB, Patel SG, Etzioni R, Eggener SE. National trends in the management of low and intermediate risk prostate cancer in the United States: SEER and NCDB et al. J Urol. 2015 Jan;193(1):95–102.
6. Serrano M. Cancer: a lower bar for senescence. Nature. 2010;464(7287):363–4.
7. Eggener S, Scardino P, Walsh P, et al. 20 year prostate cancer specific mortality after radical prostatectomy. J Urol. 2011;185(3):869–75.
8. Vellekoop A, Loeb S, Folkvaljon Y, Stattin P. Population based study of predictors of adverse pathology among candidates for active surveillance with Gleason 6 prostate cancer. J Urol. 2014;191(2):350–7.
9. Truong M, Slezak JA, Lin CP, Iremashvili V, Sado M, Razmaria AA, Leverson G, Soloway MS, Eggener SE, Abel EJ, Downs TM, Jarrard DF. Development and multi-institutional validation of an upgrading risk tool for Gleason 6 prostate cancer. Cancer. 2013;119(22): 3992–4002.
10. Albertsen PC, Hanley JA, Fine J. 20-year outcomes following conservative management of clinically localized prostate cancer. JAMA. 2005;293(17):2095–101.
11. Scott Eggener. Personal communication.
12. Ross HM, Kryvenko ON, Cowan JE, Simko JP, Wheeler TM, Epstein JI. Do adenocarcinomas of the prostate with Gleason score (GS)<=6 have the potential to metastasize to lymph nodes? Am J Surg Pathol. 2012;36(9):1346–52.
13. Esserman LJ, Thompson IM, Reid B, Nelson P, Ransohoff DF, Welch HG, Hwang S, Berry DA, Kinzler KW, Black WC, Bissell M, Parnes H, Srivastava S. Addressing overdiagnosis and overtreatment in cancer: a prescription for change. Lancet Oncol. 2014;15(6):e234–42.

14. Haffner MC, De Marzo AM, Yegnasubramanian S, Epstein JI, Carter HB. Diagnostic challenges of clonal heterogeneity in prostate cancer. J Clin Oncol. 2015;33(7):e38–40.
15. Klotz L, Zhang L, Lam A, Nam R, Mamedov A, Loblaw A. Clinical results of long-term follow-up of a large, active surveillance cohort with localized prostate cancer. J Clin Oncol. 2010;28(1):126–31.
16. Klotz L, Vesprini D, Sethukavalan P, Jethava V, Zhang L, Jain S, Yamamoto T, Mamedov A, Loblaw A. Long-term follow-up of a large active surveillance cohort of patients with prostate cancer. J Clin Oncol. 2015;33(3):272–7.
17. Bul M, Zhu X, Valdagni R, Pickles T, Kakehi Y, Rannikko A, Bjartell A, van der Schoot DK, Cornel EB, Conti GN, Boevé ER, Staerman F, Vis-Maters JJ, Vergunst H, Jaspars JJ, Strölin P, van Muilekom E, Schröder FH, Bangma CH, Roobol MJ. Active surveillance for low-risk prostate cancer worldwide: the PRIAS study. Eur Urol. 2013;63(4):597–603.
18. Dall'Era MA, Konety BR, Cowan JE, Shinohara K, Stauf F, Cooperberg MR, Meng MV, Kane CJ, Perez N, Master VA, Carroll PR. Active surveillance for the management of prostate cancer in a contemporary cohort. Cancer. 2008;112(12):2664–70.
19. Kakehi Y, Kamoto T, Shiraishi T, Ogawa O, Suzukamo Y, Fukuhara S, Saito Y, Tobisu K, Kakizoe T, Shibata T, Fukuda H, Akakura K, Suzuki H, Shinohara N, Egawa S, Irie A, Sato T, Maeda O, Meguro N, Sumiyoshi Y, Suzuki T, Shimizu N, Arai Y, Terai A, Kato T, Habuchi T, Fujimoto H, Niwakawa M. Prospective evaluation of selection criteria for active surveillance in Japanese patients with stage T1cN0M0 prostate cancer. Jpn J Clin Oncol. 2008; 38(2):122–8.
20. Tosoian JJ, Trock BJ, Landis P, et al. Active surveillance program for prostate cancer: an update of the Johns Hopkins experience. J Clin Oncol. 2011;29:2185–90.
21. Roemeling S, Roobol MJ, de Vries SH, Wolters T, Gosselaar C, van Leenders GJ, Schröder FH. Active surveillance for prostate cancers detected in three subsequent rounds of a screening trial: characteristics, PSA doubling times, and outcome. Eur Urol. 2007;51(5):1244–50.
22. Soloway MS, Soloway CT, Eldefrawy A, et al. Careful selection and close monitoring of low-risk prostate cancer patients on active surveillance minimizes the need for treatment. Eur Urol. 2010;58:831–5.
23. Patel MI, DeConcini DT, Lopez-Corona E, Ohori M, Wheeler T, Scardino PT. An analysis of men with clinically localized prostate cancer who deferred definitive therapy. J Urol. 2004;171(4):1520–4.
24. Barayan GA, Brimo F, Bégin LR, Hanley JA, Liu Z, Kassouf W, Aprikian AG, Tanguay S. Factors influencing disease progression of prostate cancer under active surveillance: a McGill University Health Center Cohort. BJU Int. 2014;114:E99–104.
25. Rubio-Briones J, Iborra I, Ramírez M, Calatrava A, Collado A, Casanova J, Domínguez-Escrig J, Gómez-Ferrer A, Ricós JV, Monrós JL, Dumont R, López-Guerrero JA, Salas D, Solsona E. Obligatory information that a patient diagnosed of prostate cancer and candidate for an active surveillance protocol must know. Actas Urol Esp. 2014;38:559–65.
26. Godtman RA, Holmberg E, Khatami A, Stranne J, Hugosson J. Outcome following active surveillance of men with screen-detected prostate cancer. Results from the Göteborg randomised population-based prostate cancer screening trial. Eur Urol. 2013;63(1):101–7.
27. Thomsen FB, Røder MA, Hvarness H, Iversen P, Brasso K. Active surveillance can reduce overtreatment in patients with low-risk prostate cancer. Dan Med J. 2013;60(2):A4575.
28. Selvadurai ED, Singhera M, Thomas K, Mohammed K, Woode-Amissah R, Horwich A, Huddart RA, Dearnaley DP, Parker CC. Medium-term outcomes of active surveillance for localised prostate cancer. Eur Urol. 2013;64:981–7.
29. Eggener SE, Mueller A, Berglund RK, Ayyathurai R, Soloway C, Soloway MS, Abouassaly R, Klein EA, Jones SJ, Zappavigna C, Goldenberg L, Scardino PT, Eastham JA, Guillonneau B. A multi-institutional evaluation of active surveillance for low risk prostate cancer. J Urol. 2013;189(1 Suppl):S19–25. discussion S25.
30. Hayes JH, Ollendorf DA, Pearson SD, Barry MJ, Kantoff PW, Stewart ST, Bhatnagar V, Sweeney CJ, Stahl JE, McMahon PM. Active surveillance compared with initial treatment for men with low-risk prostate cancer: a decision analysis. JAMA. 2010;304(21):2373–80.

31. Popiolek M, Rider JR, Andrén O, Andersson SO, Holmberg L, Adami HO, Johansson JE. Natural history of early, localized prostate cancer: a final report from three decades of follow-up. Eur Urol. 2013;63(3):428–35.

32. Kryvenko ON, Carter HB, Trock BJ, Epstein JI. Biopsy criteria for determining appropriateness for active surveillance in the modern era. Urology. 2014;83(4):869–74.

33. Porten SP, Whitson JM, Cowan JE, Cooperberg MR, Shinohara K, Perez N, Greene KL, Meng MV, Carroll PR. Changes in prostate cancer grade on serial biopsy in men undergoing active surveillance. J Clin Oncol. 2011;29(20):2795–800.

34. Dall'Era MA, Cowan JE, Simko J, Shinohara K, Davies B, Konety BR, Meng MV, Perez N, Greene K, Carroll PR. Surgical management after active surveillance for low-risk prostate cancer: pathological outcomes compared with men undergoing immediate treatment. BJU Int. 2011;107(8):1232–7.

35. Choo R, Danjoux C, Morton G, Szumacher E, Sugar L, Gardner S, Kim M, Choo CM, Klotz L. How much does Gleason grade of follow-up biopsy differ from that of initial biopsy in untreated, Gleason score 4–7, clinically localized prostate cancer? Prostate. 2007;67(15):1614–20.

36. Bratt O, Folkvaljon Y, Loeb S, Klotz L, Egevad L, Stattin P. Upper limit of cancer extent on biopsy defining very low risk prostate cancer. BJU Int. 2015 Aug;116(2):213–9.

37. Sundi D, Ross AE, Humphreys EB, Han M, Partin AW, Carter HB, Schaeffer EM. African American men with very low-risk prostate cancer exhibit adverse oncologic outcomes after radical prostatectomy: should active surveillance still be an option for them? J Clin Oncol. 2013;31(24):2991–7.

38. Odom BD, Mir MC, Hughes S, Senechal C, Santy A, Eyraud R, Stephenson AJ, Ylitalo K, Miocinovic R. Active surveillance for low-risk prostate cancer in African American men: a multi-institutional experience. Urology. 2014;83(2):364–8.

39. Zlotta AR, Egawa S, Pushkar D, Govorov A, Kimura T, Kido M, Takahashi H, Kuk C, Kovylina M, Aldaoud N, Fleshner N, Finelli A, Klotz L, Sykes J, Lockwood G, van der Kwast TH. Prevalence of prostate cancer on autopsy: cross-sectional study on unscreened Caucasian and Asian men. J Natl Cancer Inst. 2013;105(14):1050–8.

40. Stephenson A, Klotz L. Comparative propensity analysis of active surveillance vs initial treatment. AUA 2013.

41. Cooperberg MR, Cowan JE, Hilton JF, Reese AC, Zaid HB, Porten SP, Shinohara K, Meng MV, Greene KL, Carroll PR. Outcomes of active surveillance for men with intermediate-risk prostate cancer. J Clin Oncol. 2011;29(2):228–34.

42. Ploussard G, Isbacbrrn H, Briganti A, Sooriakumaran P, Surcel CI, Salomon L, Freschi M, Mirvald C, van der Poel HG, Jenkins A, Ost P, van Oort IM, Yossepowitch O, Giannarini G, van den Bergh RC. Can we expand active surveillance criteria to include biopsy Gleason 3 + 4 prostate cancer? A multi-institutional study of 2,323 patients. Urol Oncol. 2015;33:71.e1–9. pii: S1078-1439(14)00263-4.

43. Vargas HA, Akin O, Afaq A, Goldman D, Zheng J, Moskowitz CS, Shukla-Dave A, Eastham J, Scardino P, Hricak H. Magnetic resonance imaging for predicting prostate biopsy findings in patients considered for active surveillance of clinically low risk prostate cancer. J Urol. 2012;188(5):1732–8.

44. Da Rosa MR, Milot L, Sugar L, Vesprini D, Chung H, Loblaw A, Pond GR, Klotz L, Haider MA. A prospective comparison of MRI-US fused targeted biopsy versus systematic ultrasound-guided biopsy for detecting clinically significant prostate cancer in patients on active surveillance. J Magn Reson Imaging. 2015;41(1):220–5.

45. Mullins JK, Bonekamp D, Landis P, Begum H, Partin AW, Epstein JI, Carter HB, Macura KJ. Multiparametric magnetic resonance imaging findings in men with low-risk prostate cancer followed using active surveillance. BJU Int. 2013;111(7):1037–45.

46. Shakir NA, George AK, Siddiqui MM, Rothwax JT, Rais-Bahrami S, Stamatakis L, Su D, Okoro C, Raskolnikov D, Walton-Diaz A, Simon R, Turkbey B, Choyke PL, Merino MJ, Wood BJ, Pinto PA. Identification of threshold prostate specific antigen levels to optimize the detection of clinically significant prostate cancer by magnetic resonance imaging/ultrasound fusion guided biopsy. J Urol. 2014;192(6):1642–8.

47. Krakowsky Y, Loblaw A, Klotz L. Prostate cancer death of men treated with initial active surveillance: clinical and biochemical characteristics. J Urol. 2010;184(1):131–5.
48. Loblaw A, Zhang L, Lam A, Nam R, Mamedov A, Vesprini D, Klotz L. Comparing prostate specific antigen triggers for intervention in men with stable prostate cancer on active surveillance. J Urol. 2010;184(5):1942–6.
49. Vickers A. Systematic review of pretreatment PSA velocity and doubling time as PCA predictors. J Clin Oncol. 2008;27:398–403.
50. Aizer AA, Gu X, Chen MH, Choueiri TK, Martin NE, Efstathiou JA, Hyatt AS, Graham PL, Trinh QD, Hu JC, Nguyen PL. Cost implications and complications of overtreatment of low-risk prostate cancer in the United States. J Natl Compr Canc Netw. 2015;13(1):61–8.
51. Lane JA, Donovan JL, Davis M, Walsh E, Dedman D, Down L, Turner EL, Mason MD, Metcalfe C, Peters TJ, Martin RM, Neal DE, Hamdy FC, ProtecT study group. Active monitoring, radical prostatectomy, or radiotherapy for localised prostate cancer: study design and diagnostic and baseline results of the ProtecT randomised phase 3 trial. Lancet Oncol. 2014;15(10):1109–18.
52. Parsons JK, Pierce JP, Mohler J, Paskett E, Jung SH, Humphrey P, Taylor JR, Newman VA, Barbier L, Rock CL, Marshall J. A randomized trial of diet in men with early stage prostate cancer on active surveillance: rationale and design of the Men's Eating and Living (MEAL) Study (CALGB 70807). Contemp Clin Trials. 2014;38(2):198–203.
53. Bratt O, Carlsson S, Holmberg E, Holmberg L, Johansson E, Josefsson A, Nilsson A, Nyberg M, Robinsson D, Sandberg J, Sandblom D, Stattin P. The Study of Active Monitoring in Sweden (SAMS): a randomized study comparing two different follow-up schedules for active surveillance of low-risk prostate cancer. Scand J Urol. 2013;47(5):347–55.

Chapter 11
Focused Targeted Therapy in Prostate Cancer

Kevin Krughoff and Al Barqawi

Introduction

Prostate cancer is the second most common cancer in men at 28 % of all non-cutaneous malignancies and the second most common cause of cancer death in men, yet most men diagnosed with prostate cancer will not die of their disease [1, 2]. Partially accounting for this is the well-recognized stage migration that took place after the advent of PSA testing, where the proportion of metastatic prostate cancer diagnoses decreased substantially while localized disease diagnoses took precedence [3]. One large-scale study demonstrated as much as a 75 % reduction in metastatic prostate cancer diagnoses from 1993 to 2003 [4]. Given exceedingly high prostate-cancer specific survival rates for localized disease, the push for increased utilization of Active Surveillance (AS) instead of treatment is stronger than ever [5].

Despite this, overdiagnosis and overtreatment remain a problem, and non-curative initial management (NCIM) strategies, either AS or watchful waiting (WW), have for decades continued to meet minimal enrollment success [6–10]. Even though more cancers continue to be found at lower stages and are associated with lower PSA levels, epidemiological data demonstrates the opposite to be true with regard to grade, a situation that would make increases in NCIM more worrisome. An increase in Gleason $3+4$, $4+3$, or 8–10 has been noted in recent biopsies relative to

K. Krughoff, B.A.
1663 Vine St., Denver, CO 80206, USA

Division of Urology, Department of Surgery, University of Colorado Denver
School of Medicine, 12631 East 17th Ave., Room L15-5602, Aurora, CO 80045, USA
e-mail: kevin.krughoff@ucdenver.edu

A. Barqawi, M.D., F.R.C.S. (✉)
Division of Urology, Department of Surgery, University of Colorado Denver
School of Medicine, 12631 East 17th Ave., Room L15-5602, Aurora, CO 80045, USA
e-mail: Al.Barqawi@ucdenver.edu

© Springer International Publishing Switzerland 2016
N.N. Stone, E.D. Crawford (eds.), *The Prostate Cancer Dilemma*,
DOI 10.1007/978-3-319-21485-6_11

1999–2001 [11]. It's been speculated that a proposed modification to the Gleason grading system in 2005 and the increase in the number of cores taken per biopsy may account for this; however, the effect was documented prior to such recommendations [12–14]. In any event, the upward trend in Gleason grading implies trouble for the already disproportionately low AS enrollment rates as fewer men will meet eligibility criteria if grade migration continues.

Results from the more recently aggregated Michigan Urological Survey Improvement Collaborative (MUSIC) registry are encouraging for AS enrollment, and the reported 50 % AS enrollment amongst D'Amico low-risk patients may suggest a shifting tide in AS acceptance. Long-term follow-up success remains to be seen, however, given the sparse use of follow-up biopsy regimens in these patients [15]. Moreover, the MUSIC registry demonstrated that AS was still a relatively infrequent option for younger, healthier men, reflecting a not-uncommon bias against AS use in this population and a continuing problem for AS success [16]. Data from both the Surveillance, Epidemiology, and End Results Program (SEER) and the National Cancer Database (NCDB) did show that the proportion of men with Gleason ≤ 6 cancers electing NCIM strategies increased over the last 10 years, but when changes to the Gleason grading system were accounted for (i.e., looking at both Gleason 6 and 7 cancers) there was no overall significant change in the proportion of men using NCIM strategies. On the contrary, the proportion of men electing a surgical approach increased substantially over time [17].

As of today, most men who are diagnosed with clinically localized prostate cancer continue to receive radical surgical, radiation, and/or hormonal treatments, possibly due to prevailing attitudes about taking an active approach to fixing the problem, the psychological burden of living with cancer, pressure from relatives and friends, and a lack of clarity regarding clinical significance of individual cancer prognosis and impact on overall mortality [17–19]. The side effect profile from whole gland treatment arises from collateral damage to sensitive structures such as the bladder neck, neurovascular bundles, external sphincter, and rectum. Complication rates varies considerably across published data; however, the rates of urinary incontinence, erectile dysfunction, and other quality-of-life-reducing side effects and overall cost associated with these treatments remain substantial, a fact which played heavily into the recent recommendation against routine PSA screening [20–25].

Due to a high-risk side effect profile, it has been argued that such traditional treatment should be reserved only for men with significant risk of disease progression or relegated only to high-volume centers where surgical expertise can reduce complication rates [20, 26]. The difficulty in doing so lies in the sheer volume of prostatectomies that would have to be addressed by such a small proportion of surgeons. While approximately 60,000 prostatectomies take place in the USA every year, less than half of these are performed by the 7 % of surgeons that one might consider high volume (over 24 RPs per year) [27]. Robot assisted laparoscopic radical prostatectomy (RALP) became an attractive option after initial reports of less postoperative pain, less blood loss, and shorter length of stay, and since the 2000 FDA approval of the Da Vinci surgical system 42 % of high volume surgeons have adopted RALP [27, 28]. To this end, RALP has demonstrated at best equivocal continence and potency rates but with a ballooning cost increase [26].

In the face of problematic AS enrollment, the most likely scenario for men diagnosed with localized prostate cancer is the eventual pursuit of one of many treatment options with a high side effect profile and poor cost effectiveness. Given that most therapeutic options for localized cancer have virtually equivalent survival rates, it is precisely this side effect profile and the post-therapeutic quality of life (QOL) that becomes the dominant determining factor in treatment, a concept widely reflected in the literature [29–32]. Decision-making analyses find that when patients present with low grade prostate cancer, physicians place much more importance on patient preferences, and one of the most important patient concerns is how QOL is affected by treatment [33]. Of those who prefer nonsurgical options, their decision is found to be most significantly guided by concerns surrounding the impact of treatment on daily life [34].

Among the impacts to QOL from traditional treatments, most significant are urinary and sexual side effects. A systematic review of 18 randomized controlled trials and 473 observational studies found variable rates of incontinence (Table 11.1).

With regard to erectile dysfunction, results from the Prostate Cancer Outcomes Study (PCOS) found rates ranging from 33 to 86 % depending on therapeutic modality (Table 11.2).

With regard to recovery from such symptoms, a QOL evaluation of 580 patients performed over 24 months following RP, EBRT, and brachytherapy found variable results (Table 11.3).

Extended follow-up for this group was conducted out to 48 months, finding that return to sexual function remained minimal for RP patients while EBRT subjects began to demonstrate progressively worsening urinary function after 24 months but steadily improved in sexual function [36].

After 15 years following patients who received RP or EBRT for clinically localized prostate cancer, it was found that patients continue to have symptoms (Table 11.4).

Table 11.1 Incontinence rates—Wilt et al. [24]

RP	EBRT	Brachytherapy
5–35 %	2–6 %	2–32 %

RP radical prostatectomy, *EBRT* electron beam radiation therapy

Table 11.2 Erectile dysfunction rates—PCOS [23]

RP	ADT	WW
58 %	86 %	33 %

ADT androgen deprivation therapy

Table 11.3 Return to baseline following therapy—Litwin et al. [37]

	RP (%)	EBRT (%)	Brachytherapy (%)
Return to sexual function baseline	39	70	60
Return to urinary control baseline	65	95	90

Table 11.4 Complication rates 15-years following therapy—Resnick et al. [39]

	RP (%)	EBRT (%)
Frequent leakage or no control	18.3	9.4
Bowel urgency	21.9	35.8
Poor erectile quality	87	3.9

The study by Resnick et al. demonstrates that the urinary, sexual, and bowel related side effects only continue to decline after 2 years. In addition, the hypothesis that men become accustomed to these problems over the years does not hold, as bothersome indices for urinary, sexual, and bowel related side effects were shown to steadily and consistently increase over the years [37].

When considering the side effect profiles and literature on decision making in the face of localized prostate cancer, the demand for therapeutic options with minimal effects on quality of life are abundantly clear, and this is the problem that focal therapy aims to solve. By bridging the gap between surveillance and whole gland therapy, focal therapy offers the chance for cancer control while decreasing the common side effects associated with definitive therapy.

Patient Selection

The crux of successful focal therapy is proper patient selection and accurate identification and characterization of the lesion.

In regard to grade, many differing opinions exist on the ideal candidate for focal therapy and inclusion criteria was initially very limited, as established by the International Task Force on Prostate Cancer in 2007 [38]. Today, the momentum of focal therapy is moving from clinically insignificant disease and progressing towards prostate-confined intermediate disease [39]. In a meta-analysis of focal therapy covering 25 studies using focal therapy in the primary setting, 5 in the salvage setting, and 13 registered trials found that nearly half of focal therapy studies employed eligibility criteria of Gleason $\leq 4+3$, one-quarter used Gleason $\leq 3+4$, and the remaining used Gleason $\leq 3+3$ and one of Gleason ≤ 8 [40].

With regard to PSA the consensus on inclusion criteria is for a PSA value <15 ng/ mL, however, some studies have used values exceeding 20 [39, 40]. The baseline PSA may, however, be more helpful as a marker of progression rather than as a strict inclusion criterion.

It is well known that most prostate cancer is multifocal and the issue of staging warrants further discussion [41]. It has been demonstrated, for instance, that when RP specimens are closely examined approximately 80 % will harbor multifocal cancer [42–44]. As for the nature of these secondary lesions, an analysis of 100 RP specimens found that 43 % of secondary lesions are clinically significant [45]. Moreover, such secondary lesions are likely not restricted to one side of the prostate, which questions the utility of hemi-ablation. While stage migration towards unilateral disease has been documented since the PSA era, the absolute magnitude of that change and the overall proportion of unilateral prostate cancer are questionable [46]. Two large pathological studies demonstrated that 14.3 % of 3676 RP specimens from 1988 to 2006 were unilateral compared to just 21.3 % of 1467 RP specimens from 2000 to 2007 [44, 46]. There also lies a difficulty in identifying this population of unilateral cancers as unilateral cancer is extremely difficult to predict based on traditional transrectal ultrasound guided (TRUS) biopsy schemes and serum markers [47, 48].

Thus the current landscape of localized prostate cancer is one of multifocal origin, rarely limited to one side, and even if present, unlikely to be correctly identified using the traditional tools of prostate cancer screening (i.e., TRUS biopsy and serum markers). How, then, should focal therapy proceed?

Fortunately, the growing sense of utility for concept of focal therapy has ushered in an impressive array of new targeting efforts. Extensive data shows that the "gold-standard" TRUS biopsy is insufficiently accurate for the purposes of focal therapy, even when the number of biopsy cores is advanced [49–51]. To this end, new technologies emerged that demonstrate significant advances in the accuracy of prostate cancer localization, staging and grading (see Chaps. 6, 7 and 9). Chief among these are transperineal template guided mapping biopsies (TPM and multiparametric MRI (mpMRI).

The second concept of focal therapy centers around index lesion treatment rather than curative ablation of all cancer foci—a concept that has fallen out of favor amongst focal therapy experts [52]. The prevalence of index lesions was demonstrated by one evaluation of 1832 whole-mount RP specimens, in which it was found that for those with multifocal disease, 80 % of tumor burden was focused in one dominant tumor, and in those with extracapsular extension, 92 % arose from this same index lesion [53]. The literature on index lesion characteristics reveals that progression-free survival is associated with index lesion volume but not with that of the secondary tumor foci [42]. Biochemical failure was also found to be determined by index lesion characteristics and Gleason 4/5 tumor volume, whereas secondary tumors were insignificant in this regard [54, 55].

Evidence now suggests that metastatic potential can be directly related to the index tumor as well. As part of the Project to Eliminate Lethal Prostate Cancer (PELICAN), researchers analyzed single-nucleotide and copy-number polymorphism at 94 anatomically separate malignant cancer sites from 30 men who died of disseminated prostate cancer, concluding that lethal prostate cancer cells can be traced back to a common parent cell [56]. In a separate report, an extensive pathological workup of metastatic prostate cancer in one man found that metastatic foci were of the same clonal origin as a smaller secondary focus of prostate cancer. However, a nearby larger tumor of higher Gleason grade harbored the same mutation, leading the authors to believe that the clonal origin came from a small area of this larger tumor that later developed subsequent malignant potential [57].

Researchers speculate a day where the temporal sequence of genomic lesions might be tracked, and a "molecular time stamp" established whereby progression could be better defined and identification and risk stratification of the index tumor more accurately tailored [58]. This may become especially important in cases where high grade tumors exist at small volumes, which has been demonstrated in other studies [41]. If and when this may arrive is unclear, but due to the growing body of evidence relating index tumor characteristics to overall prostate cancer behavior, the consensus is that therapy should be directed towards identification and treatment of the index lesion [39, 52].

Technique

The initial phase of focal therapy is accurate cancer localization; this is best performed via 3-dimensional mapping biopsy (3DMB) with 3D-reconstruction or mpMRI.

The 3D-reconstruction is usually rendered by a specialized software program that reconstructs the cancerous foci within the prostate in three dimensions. This virtual visual representation helps the patient and physician visualize the extent and grade of cancer foci and tailor a treatment plan. Targeted focal therapy (TFT) usually takes place 8–12 weeks following 3DMB to allow sufficient time to account for reduction of swelling and allow the prostate to return to its original position and dimensions. Positioning of the prostate has been accurately obtained using at least two fiducial markers inserted at predetermined coordinates during the mapping biopsy; however, preliminary use of recent software advances and real-time imaging suggests that the same level of accuracy can be obtained without such markers. Patients can be treated with one of a variety of energies to achieve the aims of focal therapy, and a variety of approaches are used based on the patient's individual tumor characteristics. The most commonly used ablation schemes, in order of frequency, are focal/zonal ablation, hemi-ablation, or an extended "hockey-stick" approach (which includes the posterior zone of the contralateral lobe), and bilateral focal ablation [40]. Each modality has variations in approach.

During focal laser ablation patients undergo multiparametric 3.0 T prostate MRI the day before the focal laser ablation utilizing an endorectal coil and 8-channel pelvis phased array surface coil. Using proprietary software, 3D images from 3DMB ultrasound are fused with 3D rendering of the prostate by MRI to match the cancer locations from both imaging modalities. After an appropriate needle path is identified, the patient is placed under general anesthesia in lithotomy position and a urethral catheter is placed. A laser shelter with an MR-compatible titanium trocar is inserted transperineally through the appropriate template hole and advancement is monitored using ultrasound. The metal insert is then replaced with a laser applicator and the patient is transferred to the MR suite for real-time MR guided laser ablation.

In the supine position T1 weighted MR imaging of the prostate is obtained to localize and confirm the position of the laser probe and laser ablation is performed in real-time using continuously updated MR temperature mapping using MR thermometry software. Energy from the laser probe induces irreversible cell injury and coagulative necrosis at ≥ 50 °C, while the surrounding area undergoes a heat-sink

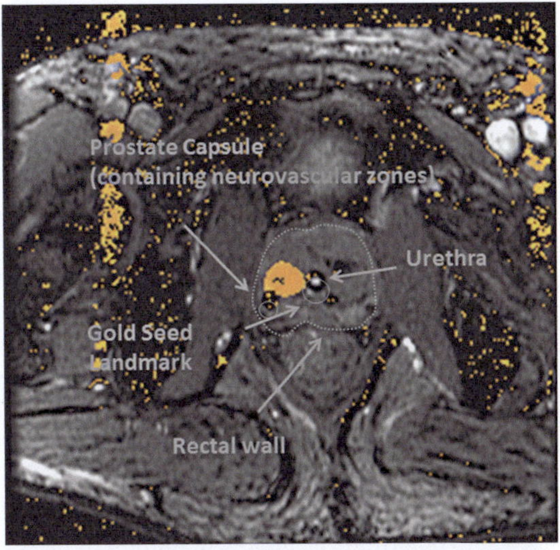

Fig 11.1 Focal laser ablation with real-time MRI thermal guidance. Borders of ablation zone are precisely visualized via MRI, critical structures are untouched

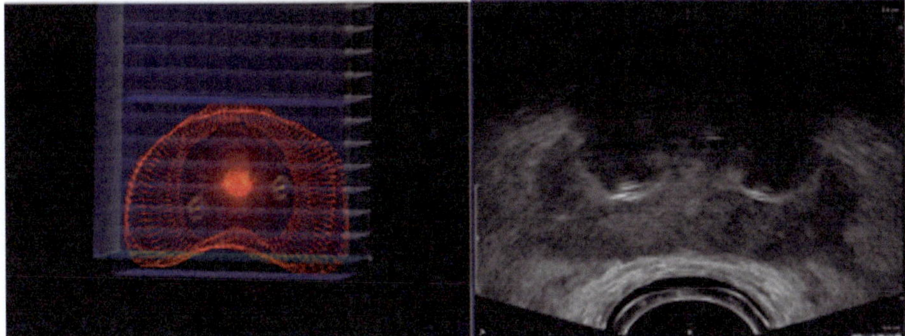

Fig 11.2 Targeted focal cryotherapy 3D reconstruction (*left*) and corresponding ablative lesion (*right*)

effect and high temperatures are dissipated. Post-procedure MRI is performed with and without IV contrast to assess ablation sites (Fig. 11.1).

Cryotherapy takes place under general anesthesia as well, and the position of the prostate is again recreated using pre-implanted fiducial markers. Thermosensors are placed at the apex, external sphincter, left and right neurovascular bundles, and Denonvilliers' fascia to monitor temperature protect these areas from damage from the cryoprobes. In addition, a urethral continued irrigation warmer is placed to protect the urethra. Cryoprobes are placed in respective cancerous zones of the prostate and ablation is performed using two cycles of argon gas freezing with helium thawing. This ensures that the targeted tissue reaches a temperature of −40 °C to ensure necrosis. Real-time monitoring with US can identify the 0 °C line, 6 mm from which exists the true −40 °C destructive zone [59]. A urethral catheter is left in place for 1 week to minimize tissue sloughing and urinary retention (Fig. 11.2).

Follow-Up

Follow-up for TFT varies by institution and there is currently no standardized follow-up regimen in regard to serum markers, biopsies, or imaging.

While many definitions for biochemical failure have been used, there has yet to be established a standardized definition of biochemical failure following focal therapy [60]. This makes sense given that various degrees of prostate tissue are ablated for each given technique and should correlate with varying levels of baseline PSA following each procedure. Some use the Phoenix (nadir + 2 ng/mL) or ASTRO (three consecutive rises in PSA) to define failure after therapy; however, these were developed for RT purposes and data exists to suggest that these may not be suitable pathological correlates for recurrence in the arena of focal therapy [61]. Focal therapy encompasses many different modalities, with options to boil, burn, freeze, necrose, or stimulate apoptosis of cancer cells, the effects of which on PSA have yet to be determined. Due to the expansive set of biochemical failure definitions in the literature, sensitivity analyses are needed to determine a suitable definition of PSA failure following focal therapy.

Technological advances in MRI have increased the sensitivity and specificity for prostate cancer to a significant degree [62]. Some advocate for the use of MRI 6 months, 2 weeks, or even immediately after surgery; however, there is again no standard approach [63]. Even though most studies employ the use of biopsy, a consensus on this has still yet to evolve. Given the wide array of treatment modalities and quantity of prostate ablated, it is possible that there may not evolve such a standard protocol that encompasses TFT as a whole (Table 11.5) and instead we find that a standard set of follow-up regimens come to light to encompass for example hemi-ablation versus focal ablation.

Future Trends and Challenges

Focal therapy seeks to achieve the trifecta of cancer control, continence, and potency, and the cornerstone of achieving this lies in accurate identification and ablation of cancerous zones. To this end more accurate imaging and biopsy schemes have been developed which identify the index lesion and a variety of primary methods of ablation are employed to eradicate such lesions. In addition, focal therapy has opened doors to new discussions on cancer management. As discussed, the aggressiveness of focal therapy varies from situation to situation. This, combined with the fact that focal therapy can be applied multiple times throughout a patient's life and/ or combined with different modalities, lends significant flexibility to the therapeutic approach. Older comorbid men who may not be suitable for whole gland treatment could instead opt for cancer *control* with a focal approach, avoiding the complications of progressive disease and the side effects of radiation therapy. At the same time, younger men could pursue more aggressive ablative options while still preserving function and living many symptom-free years.

Table 11.5 Focal Ablation and follow-up procedures

Variation in follow-up regimens for TFT			
Study	Modality	*N*	Follow-up
Barret (2013) [64]	HIFU, VTP, cryo, BT	Cryo=50 VTP=23 HIFU=21 BT=12	Serial PSA and DRE at 3, 6, and 12 months then every 6 months for 2 years, then yearly. Bx at 12 months then yearly or if BF
Nguyen (2012) [65]	MR-guided BT	MR-BT=318	PSA/DRE every 3 months for 2 years then every 6 months. Endorectal coil MRI if BF (PSA increase by 2 ng/ml above nadir when PSAV>0.75 ng/ml per year), TRUS 12 core bx if suspicious MRI
Ahmed (2012) [66]	Transrectal HIFU	HIFU=42	mpMRI 10–14 days s/p HIFU, at 6 months (w/ targeted bx) and at 12 months. PSA at 1, 3, 6, 9, 12 months
Bahn (2012) [67]	Cryo hemi-ablation	Cryo=73	PSA every 3–6 months. TRUS-Doppler imaging every 6 months. Sextant and image-targeted bx at 6–12 months, then yearly or as indicated
Truesdale (2010) [61]	Unilateral nerve-sparing cryo	Cryo=77	Physical exam and PSA at 3 and 6 months, then every 6 months. 12 core TRUS-bx if clinical suspicion of recurrence based on abnormal DRE, biochemical failure (nadir+2 ng/mL) or as otherwise indicated
Lambert (2007) [68]	US guided percutaneous cryo	Cryo=25	PE and PSA at 3, 6, and 12 months then every 6 months thereafter. 12-core bx if BF (PSA nadir plus 2 ng/mL or PSA nadir of less than 50 %)
Muto (2008) [69]	HIFU	Whole HIFU=41 Focal HIFU=29	Sextant bx and testosterone level at 6 and 12 months. PSA at 3, 6, 12, 18, 24, and 36 months. BF=3 consecutive increases in PSA after a nadir
Ellis (2007) [70]	Focal cryo	Cryo=60	PSA at 3, 6, 9, 12 months and ever 6 months thereafter. bDFS=3 successive rises in PSA

HIFU high-intensity focused ultrasound, *VTP* vascular targeted photodynamic therapy, *BT* brachytherapy, *MR-BT* magnetic resonance-guided brachytherapy, *US* ultrasound, *bx* biopsy, *BF* biochemical failure, *bDFS* biochemical disease-free status

While further refinement of focal therapy techniques continues to demonstrate improvement in the side effect profile of focal therapy, and data such as that in the COLD registry continues to demonstrate that treatment goals are being met, the methods, modalities, and follow-up regimens employed in focal therapy vary substantially across studies. For focal therapy to succeed, the multitude of practitioners involved in its use need to establish common ground for the evaluation of oncological and functional success. Until that happens, success will continue to be evaluated in a piecemeal approach, hindering consensus on the state of focal therapy. There exists a strong need for sensitivity analyses of biomarkers and/or investigation into pretest driven monitoring approaches which can more accurately guide follow-up.

In addition, the current momentum of focal therapy is to include more intermediate risk patients, and for the purposes of comparison of long-term data and analyzing outcomes, more universalized eligibility criteria should be established.

With regard to pathological aspects of focal therapy, the definition of the index lesion is still problematic. Where once it was defined simply as the largest lesion, an idea is emerging that it may not be the size so much as the dominant aggressive clone that should count as the index lesion [42, 56, 58]. Furthermore, the concept that treatment of the index lesion corresponds to treatment of the cancer as a whole has not been proven, and it remains to be seen whether or not the potentially lethal clone can be reliably identified.

Multifocality is also a concern, and while the aforementioned evidence suggests that treating the index tumor alone guides progression and prognosis, the nature of the field effect and the behavior of small lesions potentially left behind during index lesion treatment require further study, despite consensus on the appropriateness of this approach [52]. The analogy of focal therapy as "male lumpectomy" has met criticism due to the fact that a pillar of breast lumpectomy is adjuvant therapy. The argument for chemopreventative considerations following focal therapy is valid due to the multifocal nature of prostate cancer and these options should be pursued.

New markers continue to be developed that can reduce negative biopsies and help differentiate patients suitable for AS from those requiring further biopsy for focal or radical therapy [71, 72]. Others may aid in assessing the probability that high grade prostate cancer exists in a given patient, or attempt to risk stratify those with cancer into groups with less or more aggressive cancer [73, 74]. New imaging techniques like histoscanning, shear wave elastography, may also help with follow-up. Combined B-mode, Doppler, and contrast-enhanced US (CEUS) recently demonstrated an 82 % detection rate [75].

Focal therapy is not without challenges, and many steps are needed to refine this budding therapeutic option; however, the need for QOL-sparring techniques has never been stronger. As new imaging techniques, biomolecular markers, and biopsy strategies continue to advance, further consensus may be reached on appropriate patient selection and treatment regimens.

References

1. Siegel R, Naishadham D, Jemal A. Cancer statistics, 2013. CA Cancer J Clin. 2013;63(1): 11–30. doi:10.3322/caac.21166.
2. Lu-Yao GL, Albertsen PC, Moore DF, Shih W, Lin Y, DiPaola RS, et al. Outcomes of localized prostate cancer following conservative management. JAMA. 2009;302(11):1202–9. doi:10.1001/jama.2009.1348.
3. Cooperberg MR, Lubeck DP, Mehta SS, Carroll PR. CaPSURE. Time trends in clinical risk stratification for prostate cancer: implications for outcomes (data from CaPSURE). J Urol. 2003;170(6 Pt 2):S21–5. doi:10.1097/01.ju.0000095025.03331.c6. discussion S26–7.
4. Bartsch G, Horninger W, Klocker H, Pelzer A, Bektic J, Oberaigner W, et al. Tyrol Prostate Cancer Demonstration Project: early detection, treatment, outcome, incidence and mortality. BJU Int. 2008;101(7):809–16. doi:10.1111/j.1464-410X.2008.07502.x.

5. Ganz PA, Barry JM, Burke W, Col NF, Corso PS, Dodson E, et al. National Institutes of Health state-of-the-science conference: role of active surveillance in the management of men with localized prostate cancer. Ann Intern Med. 2012;156:591–5. Available at: http://annals.org/article.aspx?articleid=1103897.

6. Welch HG, Albertsen PC. Prostate cancer diagnosis and treatment after the introduction of prostate-specific antigen screening: 1986-2005. J Natl Cancer Inst. 2009;101(19):1325–9. doi:10.1093/jnci/djp278.

7. Loeb S, Bjurlin MA, Nicholson J, Tammela TL, Penson DF, Carter HB, et al. Overdiagnosis and overtreatment of prostate cancer. Eur Urol. 2014;65(6):1046–55. doi:10.1016/j.eururo.2013.12.062.

8. Cooperberg MR, Broering JM, Carroll PR. Time trends and local variation in primary treatment of localized prostate cancer. J Clin Oncol. 2010;28(7):1117–23. doi:10.1200/JCO.2009.26.0133.

9. Harlan SR, Cooperberg MR, Elkin EP, Lubeck DP, Meng M, Mehta SS, et al. Time trends and characteristics of men choosing watchful waiting for initial treatment of localized prostate cancer: results from CaPSURE. J Urol. 2003;170(5):1804–7. doi:10.1097/01.ju.0000091641.34674.11.

10. Wu X, Chen VW, Andrews PA, Chen L, Ahmed MN, Schmidit B, et al. Initial treatment patterns for clinically localized prostate cancer and factors associated with the treatment in Louisiana. J La State Med Soc. 2005;157(4):188–94.

11. Glass AS, Cowan JE, Fuldeore MJ, Cooperberg MR, Carroll PR, Kenfield SA, et al. Patient demographics, quality of life, and disease features of men with newly diagnosed prostate cancer: trends in the PSA era. Urology. 2013;82(1):60–5. doi:10.1016/j.urology.2013.01.072.

12. Weiner AB, Etzioni R, Eggener SE. Ongoing Gleason grade migration in localized prostate cancer and implications for use of active surveillance. Eur Urol. 2014;66(4):611–2. doi:10.1016/j.eururo.2014.02.051.

13. Epstein JI. An update of the Gleason grading system. J Urol. 2010;183(2):433–40. doi:10.1016/j.juro.2009.10.046.

14. Crawford ED. Epidemiology of prostate cancer. Urology. 2003;62(6):3–12. doi:10.1016/j.urology.2003.10.013.

15. Womble PR, Montie JE, Ye Z, Linsell SM, Lane BR, Miller DC, et al. Contemporary use of initial active surveillance among men in Michigan with low-risk prostate cancer. Eur Urol. 2015;67(1):44–50. doi:10.1016/j.eururo.2014.08.024.

16. Bechis SK, Carroll PR, Cooperberg MR. Impact of age at diagnosis on prostate cancer treatment and survival. J Clin Oncol. 2011;29(2):235–41. doi:10.1200/JCO.2010.30.2075.

17. Weiner AB, Patel SG, Etzioni R, Eggener SE. National trends in the management of low and intermediate risk prostate cancer in the United States. J Urol. 2015;193(1):95–102. doi:10.1016/j.juro.2014.07.111.

18. Chapple A, Ziebland S, Herxheimer A, McPherson A, Shepperd S, Miller R. Is "watchful waiting" a real choice for men with prostate cancer? A qualitative study. BJU Int. 2002;90(3):257–64.

19. Latini DM, Hart SL, Knight SJ, Cowan JE, Ross PL, Duchane J, et al. The relationship between anxiety and time to treatment for patients with prostate cancer on surveillance. J Urol. 2007;178(3):826–32. doi:10.1016/j.juro.2007.05.039.

20. Cooperberg MR. Prostate cancer: a new look at prostate cancer treatment complications. Nat Rev Clin Oncol. 2014;1:304–5. doi:10.1038/nrclinonc.2014.58.

21. Kumar RJ, Barqawi A, Crawford ED. Adverse events associated with hormonal therapy for prostate cancer. Rev Urol. 2005;7 Suppl 5:S37–43.

22. Nam RK, Cheung P, Herschorn S, Saskin R, Jiandong S, Klotz L, et al. Incidence of complications other than urinary incontinence or erectile dysfunction after radical prostatectomy or radiotherapy for prostate cancer: a population-based cohort study. Lancet Oncol. 2014;15(2):223–31. doi:10.1016/S1470-2045(13)70606-5.

23. Hoffman RM, Hunt WC, Gilliland FD, Stephenson RA, Potosky AL. Patient satisfaction with treatment decisions for clinically localized prostate carcinoma. Results from the Prostate Cancer Outcomes Study. Cancer. 2003;97(7):1653–62. doi:10.1002/cncr.11233.

24. Wilt TJ, MacDonald R, Rutks I, Shamliyan TA, Taylor BC, Kane RL. Systematic review: comparative effectiveness and harms of treatments for clinically localized prostate cancer. Ann Intern Med. 2008;148(6):435–48.

25. Chou R, Croswell JM, Dana T, Bougatsos C, Blazina I, Fu R, et al. Screening for prostate cancer: a review of the evidence for the U.S. Preventive Services Task Force. Ann Intern Med. 2011;155(11):762. doi:10.7326/0003-4819-155-11-201112060-00375.

26. Coelho RF, Rocco B, Patel MB, Orvieto MA, Chauhan S, Ficarra V, et al. Retropubic, laparoscopic, and robot-assisted radical prostatectomy: a critical review of outcomes reported by high-volume centers. J Endourol. 2010;24(12):2003–15. doi:10.1089/end.2010.0295.

27. Chang SL, Kibel AS, Brooks JD, Chung BI. The impact of robotic surgery on the surgical management of prostate cancer in the USA. BJU Int. 2015;115:929. doi:10.1111/bju.12850.

28. Nelson B, Kaufman M, Broughton G, Cookson MS, Chang SS, Herrell SD, et al. Comparison of length of hospital stay between radical retropubic prostatectomy and robotic assisted laparoscopic prostatectomy. J Urol. 2007;177(3):929–31. doi:10.1016/j.juro.2006.10.070.

29. D'Amico AV, Whittington R, Malkowicz SB, Cote K, Loffredo M, Schultz D, et al. Biochemical outcome after radical prostatectomy or external beam radiation therapy for patients with clinically localized prostate carcinoma in the prostate specific antigen era. Cancer. 2002;95(2):281–6. doi:10.1002/cncr.10657.

30. Birkhahn M, Penson DF, Cai J, Groshen S, Stein JP, Lieskovsky G, et al. Long-term outcome in patients with a Gleason score ≤6 prostate cancer treated by radical prostatectomy. BJU Int. 2011;108(5):660–4. doi:10.1111/j.1464-410X.2010.09978.x.

31. Sylvester JE, Grimm PD, Blasko JC, Millar J, Orio 3rd PF, Skoglund S, et al. 15-Year biochemical relapse free survival in clinical Stage T1-T3 prostate cancer following combined external beam radiotherapy and brachytherapy; Seattle experience. Int J Radiat Oncol Biol Phys. 2007;67(1):57–64. doi:10.1016/j.ijrobp.2006.07.1382.

32. Alicikus ZA, Yamada Y, Zhang Z, Pei X, Hunt M, Kollmeier M, et al. Ten-year outcomes of high-dose, intensity-modulated radiotherapy for localized prostate cancer. Cancer. 2011;117(7):1429–37. doi:10.1002/cncr.25467.

33. Song L, Chen RC, Bensen JT, Knafl GJ, Nielsen ME, Farnan L, et al. Who makes the decision regarding the treatment of clinically localized prostate cancer-the patient or physician? Cancer. 2012;119(2):421–8. doi:10.1002/cncr.27738.

34. Zeliadt SB, Moinpour CM, Blough DK, Penson DF, Hall IJ, Smith JL, et al. Preliminary treatment considerations among men with newly diagnosed prostate cancer. Am J Manag Care. 2010;16(5):e121–30.

35. Litwin MS, Gore JL, Kwan L, Brandeis JM, Lee SP, Withers HR, et al. Quality of life after surgery, external beam irradiation, or brachytherapy for early-stage prostate cancer. Cancer. 2007;109(11):2239–47. doi:10.1002/cncr.22676.

36. Gore JL, Kwan L, Lee SP, Reiter RE, Litwin MS. Survivorship beyond convalescence: 48-month quality-of-life outcomes after treatment for localized prostate cancer. J Natl Cancer Inst. 2009;101(12):888–92. doi:10.1093/jnci/djp114.

37. Resnick MJ, Koyama T, Fan K-H, Albertsen PC, Goodman M, Hamilton AS, et al. Long-term functional outcomes after treatment for localized prostate cancer. N Engl J Med. 2013;368(5):436–45. doi:10.1056/NEJMoa1209978.

38. Eggener SE, Scardino PT, Carroll PR, Zelefsky MJ, Sartor O, Hricak H, et al. Focal therapy for localized prostate cancer: a critical appraisal of rationale and modalities. J Urol. 2007;178(6):2260–7. doi:10.1016/j.juro.2007.08.072.

39. van den Bos W, Muller BG, Ahmed H, Bangma CH, Barret E, Crouzet S, et al. Focal therapy in prostate cancer: international multidisciplinary consensus on trial design. Eur Urol. 2014;65(6):1078–83. doi:10.1016/j.eururo.2014.01.001.

40. Valerio M, Ahmed HU, Emberton M, Lawrentschuk N, Lazzeri M, Montironi R, et al. The role of focal therapy in the management of localised prostate cancer: a systematic review. Eur Urol. 2014;66(4):732–51. doi:10.1016/j.eururo.2013.05.048.

41. Epstein JI, Carmichael MJ, Partin AW, Walsh PC. Small high grade adenocarcinoma of the prostate in radical prostatectomy specimens performed for nonpalpable disease: pathogenetic and clinical implications. J Urol. 1994;151(6):1587–92.

42. Wise AM, Stamey TA, McNeal JE, Clayton JL. Morphologic and clinical significance of multifocal prostate cancers in radical prostatectomy specimens. Urology. 2002;60(2):264–9.

43. Mouraviev V, Mayes JM, Sun L, Madden JF, Moul JW, Polascik TJ. Prostate cancer laterality as a rationale of focal ablative therapy for the treatment of clinically localized prostate cancer. Cancer. 2007;110(4):906–10. doi:10.1002/cncr.22858.
44. Tareen B, Sankin A, Godoy G, Temkin S, Lepor H, Taneja SS. Appropriate candidates for hemiablative focal therapy are infrequently encountered among men selected for radical prostatectomy in contemporary cohort. Urology. 2009;73(2):351–4. doi:10.1016/j.urology.2008.08.504. discussion 354–5.
45. Bott SRJ, Ahmed HU, Hindley RG, Abdul-Rahman A, Freeman A, Emberton M. The index lesion and focal therapy: an analysis of the pathological characteristics of prostate cancer. BJU Int. 2010;106(11):1607–11. doi:10.1111/j.1464-410X.2010.09436.x.
46. Polascik TJ, Mayes JM, Sun L, Madden JF, Moul JW, Mouraviev V. Pathologic stage T2a and T2b prostate cancer in the recent prostate-specific antigen era: implications for unilateral ablative therapy. Prostate. 2008;68(13):1380–6. doi:10.1002/pros.20804.
47. Isbarn H, Karakiewicz PI, Vogel S, Jeldres C, Lughezzani G, Briganti A, et al. Unilateral prostate cancer cannot be accurately predicted in low-risk patients. Int J Radiat Oncol Biol Phys. 2010;77(3):784–7. doi:10.1016/j.ijrobp.2009.05.068.
48. Briganti A, Tutolo M, Suardi N, Gallina A, Abdollah F, Capitanio U, et al. There is no way to identify patients who will harbor small volume, unilateral prostate cancer at final pathology. Implications for focal therapies. Prostate. 2012;72(8):925–30. doi:10.1002/pros.21497.
49. Berg KD, Toft BG, Røder MA, Brasso K, Vainer B, Iversen P. Is it possible to predict low-volume and insignificant prostate cancer by core needle biopsies? APMIS. 2013;121(4):257–65. doi:10.1111/j.1600-0463.2012.02965.x.
50. Gallina A, Maccagnano C, Suardi N, Capitanio U, Abdollah F, Raber M, et al. Unilateral positive biopsies in low risk prostate cancer patients diagnosed with extended transrectal ultrasound-guided biopsy schemes do not predict unilateral prostate cancer at radical prostatectomy. BJU Int. 2012;110(2 Pt 2):E64–8. doi:10.1111/j.1464-410X.2011.10762.x.
51. Sinnott M, Falzarano SM, Hernandez AV, Jones JS, Klein EA, Zhou M, et al. Discrepancy in prostate cancer localization between biopsy and prostatectomy specimens in patients with unilateral positive biopsy: implications for focal therapy. Prostate. 2012;72(11):1179–86. doi:10.1002/pros.22467.
52. Donaldson IA, Alonzi R, Barratt D, Barret E, Berge V, Bott S, et al. Focal therapy: patients, interventions, and outcomes - a report from a consensus meeting. Eur Urol. 2015;67:771. doi:10.1016/j.eururo.2014.09.018.
53. Ohori M, Eastham JA, Koh H. Is focal therapy reasonable in patients with early stage prostate cancer (CaP): an analysis of radical prostatectomy (RP) specimens. J Urol. 2006;175(Suppl):507. doi:10.1002/cncr.22858/full.
54. Stamey TA, McNeal JM, Wise AM, Clayton JL. Secondary cancers in the prostate do not determine PSA biochemical failure in untreated men undergoing radical retropubic prostatectomy. Eur Urol. 2001;39 Suppl 4:22–3. doi:10.1159/000052577.
55. Masterson TA, Cheng L, Mehan RM, Koch MO. Tumor focality does not predict biochemical recurrence after radical prostatectomy in men with clinically localized prostate cancer. J Urol. 2011;186(2):506–10. doi:10.1016/j.juro.2011.03.106.
56. Liu W, Laitinen S, Khan S, Vihinen M, Kowalski J, Yu G, et al. Copy number analysis indicates monoclonal origin of lethal metastatic prostate cancer. Nat Med. 2009;15(5):559–65. doi:10.1038/nm.1944.
57. Haffner MC, Mosbruger T, Esopi DM, Fedor H, Heaphy CM, Walker DA, et al. Tracking the clonal origin of lethal prostate cancer. J Clin Invest. 2013;123(11):4918–22. doi:10.1172/JCI70354.
58. Barbieri CE, Demichelis F, Rubin MA. The lethal clone in prostate cancer: redefining the index. Eur Urol. 2014;66(3):395–7. doi:10.1016/j.eururo.2013.12.052.
59. Georgiades C, Rodriguez R, Azene E, Weiss C, Chaux A, Gonzalez-Roibon N, et al. Determination of the nonlethal margin inside the visible "ice-ball" during percutaneous cryoablation of renal tissue. Cardiovasc Intervent Radiol. 2013;36(3):783–90. doi:10.1007/s00270-012-0470-5.

60. Phillips JM, Catarinicchia S, Krughoff K, Barqawi AB. Cryotherapy in prostate cancer. J Clin Urol. 2014;7(5):308–17. doi:10.1177/2051415814521806.
61. Truesdale MD, Cheetham PJ, Hruby GW, Wenske S, Conforto AK, Cooper AB, et al. An evaluation of patient selection criteria on predicting progression-free survival after primary focal unilateral nerve-sparing cryoablation for prostate cancer. Cancer J. 2010;16(5):544–9. doi:10.1097/PPO.0b013e3181f84639.
62. Heijmink SWTPJ, Fütterer JJ, Hambrock T, et al. Prostate cancer: body-array versus endorectal coil MR imaging at 3 T--comparison of image quality, localization, and staging performance. Radiology. 2007;244(1):184–95. doi:10.1148/radiol.2441060425.
63. Muller BG, Fütterer JJ, Gupta RT, Takahashi S, Scheenen TW, Huisman HJ, et al. The role of magnetic resonance imaging (MRI) in focal therapy for prostate cancer: recommendations from a consensus panel. BJU Int. 2014;113:218–27. doi:10.1111/bju.12243.
64. Barret E, Ahallal Y, Sanchez-Salas R, Galiano M, Cosset JM, Validire P, et al. Morbidity of focal therapy in the treatment of localized prostate cancer. Eur Urol. 2013;63(4):618–22. doi:10.1016/j.eururo.2012.11.057.
65. Nguyen PL, Chen M-H, Zhang Y, Tempany CM, Cormack RA, Beard CJ, et al. Updated results of magnetic resonance imaging guided partial prostate brachytherapy for favorable risk prostate cancer: implications for focal therapy. J Urol. 2012;188(4):1151–6. doi:10.1016/j.juro.2012.06.010.
66. Ahmed HU, Hindley RG, Dickinson L, Freeman A, Kirkham AP, Sahu M, et al. Focal therapy for localised unifocal and multifocal prostate cancer: a prospective development study. Lancet Oncol. 2012;13(6):622–32. doi:10.1016/S1470-2045(12)70121-3.
67. Bahn D, de Castro Abreu AL, Gill IS, Hung AJ, Silverman P, Gross ME, et al. Focal cryotherapy for clinically unilateral, low-intermediate risk prostate cancer in 73 men with a median follow-up of 3.7 years. Eur Urol. 2012;62(1):55–63. doi:10.1016/j.eururo.2012.03.006.
68. Lambert EH, Bolte K, Masson P, Katz AE. Focal cryosurgery: encouraging health outcomes for unifocal prostate cancer. Urology. 2007;69(6):1117–20. doi:10.1016/j.urology.2007.02.047.
69. Muto S, Yoshii T, Saito K, Kamiyama Y, Ide H, Horie S. Focal therapy with high-intensity-focused ultrasound in the treatment of localized prostate cancer. Jpn J Clin Oncol. 2008;38(3):192–9. doi:10.1093/jjco/hym173.
70. Ellis DS, Manny TB, Rewcastle JC. Focal cryosurgery followed by penile rehabilitation as primary treatment for localized prostate cancer: initial results. Urology. 2007;70(6 Suppl):9–15. doi:10.1016/j.urology.2007.07.036.
71. Loeb S, Catalona WJ. The Prostate Health Index: a new test for the detection of prostate cancer. Ther Adv Urol. 2014;6(2):74–7. doi:10.1177/1756287213513488.
72. Crawford ED, Rove KO, Trabulsi EJ, Qian J, Drewnowska KP, Kaminetsky JC, et al. Diagnostic performance of PCA3 to detect prostate cancer in men with increased prostate specific antigen: a prospective study of 1,962 cases. J Urol. 2012;188(5):1726–31. doi:10.1016/j.juro.2012.07.023.
73. Parekh DJ, Punnen S, Sjoberg DD, Asroff SW, Bailen JL, Cochran JS, et al. A multi-institutional prospective trial in the USA confirms that the 4kscore accurately identifies men with high-grade prostate cancer. Eur Urol. 2014. pii: S0302-2838(14)01035-5. doi: 10.1016/j.eururo.2014.10.021. [Epub ahead of print]
74. Cooperberg MR, Simko JP, Cowan JE, Reid JE, Djalilvand A, Bhatnagar S, et al. Validation of a cell-cycle progression gene panel to improve risk stratification in a contemporary prostatectomy cohort. J Clin Oncol. 2013;31(11):1428–34. doi:10.1200/JCO.2012.46.4396.
75. Xie SW, Li HL, Du J, Xia JG, Guo YF, Xin M, et al. Contrast-enhanced ultrasonography with contrast-tuned imaging technology for the detection of prostate cancer: comparison with conventional ultrasonography. BJU Int. 2012;109(11):1620–6. doi:10.1111/j.1464-410X.2011.10577.x.

Chapter 12
Technologies and Methods in Primary Ablation with Focal Therapy

Gary Onik

Introduction

The introduction of breast-sparing surgery (i.e., "lumpectomy") revolutionized the management of breast cancer. The use of lumpectomy showed that quality of life could be optimized without compromising treatment efficacy. In 2002, Onik et al. introduced the concept of focal therapy for prostate cancer utilizing cryosurgery, i.e., a male lumpectomy [1]. Following the lead of breast cancer management, the intention was to limit prostate cancer treatment morbidity while maintaining good cancer results. A number of short term studies regarding focal therapy using a variety of ablation methods have been reported confirming that incontinence can be virtually eliminated as a complication of prostate cancer treatment and that potency can be maintained in up to 85 % of patients [2–5].

These results have now established focal therapy as a major trend in prostate cancer management, resulting in the publication of scientific articles and topical textbooks, and the convening of international scientific forums and consensus conferences of experts to define the approach [6–8].

Until recently long-term data on patients who have undergone focal therapy has not been available. The two seminal questions associated with the strategy have always been (1) the cancer control efficacy of focal therapy compared to radical treatments, and (2) which patients might benefit from this conservative approach. A recent study published by Onik et al. [9] following 70 patients treated with focal cryoablation for an average of 10 years has shown that the results of focal therapy can be successfully used in even medium- and high-risk patients suggesting that better biochemical disease-free survival are obtainable in these

G. Onik, M.D. (✉)
Center for High Risk and Recurrent Prostate Cancer, Carnegie Mellon University,
401 East Las Olas Blvd Suite 130-407 Ft, Lauderdale, FL 33301, USA
e-mail: onikcryo@gmail.com

© Springer International Publishing Switzerland 2016
N.N. Stone, E.D. Crawford (eds.), *The Prostate Cancer Dilemma*,
DOI 10.1007/978-3-319-21485-6_12

patient groups than with traditional treatments, such as robotic radical prostatectomy and IMRT [10, 11].

This chapter which deals with the methods of primary ablation used in focal therapy, in its narrowest terms could be a listing and discussion of the various tissue destructive technologies now being used for focal therapy, but the real issue to be dealt with is whether there are any lessons that can be learned from the literature as to how to optimize the results of focal therapy in respect to whatever technology is used. The recommendations to be made are based on my own 18-year experience doing focal therapy. The chapter therefore proceeds as follows:

1. A review of the methods that are common to all the technologies under investigation for performing focal therapy that might be optimized for success,
2. The techniques particular to cryoablation, as this is the only method that is generally available for anyone contemplating starting to utilize focal therapy clinically, and
3. A review of what the ideal technology for prostate ablation might be and a comparison of the various technologies available.

General Issues for Optimizing Focal Therapy

Patient Population for Focal Therapy

Focal therapy has been suggested as a middle ground between active surveillance and radical whole gland treatment. The ideal candidate according to this thinking would therefore be the patient who has low-risk prostate cancer who chooses not to undergo active surveillance or the patient who has eventually progressed on an active surveillance program and seeks treatment. There are various methods of stratifying patients as to risk levels based on pathology, genetic profile of the cancer, and a combination pathologic (Gleason score), PSA, and stage (the D'Amico stratification).

From the very start of my experience with this modality I felt that focal therapy should not be limited to patients with low grade and low volume disease but rather it should be considered in many cases of higher grade and volume tumors. The majority of patients who experience systemic relapse are those with higher risk disease and were treated by IMRT or EBRT [12]. Application of focal therapy in this patient group grew out of my experience treating patients with unresectable terminal cancer in whom focal therapy resulted in long-term disease-free survival [13].

In a recent publication of long term which followed patients for a mean of 10 years results of focal therapy the patient population treated with focal therapy was representative of all risk levels of disease (Table 12.1). The majority of patients that had focal therapy had intermediate- and high-risk disease (57 %). This distribution is similar to patients in other long-term series with other treatments [10, 11]. The survival curves demonstrate show that no statistically significant difference between the risk levels in these long-term results by risk level (Fig. 12.1). Our updated latest survival statistics are shown in Table 12.2.

Table 12.1 Patient demographics for a representative focal therapy series

	Patient demographics	
Patients	70	
Follow-up	8–18 years	Mean 10.1 years
D'Amico risk level		
Low	29	
Medium	32	
High	9	
Gleason score		
Gleason 6 or less	41	
Gleason 7	24	
Gleason 8 or greater	5	
Stage		
T1c	56	
T2a	6	
T2b	3	
T2c	4	
T4	1	
PSA level at DX		
Less than 10	54	
10–20	13	
Greater than 20	2	

Adapted from Onik Gary, et al. Long-term results of optimized focal therapy for prostate cancer: average 10-year follow-up in 70 patients. J Mens Health. 2014;11(2):64–74

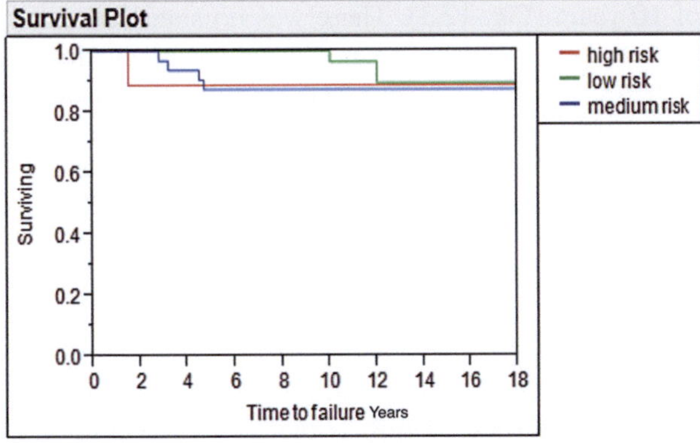

Fig 12.1 Shows the Kaplan–Meier curves of 70 patients treated with focal cryoablation followed for 10 years. There is no significant difference in BDFS between the risk groups. Adapted from Onik G, et al. Long-term results of optimized focal therapy for prostate cancer: average 10-year follow-up in 70 patients. J Mens Health. 2014;11(2):64–74

Table 12.2 The results of 75 patients treated with focal therapy with cryoablation follow-up between 8–18 years with average 10-year follow-up

		Results
Overall actuarial survival	$N=75$	71/75 (94.6 %)
Disease-specific survival	$N=71$	71/71 (100 %)
Biochemical disease-free survival	$N=75$	67/75 (90 %)
BDFS high risk (D'Amico)	$N=10$	9/10 (89 %)
BDFS med risk (D'Amico)	$N=33$	29/33 (88 %)
BDFS low risk (D'Amico)	$N=32$	29/32 (90 %)
		$P=.965$ no difference risk levels
Bilateral multi focal	$N=20$	19/20 (95 %)
Local recurrence	$N=10$	9/10 (90 %)
Complications		
Continent after primary procedure	$N=75$	75/75 100 %)—no pads
Retained potency after first treatment	$N=58$	53/58 (94 %)

When historical controls are examined from other long-term series reported for RP and IMRT focal cryoablation shows at least equivalent results to traditional therapies for all risks levels but actually improved results in medium- and high-risk patients [10, 11]. Why this might be is discussed later in the chapter since it has implications for the various technologies utilized for focal therapy but suffice to say all risk levels should be considered when applying focal therapy, particularly in an investigative setting.

A subset of high-risk patients has gross extra-capsular extension. These patients are particularly well suited to focal ablation since ablation carried outside the margins into the peri-prostatic tissue is not difficult to accomplish (Fig. 12.2).

What about those patients that have bilateral multifocal disease? In our series we treated 20 patients with bilateral multifocal disease with 19 of them being BDFS at an average of 10 years (Fig. 12.3). There was no statistical difference between bilateral multifocal and the unifocal group. Considering inclusion of these patients it has been estimated that over 90 % of patients could be considered candidates for focal therapy [14]. Thus it appears that focal therapy is not a marginally applicable technique for a narrow group of patients but potentially competitive to all whole gland radical treatments in a diverse patient population.

Patient Staging for Focal Therapy

The staging of a patient for focal therapy is the most critical issue associated with focal therapy. Long-term results are going to be dependent on knowing the full extent and location of a patient's disease and adequately treating it. The more accurate the localization the more targeted the approach can be applied whatever the ablation technology being used. This ultimately will apply the destructive energy

Fig. 12.2 (**a**) MRI showing a large extra-capsular tumor (*arrow*) invading the bladder base and left SV. Tumor was a Gleason 10. The patient had failed androgen deprivation therapy. (**b**) CT scan 3 years later shows the mass is gone with residual scar remaining. The patient remained disease free 8 years later

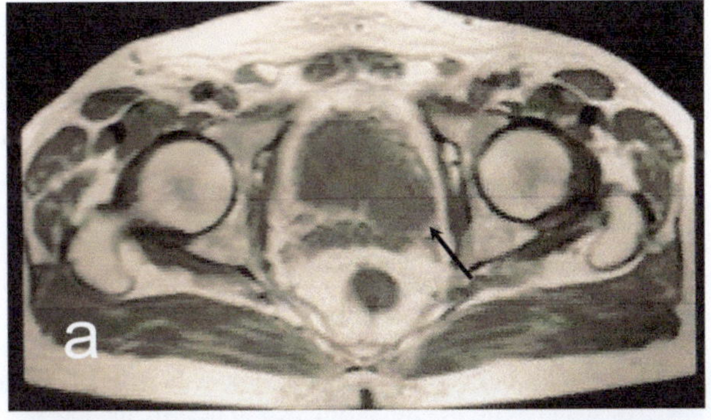

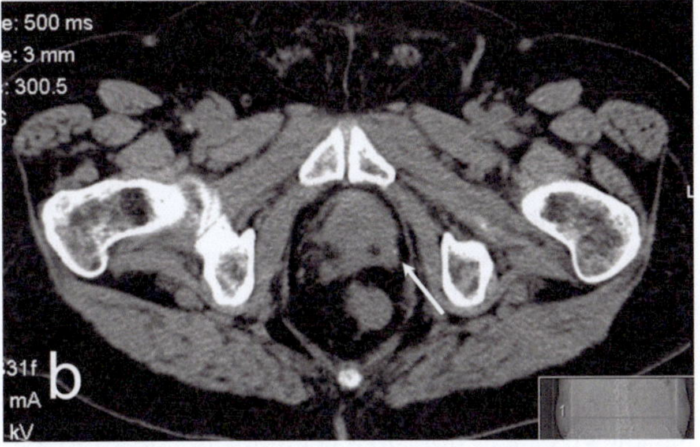

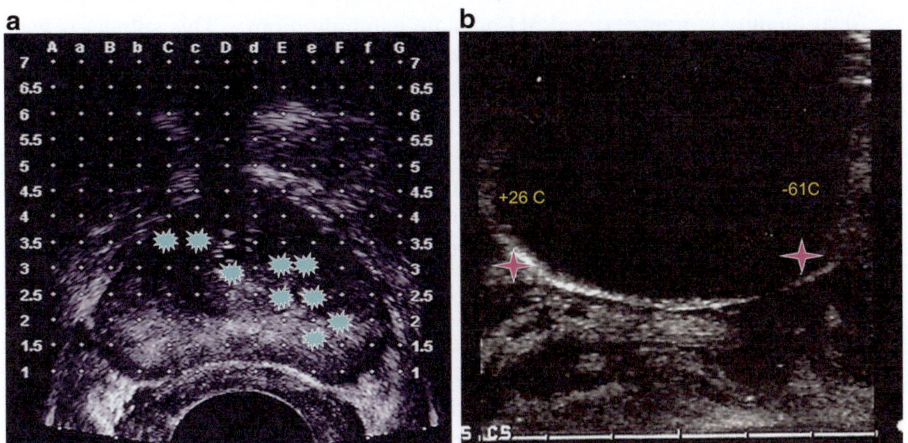

Fig. 12.3 (**a**) The image on the *left* shows a patient with bilateral multifocal disease with the positive areas indicated on the US image taken at the time of 3D Prostate Mapping Biopsy. (**b**) The image on the *right* taken during the freezing showing a temp of +26 °C at the Neurovascular bundle on the *right* and a temp of −61 °C at the *left* Neurovascular bundle

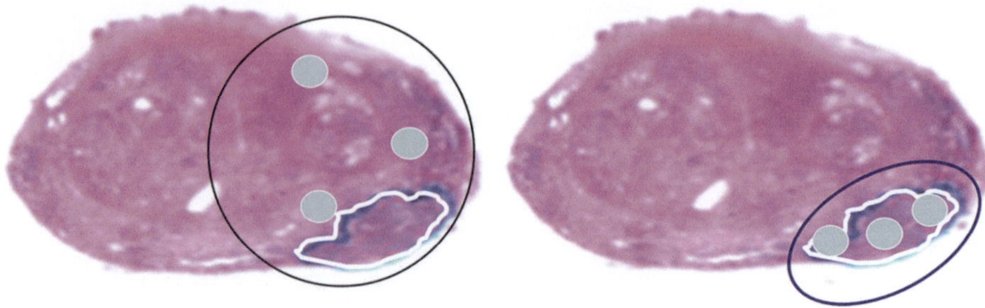

Fig. 12.4 On the *left* is a whole mount slide with a tumor outlined in white in the left peripheral zone. The ablation probes are positioned to destroy the left side of the gland in a hemi-ablation. Note that the probes are not optimally placed to destroy the tumor. On the *right side* is the same tumor now with the probes optimally grouped to focally destroy the tumor. The power of the 3D-Mapping biopsy is the ability to target the tumor as in the *right hand slide*

where it is needed most improving results and limiting the extent of the ablation needed and therefore minimizing side effects (Fig. 12.4). This is why hemi-ablation while it seems the more conservative approach will ultimately yield poorer results than a targeted approach.

Based on our experience the use of TRUS biopsy, even in a saturation fashion is not adequate for staging and locating tumors for focal therapy. Our experience with TRUS biopsy, even with an additional staging biopsy obtained on the side opposite the known cancer prior to a hemi-ablation leads to a long-term recurrence a recurrence rate of 33 %. Even with a high level of expertise in TRUS with color Doppler a recurrence rate of 25 % [3] can be expected.

The most accurate modality for staging and localization of cancer for targeting by focal therapy is transperineal 3D-prostate mapping biopsy. This subject is well covered in other sections of this book; however, our experience confirms that when applied in this setting 3D-PMB lowers the long-term local recurrence rate from 33 % to just 4 %. This is consistent with the theoretical sensitivity of 95 % shown for significant cancers in previous studies [15, 16].

I know that the major trend at academic centers is to use mpMRI and fusion directed biopsies as the standard for guiding focal therapy but based on our experience and a review of the mpMRI literature in which mpMRI was compared to the gold standard of RP specimens, mpMRI as it stands now, the role for mpMRI for staging and guiding focal therapy should be approached with caution at this time. The excellent studies by Delongchamps et al. and Bratan et al. compare mpMRI to the gold standard of whole mount radical prostatectomy specimens [17, 18]. Delongchamps et al. show that its sensitivity for picking up clinically significant tumors in the peripheral zone of the prostate was 85 % and just 62 % in the transition zone. These results were confirmed in a study by Bratan et al. comparing mpMRI in 175 patients with radical prostatectomy specimens.

Focal abnormalities observed on mpMRI were localized using a 27-point grid diagram. RP whole mount sections were digitized, and regions of cancer were highlighted. Focal abnormalities on mpMRI were considered true positives if their diameters corresponded to 50–150 % with a histologic cancer in an overlapping region. The lesson here is that based on this data there is not a 1 to 1 correlation to prostate cancer on pathology to the lesion seen on mpMRI. This theoretically could lead to over or under treatment of lesions based on mpMRI lesion borders.

In addition, overall mpMRI detected only 25, 48, and 71 % of Gleason 6 diameter tumors <0.5, 0.5–2, and >2 cm, respectively. Taking the traditional definition of a tumor that is 0.5 mm [19] in diameter being clinically significant, mpMRI is missing 50 % of tumors 0.5–2 cm and 30 % of those over 2 cm. Caution should be used in discounting such large tumors even though they may be Gleason 6 now that they may be further characterized with genetic profiling. For Gleason 7 tumors, mpMRI detected 63, 85, and 97 % of Gleason 7 tumors, diameter tumors <0.5, 0.5–2, and >2 cm, respectively; and 80, 93, and 100 % of Gleason 8 or greater.

At this time the use of mpMRI as the sole means of guidance for focal therapy is most likely inadequate for reproducing the long-term results recently published using the 3D-mapping biopsy.

The Immune Response Associated with Tumor Ablation

There is a growing body of evidence that there is a tumor-specific immune response associated with tumor ablation particularly cryoablation. This response was first described by Ablin et al. [20] in relation to cryoablation, who reported the spontaneous remission of metastatic prostate cancer after freezing of the primary tumor for palliation. There is a growing body of literature describing this phenomenon. The essential concept is that the dead tumor left in situ exposes unique tumor antigens to the patient's immune system, acting as an in vivo tumor vaccine. The belief is that cryoablation, since it does not denature proteins such as heat based ablation modalities is able to elicit this response. Whether cryoablation acts as an immune stimulator or actual suppressant is a complex interplay of many factors which is covered very well by Sabel [21]. An indication that cryoablation might be having such an effect can be appreciated by the whole gland cryoablation data published by Bahn [22] which compared favorably to our own survival data and in which the failure rates were the same regardless of risk category. This is in contrast to radiation and RP series whose survival curves have an ongoing downward trend over time [23].

Literature is now emerging showing that cryoablation in combination with other immune enhancing approaches, such as CTLA-4 blockade with drugs such as Ipilimumab, Treg suppression with cyclophosphamide, or autologous dendritic cell therapy, work synergistically to prevent metastatic disease or even treat existing metastatic disease in both animals and humans [24–26].

This is perhaps the most exciting and profound aspect of focal therapy. Might the biology of prostate cancer be manipulated by treating the primary cancer with an immune enhancing ablation to improve overall survival?

Technical Considerations for Optimizing Focal Therapy Using Cryoablation

Cryoablation is the ablation modality most practitioners are going to have access to so it behooves us to consider some technical aspects of the technology that are critical to consistently good results.

Since no imaging modality can reliably determine microscopic extra-capsular extension, when a tumor is adjacent to structures that are known weaknesses in the capsule, tumor destruction should be planned to prophylactically include areas of potential extension. Such areas include the NVB or the central seminal vesicles when cancer is in the midline and has access to the ejaculatory ducts and the apex of the gland. This is designed to prevent local recurrences particularly in intermediate- and high-risk patients.

Another critical technical adjunct is to separate the rectum from the prostate with a saline injection into Denonvilliers' fascia [27] (Fig. 12.5). This technique, which many cryosurgeons do not employ, ensures that tumors in the posterior peripheral zone can be adequately frozen without stopping the freezing prematurely for fear of causing rectal damage and potential urethrorectal fistula, the occurrence of which can be virtually eliminated with this technique.

The freezing process itself has a number of important technical issues that have to be followed for optimal results. Two freeze–thaw cycles to −40 °C has been the standard recommended protocol [28]. However, over time we have modified our approach and now use three freeze–thaw cycles to −10 °C. This provides equivalent tumor destruction while minimizing the area that needs to be frozen. Cryosurgical literature confirms that the parameters for optimal tissue destruction include a slow passive thaw. Current cryoprobes have a warming feature to disengage them from the tissue at the end of the last freeze. Most surgeons now use this feature to actively

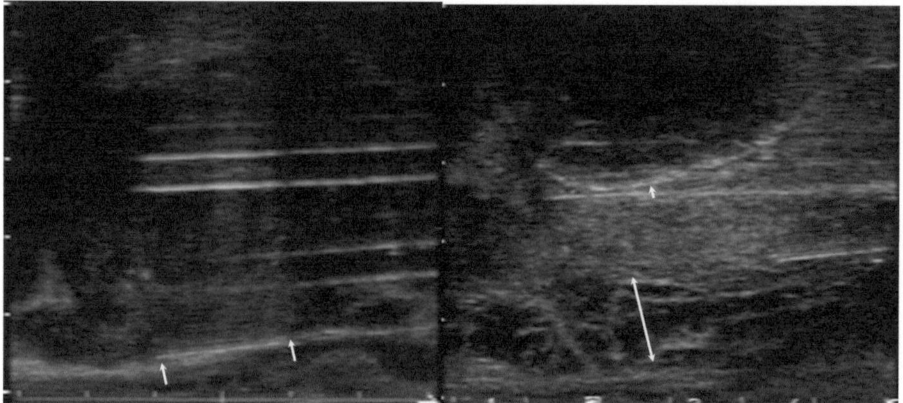

Fig. 12.5 On the *left* is an ultrasound showing a needle placed into Denonvilliers' fascia (*arrowheads*). On the *right* saline has been injected markedly increasing the space between the rectum and the prostate

thaw the tissue to save time during the procedure, a technique which might possibly compromise long-term results.

More than a few physicians carrying out cryoablation do not monitor temperatures using just US imaging to determine the adequacy of freezing. Based on the fact that the certain goals of temperature have to be met in order to reliably kill prostate cancer [29] and to prevent injury to the external sphincter, temperature monitoring is essential. Adequate temp robe monitoring is one of the most challenging technical aspects of cryoablation and literally differences of millimeters can mean the difference between success and failure.

The Technologies of Tumor Ablation for Focal Therapy

Once the patient has been chosen and staged and the tumor is ready to be targeted there are a number of technologies that can be used to ablate the tumor. The ideal ablation modality should have the following characteristics:

1. Clinical evidence of efficacy,
2. Reliable tissue destruction,
3. Accurate monitoring to confirm tissue destruction and prevent complications,
4. General availability and cost effective, and
5. Ability to stimulate a tumor-specific immune response.

The main tumor ablation modalities that are available for focal therapy can be grouped by those readily available in the USA with FDA approval and those that are considered experimental. The former group includes cryoablation, irreversible electroporation, laser ablation, and radiation. Experimental therapies include HIFU and photodynamic therapy.

Cryoablation

Technological advances in prostate cryoablation, such as the addition of the urethral warmer and argon based cryosurgical systems with greater freezing control helped propel the procedure to an effective and safe alternative in treating prostate cancer. In July 1999, prostate cryoablation was approved by Medicare as a treatment for primary prostate cancer (removing it from the investigational category) and it is paid for by all insurance companies.

Level one evidence is now available on the efficacy of cryoablation. Donnelly et al. reported in 2010 a randomized study of 244 patients to either cryoablation or external beam radiation therapy [30]. The median follow-up was 100 months. 92 % of patients had intermediate to high-risk disease. Disease progression at 36 months was observed in 23.9 % (PSA nadir + 2 ng/mL) of men in the cryoablation arm and in 23.7 % (PSA nadir + 2 ng/mL) of men in the radiotherapy arm. No differences in overall or disease-specific survival were observed. At 60 months, the observed failure rates in the two groups were equal; but at 84 months, the observed difference was in favor of cryoablation. At 36 months, more patients in the radiotherapy arm had a cancer-positive biopsy (28.9 %) compared with patients in the cryoablation arm (7.7 %). It should also be noted that in the cryoablation arm six patients remained disease free 7–9 years later after a re-treatment with cryoablation (one of the major advantages of this type of therapy) but were counted as failures based on the criteria accepted at the start of the study. The authors concluded that the long-term trend in the data favored cryoablation.

Using cryoablation a number of focal therapy series have been published and a recent review of the focal cryo literature by Shah et al. showed 9 series of focal cryoablation published with a total of 1582 patients treated [31]. The BDFS ranged from 71 to 93 % at 9–70 months follow-up. Incontinence rates were 0–3.6 % and potency rates were 58–100 %. Urethrorectal fistula occurred in three patients (0.2 %). Ward et al. [32] recently published data accumulated from the COLD registry, a cooperative collection of outcomes from several clinicians. These data showed a marked increase in the use of focal therapy vs whole gland cryo between 2004 and 2007. Low-risk disease was present in 541 (47 %), intermediate risk in 473 (41 %) and 143 (12 %) had high risk, clearly indicating that practitioners felt that medium- and high-risk patients were candidates for focal therapy. The biochemical disease-free rate at 36 months was 75.7 % using the ASTRO criteria. There was no significant difference in results between the risk levels. In addition there was no significant difference between whole gland cryosurgery and focal therapy (Fig. 12.6). A look at the KM

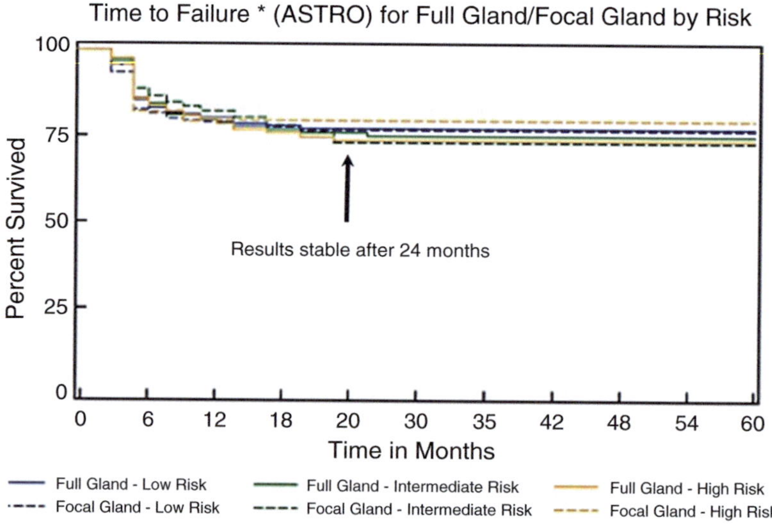

Fig. 12.6 This shows the Kaplan–Meier curves reported from the COLD registry for both focal and whole gland cryoablation. Note that there is no difference in the results between risk groups for either the full gland cryo or the focal cryo. Also note the similarities of these curves to the curves in Fig. 12.1, where after approximately 2 years the curves flatten and maintain the same level of success. This is a unique characteristic that has been demonstrated in all the long-term cryo results. Adapted from Ward JF, Jones JS. Focal cryotherapy for localized prostate cancer a report from the National Cryo On-Line database. BJU Int 2012;109:1648–1654

curves for the various groups demonstrate stable results after 24 months, a finding characteristic of cryoablation. The positive biopsy rate for the whole cohort was only 3.7 %. Urinary continence defined as 0 pads was 98.4 % and potency was 58.1 %.

The reliability of cryo tissue destruction is very high. In Ward et al. the overall positive biopsy rate was just 3.7 % of 1160 patients treated. In our series we did not have a positive biopsy in any of the frozen regions, local recurrences were found only in previously unfrozen tissue [1]. The reliability of cryo is, however, greatly dependent on placement of probes correctly into the cancer focus (targeted focal vs hemi-gland ablation), the use and accuracy of temperature monitoring, the routine use of hydro dissection of Denonvilliers' fascia, and the freezing protocol (2–3 freezes).

Cryoablation is widely available, relatively cheap, and any practitioner can start a cryoablation program with few barriers. Specific CPT codes for cryoablation are available and mobile services can provide equipment on a per case basis. With US guidance and a relatively cheap per probe cost, cryoablation is extremely cost effective.

Irreversible Electroporation (IRE)

IRE is a non-thermal ablation modality that uses microsecond pulses of DC electrical current to perforate the cell membrane. The animal work on prostate IRE showed it had certain advantages in relation to prostate ablation including rapid resolution of ablated tissue [33]. IRE being a non-thermal ablation modality spares tissue structures such as the rectum, urethra, ejaculatory ducts, and nerves (Figs. 12.7 and 12.8).

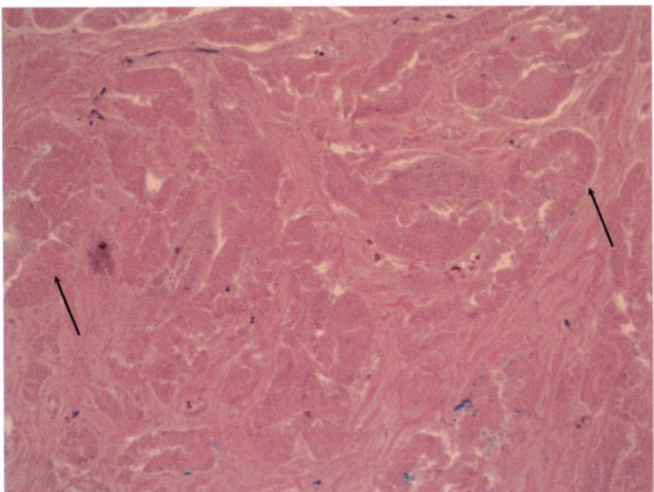

Fig. 12.7 Pathology of the prostate taken after an IRE treatment. The *arrows* indicate glands that still have their basic morphology. Ghosts of the cell nucleus can still be seen. IRE is a structure sparing non thermal ablation which causes cell death by apoptosis

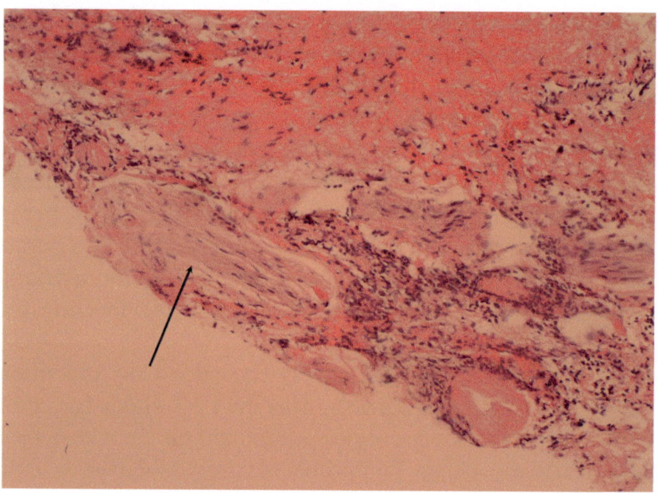

Fig. 12.8 Pathology showing an intact nerve (*arrow*) after an IRE treatment

There is little clinical data associated with prostate IRE; most information comes from the treatment of pancreatic carcinoma where IRE'S structure sparing qualities has allowed safe ablation of this disease [34]. A single study recently published by Valerio et al. [35] reports initial results on 34 patients the majority of whom had intermediate-risk disease (74 %). The median follow-up was 6 months. Seventeen percent of the patients failed and went on to another therapy. Continence was 100 % and potency was 95 % in those who were potent before treatment.

My personal unpublished experience comprises 17 patients. All were staged with 3D-PMB and 16 of the 17 had a post-op 3D-PMB to cover the area of treatment and a 5 mm margin around it. Of the 16 patients biopsied 15 of the 16 were negative for cancer and 1 had a residual microscopic focus. Continence was 100 % and potency was maintained in the 14 patients who were potent preoperatively. Of interest is that one of the patients treated was actually a whole gland treatment (Fig. 12.9) and he regained full potency at 7 months post-IRE which would be highly unlikely if he had been treated by whole gland cryoablation based on my experience.

IRE is a challenging technology since there is a complex interplay between the electrical parameters such as pulse number, pulse width, voltage and the arrangement and the length of the conducting portion of the probe exposed. The inability to monitor and confirm an adequate treatment at the time of the procedure is the biggest inadequacy of the technology although parameters for an adequate treatment have been elucidated in prostate cancer cell studies allowing some degree of pre-procedure planning [36].

I currently use IRE in those patients in whom the tissue sparing aspects of IRE are important (such as patients with bilateral disease adjacent to the NVB's) or disease adjacent to the urethra in which I am worried that the urethral warmer would spare cancer in a cryoablation. In these setting I often combine using cryo and IRE in the same procedure.

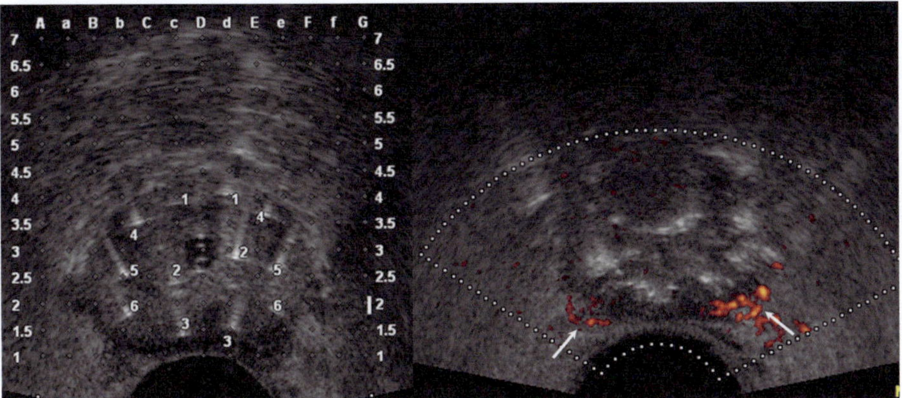

Fig. 12.9 The image on the left shows a ultrasound with 12 IRE probes in place ready to treat the whole gland in a patient with diffuse Gleason 4 + 3 cancer throughout both lobes. The image on the *right* shows post IRE the gland is obscured by gas created during the treatment but color Doppler shows the neuro vascular bundles are intact with flow still occurring (*arrows*). The patient had full potency return and 7 years later maintains a PSA of .1

Compared to cryoablation the equipment is very expensive (approximate cost $250,000) and the probe cost of $2,000/probe (2–6 probes per case) is almost prohibitive. If you want to take advantage of IRE the best strategy is to create a program where it is used for multiple areas of the body.

Lastly while we originally thought that IRE would provide an immunologic response similar to cryoablation, IRE's main cell destructive mechanism of apoptosis is not an optimal immunologic stimulatory method and studies looking at this aspect of IRE has been mixed.

Laser Ablation

Studies are now just emerging using laser ablation for focal therapy. The technology is approved for general tissue ablation but not specifically for prostate and there are currently no CPT codes for payment. The first series published with over ten patients was reported by Lindner et al. [37]. In this study the area to be ablated was confirmed and targeted using MR imaging with US MRI fusion software. The procedure was monitored using contrast enhanced ultrasound. Twelve patients were treated. The procedure was well tolerated with 75 % of the patients were discharged home without a catheter the same day. There were no perioperative complications and minimal morbidity. All patients who were potent before the procedure maintained potency after the procedure. Continence was 100 %. Based on multicore total prostate biopsy carried out at 6 months, however, only 67 % of patients were free of tumor in the targeted area and 50 % were free of disease overall.

Laser therapy is now being carried out under MRI guidance and monitoring. By using special MR sequences such as proton-resonance frequency (PRF) shift MR thermometry, near real-time quantification of temperature using changes in the phase of gradient-recalled echo (GRE) images to estimate relative temperature changes can be made [38]. The laser being used is 980-nm diode surrounded by a 1.65-mm cooling catheter manufactured by Visualase, Inc. (Houston, TX). The technical considerations are well beyond the scope of this chapter but I refer the reader to the excellent review on the subject by Lee et al. [39]. In this article they also report their first series of 23 patients of laser ablated focal therapy. The inclusion criteria for the study included, a 10-year life expectancy, between one to two focal abnormalities on mpMRI consistent with prostate cancer, no dominant Gleason pattern 4 disease on random TRUS-guided biopsies of the normal appearing prostate on mpMRI, focal abnormality on MRI <15 mm, and no Gleason score over 7.

The procedures were well tolerated with 100 % continence and no change in sexual function. Follow-up was very short with only 14 of the patients reaching 6 month follow-up. Of the 14 patients 2 were noted to have positive biopsies (one Gleason 6 and one Gleason 7 (3 + 4).

The trend in focal therapy as indicated by the above study is toward using MRI guided biopsies followed by MRI guided ablation. Based on the previous discussion of multiparametric MRI the investigators using this modality may in the end be biasing the results against laser ablation. With that said each investigator and practitioner will have to make their own judgment as to whether mpMRI guided biopsy as the sole staging and guidance method for focal therapy is sufficient. From a cost effectiveness and availability standpoint mpMRI guidance of focal therapy is obviously problematic. Our approach to focal therapy has always been and remains to stage as accurately as possible and leave no known cancer untreated.

From an immunologic standpoint heating lesions are least likely to illicit a therapeutic immunologic response due to the denaturing of the unique cancer protein/antigens.

As with all other focal therapy modalities, laser ablation appears to have an excellent morbidity profile.

Focal Radiation Therapy

There is minimal data relating to the use of focal radiation therapy as the primary treatment for prostate cancer. No studies have been carried relating to any external beam technology for focal therapy although it appears to be technically feasible [40]. Only a few have been published on focal brachytherapy with the largest series by Nguyen et al. [41] with 318 patients. In this study, however, there was not targeting of specific lesion but partial treatment of the gland by just treating the peripheral zone. With a median follow-up of 5.1 years, the BDSF for intermediate-risk cases was 73 % at 5 years and 66 % at 8 years. High recurrence rates would be expected with such an approach since 30 % of tumors are expected to be found in the transition zone of the gland and would not be adequately treated with such an approach. No other series reporting the cancer control results of primary brachytherapy have been published as yet. For further considerations on this topic I refer the reader to an excellent review of the theoretical considerations of the subject by Kovacs et al. [40].

Clearly with the advent of new technologies such a proton beam therapy and the Cyberknife trials with focal therapy using radiation will be pursued. Just as clearly, however, the major limitations to radiation therapy, including radiation scatter, variable effectiveness in high Gleason grade tumors, the delayed effect of radiation, and dose limitations for re-treatment, make the competitiveness of this modality questionable.

Photodynamic Therapy

Vascular-targeted photodynamic (VTP) therapy comprises three elements: a photosensitizing agent to enhance the sensitivity of tumor vasculature to light energy; light of a specific wavelength; and sufficient oxygen to drive the reaction. VTP uses an intravenous administered photo sensitizer. TOOKAD® Soluble (WST11) (padeliporfin; palladium bacteriopheophorbide monolysotaurine) is the drug currently being studied for prostate ablation. Optical fibers within hollow plastic needles allow accurate positioning in the prostate. The light activates the TOOKAD within the prostate, which creates reactive oxygen species that cause thrombosis within the vessels. This results in destruction of the microvasculature with resultant deprivation of oxygen and destruction of the prostate cancer cells.

Azzouzi et al. [42] reported the results of 83 patients treated with VTP with TOOKAD. The patients were divided into two main groups those treated with 4 mg/kg and those with 6 mg/kg doses. Approximately a quarter of the patients were treated bilaterally. At the 6-month follow-up, 61/83 (74 %) patients had negative biopsies. The most successful group were the patients treated with 4 mg/kg TOOKAD® Soluble and 200 J/cm light (unilateral), 38/46 of which (83 %) patients had negative biopsies at the 6-month follow-up. Complications were in general minor and self-limited and were felt to be related to the procedure; however, there were two complications felt to be related to the drug itself, one of which was ischemic optic neuropathy resulting in a visual field defect for the patient. Being dependent on a drug given systemically creates added regulatory hurdles making the availability of VTP in the near future not likely. With many excellent alternatives for thermal and non-thermal ablation available, VTP is unlikely to gain significant interest.

High Intensity Focused US-HIFU

HIFU has a long history only second to cryoablation in follow-up and volume of patients treated. HIFU uses sound waves to achieve coagulative necrosis and destruction of the targeted tissue by heating which denatures proteins and destroys cellular membranes. This results in instantaneous and irreversible coagulative necrosis. At the present time two systems are available the Sonoblate-500 produced by Focus Surgery (Indianapolis, IN) and Ablatherm produced by EDAP TMS (Lyons, France) for treating prostate cancer. Neither system has been approved for use in the USA, and patients who want the treatment are taken to centers outside of the country. Due to the limits of the ultrasound wave depth penetration there can be difficulty in ablating anterior cancers [43].

No level one data is available for HIFU but several studies treating the whole gland report on the technology's efficacy. A multicenter trial using the Ablatherm was reported in 2003 [43]. Although 28 % of the patients required two treatment sessions, 87 % of the patients had a negative biopsy with 92, 86, and 82 % in the low-, intermediate-, and high-risk groups, respectively. Gelet et al. [44] analyzed the long-term results in patients with low-risk disease. Patients demonstrated negative biopsy of 78 % and 5-year disease-free survivals of 83 %, but for those in intermediate- and high-risk groups, the disease-free survival rate was just 53 and 36 %, respectively. Blana et al. [45] reported a large group of patients with low- and intermediate-risk disease. The overall 5-year disease-free probability was 66 %.

A number of small series have been published using HIFU as focal therapy. In 2008, Muto et al. [46] compared the results of whole gland to hemi gland HIFU. 57 % of the patients had whole gland therapy and 45 % focal therapy. At 12 months post procedure whole gland patients had an 84.4 % negative biopsy rate and in the focal therapy group 76.5 % had negative biopsy rate. The 2-year biochemical DFS rates in patients at low, intermediate and high-risk were 85.9, 50.9 and 0 %, respectively. No significant differences were noted in the 2-year biochemical DFS rates for the patients at low and intermediate risk treated for the whole and hemi treated patients. All patients were continent. Sexual potency was not evaluated. There were no major complications.

In 2011, El Fegoun et al. [47] presented a series of 12 cases of low and intermediate risk treated with hemiablation by HIFU. The mean follow-up was 10 years. BDFS at 5 and 10 years was 90 and 38 % with 4 of the 12 patients on hormonal therapy. All patients were continent. Sexual function was not reported. Finally, Ahmed et al. published two series [48, 49]. The first was in 2011, where he evaluated 20 low- and intermediate-risk patients over 12 months. The protocol included the use of MRI and transperineal biopsies with template mapping. The recurrence in the follow-up biopsy at 6 months was 11 %, 2 of the 20 patients were incontinent and required use of pads and 95 % maintained potency. Another series by Ahmed et al. was published in 2012 using the Sonoblate machine [49]. 41 low- and intermediate-risk patients were assessed during a period of 12 months. The positive biopsy rate at 6 months was 23 %. Continence was ultimately 100 % but at 1 month 30 % of the patients were using pads and full continence was not achieved by all the patients until 9 months post-op. In all, the focal therapy experience with HIFU is fairly limited in numbers and follow-up. Short term positive biopsy rates appear rather high, but the most disturbing factor is the tendency toward incontinence requiring pads in both the short and long term.

Being a heat based ablation there would minimal positive immunologic effect expected from HIFU treatment.

Conclusion

Based on the current available data, focal therapy appears to offer consistent if not superior cancer control results, compared with whole gland ablation. It accomplishes this with extremely low morbidity. The long-term results that are just being reported with focal therapy can give some degree of comfort that patient outcomes are not compromised. Many technologies are being investigated for focal therapy and time will tell the utility of each. The most exciting future possibility associated with focal therapy is the harnessing of a specific tumor immune response to improve results in the high-risk patients.

References

1. Onik G, Narayan P, Vaughan D, Dineen M, Brunelle R. Focal "nerve-sparing" cryosurgery for treatment of primary prostate cancer: a new approach to preserving potency. Urology. 2002;60:109–14.
2. Bahn DK, Silverman P, Lee Sr F, Badalament R, Bahn ED, Rewcastle JC. Focal prostate cryoablation: initial results show cancer control and potency preservation. J Endourol. 2006;20:688–92.
3. Bahn D, de Castro Abreu AL, Gill IS, Hung AJ, Silverman P, Gross ME. Focal cryotherapy for clinically unilateral, low-intermediate risk prostate cancer in 73 men with a median follow-up of 3.7 years. Eur Urol. 2012;62:55–63.
4. de Castro Abreu AL, Bahn D, Leslie S, et al. Salvage focal and salvage total cryoablation for locally recurrent prostate cancer after primary radiation therapy. BJU Int. 2013;112:298–307.
5. Hale Z, Miyake M, Palacios DA, Rosser CJ. Focal cryosurgical ablation of the prostate: a single institute's perspective. BMC Urol. 2013;13:2.
6. Ahmed HU, Arya M, Carroll PR, Emberton M, editors. Focal therapy in prostate cancer. Chichester, West Sussex: Wiley-Blackwell; 2012.
7. van den Bos W, Muller BG, Ahmed H, et al. Focal therapy in prostate cancer: international multidisciplinary consensus on trial design. Eur Urol. 2014;65:1084–5.
8. Bostwick DG, Waters DJ, Farley ER, et al. Group consensus reports from the Consensus conference on focal treatment of prostatic carcinoma, Celebration, Florida, February 24, 2006. Urology. 2007;70:42–4.
9. Gary O, Karen B, Matthew M, David B, David V, Jeff B, et al. Long-term results of optimized focal therapy for prostate cancer: average 10-year follow-up in 70 patients. J Mens Health. 2014;11(2):64–74.
10. Alicikus ZA, Yamada Y, Zhang Z, et al. Ten-year outcomes of high-dose, intensity-modulated radiotherapy for localized prostate cancer. Cancer. 2011;117:1429–37.
11. Ginzburg S, Nevers T, Staff I, et al. Prostate cancer biochemical recurrence rates after robotic-assisted laparoscopic radical prostatectomy. JSLS. 2012;16:443–50.
12. Onik G, Vaughan D, Lotenfoe R, Dineen M, Brady J. "Male lumpectomy": focal therapy for prostate cancer using cryoablation. Urology. 2007;70(6 Suppl):16–21.
13. Onik G, Rubinsky B, Zemel R, et al. Ultrasound guided hepatic cryosurgery in the treatment of metastatic colon carcinoma: Preliminary results. Cancer. 1991;67:901–7.
14. Singh PB, Anele C, Dalton E, et al. Prostate cancer tumour features on template prostate mapping biopsies: implications for focal therapy. Eur Urol. 2014;66(1):12–9.
15. Crawford ED, Wilson SS, Torkko KC, et al. Clinical staging of prostate cancer: a computer-simulated study of transperineal prostate biopsy. BJU Int. 2005;96:999–1004.

16. Crawford ED, Rove KO, Barqawi AB, et al. Clinical-pathologic correlation between transperineal mapping biopsies of the prostate and three-dimensional reconstruction of prostatectomy specimens. Prostate. 2013;73:778–87.

17. Delongchamps NB, Beuvon F, Eiss D, et al. Multiparametric MRI is helpful to predict tumor focality, stage, and size in patients diagnosed with unilateral low-risk prostate cancer. Prostate Cancer Prostatic Dis. 2011;14:232–7.

18. Bratan F, Niaf E, Melodelima C, et al. Influence of imaging and histological factors on prostate cancer detection and localisation on multiparametric MRI: a prospective study. Eur Radiol. 2013;23:2019–29.

19. Noguchi M, Stamey TA, McNeal JE, Nolley R. Prognostic factors for multifocal prostate cancer in radical prostatectomy specimens: lack of significance of secondary cancers. J Urol. 2003;170:459–63.

20. Ablin RJ, Fontana G. Cryoimmunotherapy: continuing studies toward determining a rational approach for assessing the candidacy of the prostatic cancer patient for cryoimmunotherapy and postoperative responsiveness. An interim report. Cryobiology. 1980;17:170–7.

21. Sabel MS. Cryo-immunology: a review of the literature and proposed mechanisms for stimulatory versus suppressive immune responses. Cryobiology. 2009;58:1–11.

22. Bahn DK, Lee F, Badalament R, Kumar A, Greski J, Chernick M. Targeted cryoablation of the prostate: 7-year outcomes in the primary treatment of prostate cancer. Urology. 2002;60:3–11.

23. Grimm P, Billiet I, Bostwick D, et al. Comparative analysis of prostate-specific antigen free survival outcomes for patients with low, intermediate and high risk prostate cancer treatment by radical therapy. Results from the Prostate Cancer Results Study Group. BJU Int. 2012;109:22–9.

24. Waitz R, Solomon SB, Petre EN, et al. Potent induction of tumor immunity by combining tumor cryoablation with anti-CTLA-4 therapy. Cancer Res. 2012;72:430–9.

25. Kawano M, Nishida H, Nakamoto Y, Tsumura H, Tsuchiya H. Cryoimmunologic antitumor effects enhanced by dendritic cells in osteosarcoma. Clin Orthop Relat Res. 2010;46.

26. Niu L-Z, Li J-L, Zeng J-Y, Feng M, et al. Combination treatment with comprehensive cryoablation and immunotherapy in metastatic hepatocellular cancer. World J Gastroenterol. 2013;19(22):3473–80.

27. Onik G, Narayan P, Brunelle R, Vaughn D, Dineen M, Brown T. Saline injection into Denonvilliers' fascia during prostate cryosurgery. J Min Inv Ther Relat Tech. 2000;6:423–7.

28. Tatsutani K, Rubinsky B, Onik G, Dahiya R, Narayan P. The effect of thermal variables on frozen human primary prostatic adenocarcinoma cells. Urology. 1996;48(3):441–7.

29. Larson TR, Rrobertson DW, Corica A, Bostwick DG. In vivo interstitial temperature mapping of the human prostate during cryosurgery with correlation to histopathologic outcomes. Urology. 2000;55(4):547–52.

30. Donnelly BJ, Saliken JC, Brasher PM, et al. A randomized trial of external beam radiotherapy versus cryoablation in patients with localized prostate cancer. Cancer. 2010;116:323–30.

31. Shah TT, Ahmed H, Kanthabalan A, Lau B, Ghei M, Maraj B, et al. Focal cryotherapy of localized prostate cancer: a systematic review of the literature. Expert Rev Anticancer Ther. 2014;14(11):1337–47.

32. Ward JF, Jones JS. Focal cryotherapy for localized prostate cancer a report from the National Cryo On-Line database. BJU Int. 2012;109:1648–54.

33. Onik G, Mikus P, Rubinsky B. Irreversible electroporation: implications for prostate ablation. Technol Cancer Res Treat. 2007;6:295–300.

34. Martin 2nd RC, McFarland K, Ellis S, Velanovich V. Irreversible electroporation therapy in the management of locally advanced pancreatic adenocarcinoma. J Am Coll Surg. 2012;215(3):361–9.

35. Valerio M, Stricker PD, Ahmed HU. Dick Initial assessment of safety and clinical feasibility of irreversible electroporation in the focal treatment of prostate cancer. Prostate Cancer Prostatic Dis. 2014;17(4):343–7.

36. Rubinsky B, Onik G, Mikus P. Irreversible electroporation: a new ablation modality—clinical implications. Technol Cancer Res Treat. 2007;6(1):37–48.

37. Lindner U, Weersink RA, Haider MA, Gertner MR, Davidson SR, Atri M, et al. Image guided photothermal focal therapy for localized prostate cancer: phase I trial. J Urol. 2009;182(4):1371–7.
38. Rieke V, Vigen KK, Sommer G, et al. Referenceless PRF shift thermometry. Magn Reson Med. 2004;51:1223–31.
39. Lee T, Mendhiratta N, Sperling D, Lepor H. Focal laser ablation for localized prostate cancer: principles, clinical trials, and our initial experience. Rev Urol. 2014;16(2):55–66.
40. Kovács G, Cosset JM, Carey B. Focal radiotherapy as focal therapy of prostate cancer. Curr Opin Urol. 2014;24:231–5.
41. Nguyen PL, Chen MH, Zhang Y, et al. Updated results of magnetic resonance imaging guided partial prostate brachytherapy for favorable risk prostate cancer: implications for focal therapy. J Urol. 2012;188:1151–6.
42. Azzouzi AR, Barret E, Moore CM, Villers A, Allen C, Scherz A, et al. TOOKAD(®) Soluble vascular-targeted photodynamic (VTP) therapy: determination of optimal treatment conditions and assessment of effects in patients with localised prostate cancer. BJU Int. 2013;112(6):766–74. doi:10.1111/bju.12265.
43. Thüroff S, Chaussy C, Vallancien G, et al. High-intensity focused ultrasound and localized prostate cancer: efficacy results from the European multicentric study. J Endourol. 2003;17(8):673–7.
44. Gelet A, Chapelon JY, Poissonier L, et al. Prostate cancer control with transrectal HIFU in 242 consecutive patients: 5-year results. Eur Urol. 2004;3(Suppl):214.
45. Blana A, Murat FJ, Walter B, et al. First analysis of the long-term results with transrectal HIFU in patients with localised prostate cancer. Eur Urol. 2008;53(6):1194–203.
46. Muto S et al. Focal therapy with high-intensity focused ultrasound in the treatment of localized prostate cancer. Jpn J Clin Oncol. 2008;38:192–9.
47. Fegoun E et al. Focal therapy with high intensity focused ultrasound for prostate cancer in the elderly. A feasibility study with 10 years follow-up. Int Braz J Urol. 2011;37:213–22.
48. Ahmed HU et al. Focal therapy for localized prostate cancer: a phase I/II trial. J Urol. 2010;185:1246–54.
49. Ahmed HU, Hindley RG, Dickinson L, et al. Focal therapy for localised unifocal and multifocal prostate cancer: a prospective development study. Lancet Oncol. 2012;13(6):622–32.

Chapter 13
Multiparametric MRI (mpMRI): Guided Focal Therapy

Michele Fascelli, Amichai Kilchevsky, Arvin K. George, and Peter A. Pinto

Introduction

Approximately one in seven men will be diagnosed with prostate cancer (PCa) during his lifetime, with roughly 50 % of newly diagnosed patients presenting with low-risk disease features [1]. The ubiquitous use of PSA screening has been responsible for increased rates of cancer detection, with concurrent increase of definitive therapy, namely radical prostatectomy (RP) and radiation therapy (RT). Increasing rates of treatment for clinically localized prostate cancer via RP or RT have caused both escalating healthcare costs and patient morbidity, including erectile dysfunction, urinary incontinence, and anxiety associated with decreased quality of life [2]. Approximately half of all men enrolled in the European Randomized Study for Screening Prostate Cancer (ERSPC) trial underwent surgery for cancers found to meet criteria for "clinically indolent disease" (<0.5 cm^3 tumor volume, organ confined, and Gleason score ≤ 6) [3]. Focal therapy thus emerged as a safe treatment alternative to spare patients the morbidity of established definitive treatment methods while preserving oncologic control.

The Prostate Intervention Versus Observation Trial (PIVOT) was among the first studies to reveal a limited benefit of treatment in the subset of patients identified by PSA

Electronic supplementary material: The online version of this chapter (doi:10.1007/978-3-319-21485-6_13) contains supplementary material, which is available to authorized users. Videos can also be accessed at http://link.springer.com/chapter/10.1007/978-3-319-21485-6_13.

M. Fascelli, B.A. • A. Kilchevsky, M.D. • A.K. George, M.D.
Urologic Oncology Branch, National Cancer Institute—National Institutes of Health,
9000 Rockville Pike, Building 10, Room 1-5940, Bethesda, MD 20892, USA
e-mail: mfascelli@gmail.com; akilchev@gmail.com; arvin.george@nih.gov

P.A. Pinto, M.D. (✉)
Prostate Cancer Division, Urologic Oncology Branch, National Cancer Institute,
10 Center Drive, MSC 1210, Bethesda, MD 20892-1210, USA
e-mail: pintop@mail.nih.gov

© Springer International Publishing Switzerland 2016
N.N. Stone, E.D. Crawford (eds.), *The Prostate Cancer Dilemma*,
DOI 10.1007/978-3-319-21485-6_13

and TRUS biopsy [4]. PIVOT elucidated the role of observation in the management of patients with low-grade, low-volume disease, discouraging unnecessary biopsies and treatment-related morbidity without tangible benefit; however, many patients ultimately go on to definitive therapy because of uncertainty regarding the reliability of PSA and random biopsies for detecting lethal cancers and reluctance to defer treatment.

Fundamental to the application of focal therapy is reliable and accurate imaging to patient selection, treatment guidance, and patient follow-up while preserving oncologic efficacy, sexual potency, and urinary continence. Multiparametric magnetic resonance imaging (mpMRI), an imaging modality demonstrating improved detection rates of prostate cancer, has been utilized to guide clinical decision-making, touting accurate tumor localization and improved staging of disease [5–8]. The parameters of mpMRI include: T2-weighted imaging (T2W), dynamic contrast enhancement (DCE), apparent diffusion coefficient (ADC) on diffusion weighted imaging (DWI), and MR spectroscopic imaging (MRSI) (Fig. 13.1). T2W imaging,

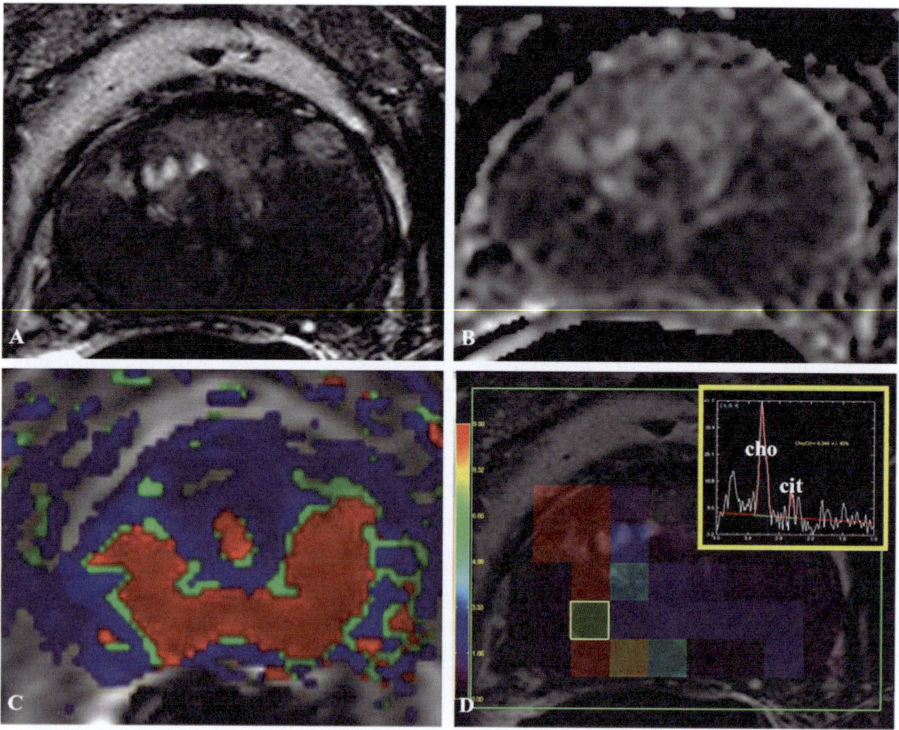

Fig. 13.1 Example of multiparametric MRI and all parameters. A 78-year-old male was referred to our institution for elevating PSA, measured at 6.21 ng/mL at time of biopsy. Multiparametric MRI revealed a 4.8 cm lesion encompassing most of the peripheral zone, positive on all mpMRI parameters: T2 (**a**), diffusion weighted imaging (**b**), permeability mapping on dynamic contrast enhancement (**c**), and MR spectroscopy (**d**). In (**d**), the *yellow box* in the *upper right corner* depicts the choline (cho) and citrate (cit) peaks measured for the *yellow/green square* highlighted in the prostate imaged. This patient had a high choline–citrate ratio, consistent with a positive MR spectroscopy parameter

reflecting tissue water content, provides the highest spatial resolution and zonal anatomy. DWI reflects the diffusion of water within tissue and is given an order of magnitude, referred to as the apparent diffusion coefficient (ADC); diffusion of water is restricted within tumors representing hypercellularity, making DWI very sensitive for detecting cancers, especially in the peripheral zone of the prostate. Moreover, lower ADC values on DWI correlate with higher Gleason grade at histology, allowing for risk stratification of patients. Dynamic contrast enhanced MRI consists of a series of fast T1-weighted sequences before and after injection of contrast, assessing the focal kinetics of enhancement within prostatic lesions. Lastly, MRSI detects relative levels of the prostate metabolites, choline and citrate, in which altered concentrations exist in benign and malignant disease. Among these parameters, MRSI is the least often employed, and current protocols have moved away from it due to limited additional benefits when accounting for time and cost.

MpMRI has reliably shown diagnostic accuracy with an ability to localize disease and correctly characterize and identify multifocal disease using its multiple parameters. Success utilizing mpMRI stems from accurate disease localization and subsequent histopathological correlation, reliable identification of index lesions, and matching the tumor volumes of these suspicious lesions to their final pathology, therein providing ample measurement when applying therapies.

MpMRI may specifically identify those patients harboring intermediate–high-grade, high-volume disease who would benefit from definitive treatment, simultaneously reducing unnecessary detection of patients with low-grade, low-volume disease. Correlating histological lesions and MRI findings had been previously difficult to determine as angles varied between section intervals on MRI images and prostatectomy specimens. Despite this hurdle, the Turkbey et al. group corrected for this variability with a shrinkage factor as well as co-registration between histology and imaging; furthermore, in order to confirm the accuracy of mpMRI targeted lesions, the group assessed cancer detection using whole mount sectioning from customized three-dimensional prostatic molds to register specimen pathology and MRI [9]. Cancer detection using whole mount sectioning from the 3D prostatic molds allowing registration between specimen pathology and MRI found that mpMRI had high sensitivity for tumors larger than 5 mm in diameter and with Gleason scores greater than $3+4=7$, while low suspicious lesions identified on MRI reliably represented benign tissue or low-grade prostate cancer [9, 10]. Additionally, mpMRI has shown superiority in predicting active surveillance eligibility (no tumor larger than 0.5 cc or possessing any Gleason 4 or 5 pattern disease) with sensitivity and overall accuracy of 93 and 92 %, respectively [8]. These findings suggest that imaging supplements clinicopathologic criteria and improves disease identification in patients while encouraging a potential union of mpMRI and focal therapy.

Focal therapy operates on the pathophysiologic principle of prostate cancer existing as a multifocal disease, wherein the highest suspicious lesions identified on imaging can be defined as index lesions, or those responsible for driving disease biology, and thus targeted for curative treatment. Targeted biopsy of MR-identified lesions is becoming the new standard technique for diagnosis of any prostate cancer and of clinically significant prostate cancer [11]. Baco and colleagues posited that index lesions could be precisely identified on multiparametric MRI in comparison to radical prostatectomy specimen, yielding successful characterization of 95 % (128/135) of males with high concordance ($\kappa=0.76$) between primary Gleason pattern on targeted biopsy and RP specimen, and suggesting there exist means to identify disease using diagnostic imaging to provide pertinent prognostic information [12]. Several groups have shown mpMRI does reliably estimate index lesion tumor volumes and these mpMRI estimates correlated with histopathologic volumes [13, 14].

Different focal therapy techniques for localized disease have emerged as potential means to eradicate these foci of cancer, including cryotherapy, high-intensity focused ultrasound (HIFU), and laser interstitial therapy. The objective of this chapter is to review the current status and role of multiparametric magnetic resonance imaging in these focal therapy techniques.

Cryotherapy

Cryotherapy, also known as cryoablation or cryosurgery, is a thermoablative technique using rapid cycles of freezing and thawing of cells to induce coagulative necrosis at targeted areas. First described in the 1850s when James Arnott used ice-salt mixtures to treat cancers, cryoablation underwent drastic modernization by Irving Cooper in the 1960s when the use of liquid nitrogen was adopted [15, 16]. By 2008, the American Urologic Association acknowledged cryotherapy as a treatment option for newly diagnosed or recurrent organ-confined prostate cancer [17]. Typically, cryotherapy is performed using transrectal ultrasound (TRUS)-guided needles inserted via a transperineal approach. Pressurized gases that freeze (argon) and actively warm (helium) are used, operating under the Joule–Thompson effect wherein different gases undergo temperature changes when depressurized. Ice crystals form in targeted cells surrounding argon-based probes, reaching temperatures lower than −40 °C, and causing rapid thermal expansion. Thawing of the ice crystals induces cell damage and death by dehydration, protein denaturation, and cell membrane rupture; localized glandular ischemia and microthrombi also occur as a result of vascular stasis [18].

More recently, improved control of freezing and thawing has been coupled with MRI thermometry. MRI thermometry serves a unique advantage over ultrasound, accurately detecting temperature changes in real-time and allowing intraoperative assessment of tissue damage (Fig. 13.2). During the freezing, the location of the probe tip is considered the most effective region for therapy and therefore depends upon accurate visualization of technique and treatment. On real-time MRI, "iceballs" formed by application of cryoprobe tips to cancerous lesions can be seen as a signal void due to the absence of free hydrogen atoms in frozen tissue water. This tracking information allows the cryotherapy operator to determine the distance and extent of treatment coverage. The iceball needs to extend beyond the border of the tumor in order to fully treat all margins of disease [19]. Should the iceball configuration inadequately cover the area of gland in question, the probe position could be

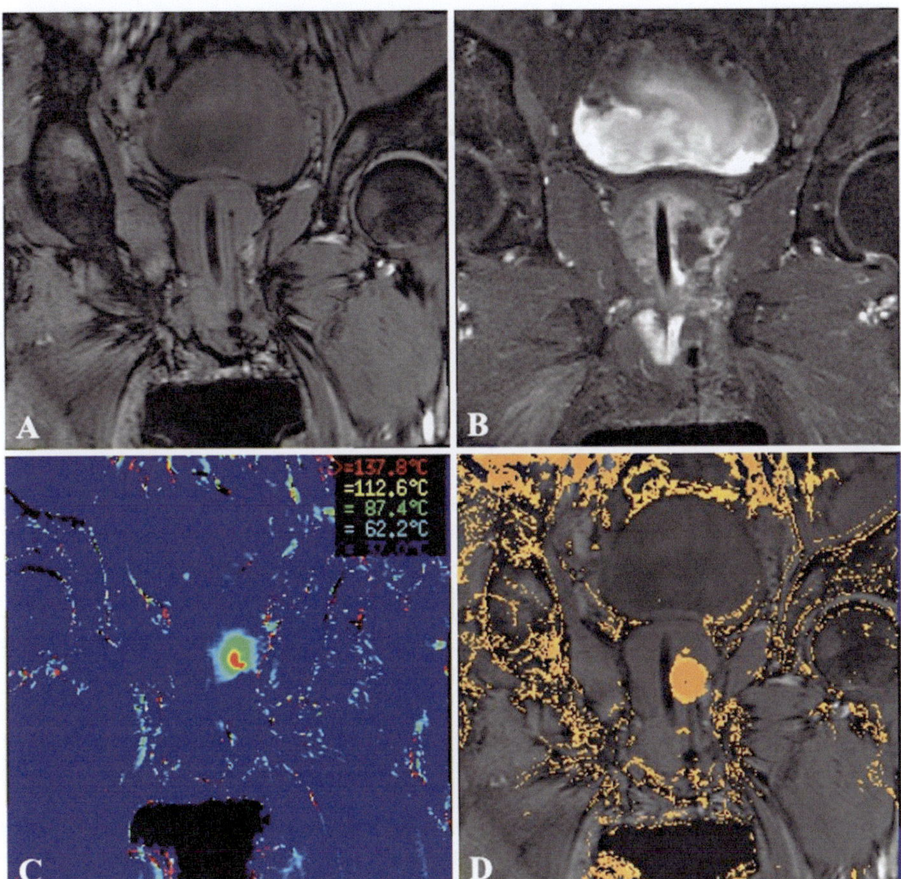

Fig. 13.2 Sagittal view of MR thermometry. Sagittal view of T2 MR pre-ablation (**a**) with the laser probe visible in the prostate and post-ablation (**b**). MR thermometry allows real-time temperature mapping during this focal laser ablation (**c**), later providing a post-ablation tissue damage map (**d**)

readjusted in real-time. Moreover, if the ice ball is seen approaching the rectal wall, then the corresponding cryoprobe could be slowed down or stopped [20].

MRI compatible cryoprobes used in liver and kidney cancer treatment, as well as experimental robots used to insert needles into the prostate, have allowed for more development of MRI-real time monitoring and technique application to patients [21, 22]. Early work done in canine models using 0.5 T MRI showed technically feasible MRI-guided cryosurgery, but initial cryoprobes scattered T1 and T2 signals [23, 24]. Information from canine models revealed that T1 sequences of MRI did not reliably correlate tissue necrosis volume with that induced. Rather, contrast-enhanced sequences were more consistent at predicting tissue damage after cryosurgery with an accuracy rate of 91 % (Pearson $r^2 = 0.97$) [24].

Initial work done in 29 patients with prostate cancer using MRI-guided cryosurgery has revealed minor complications, including hematuria, dysuria, scrotal pain, and urinary retention [20, 25] while reporting one major instance of urethrorectal fistula that healed within 3 months of surgery [20]. MRI guidance instead of transrectal ultrasound allows for insertion of a rectal balloon with warm saline to protect the rectal wall from freezing. Additionally, published follow-up literature has shown these initial cohorts had no change in erectile function but worsening incontinence in three of 18 patients [25].

There is a paucity of long-term follow-up in patients receiving prostate cryoablation with MRI guidance as primary treatment for prostate cancer thereby making long-term outcomes difficult to assess. In fact, only Gangi et al. looked at cancer recurrence in this patient population. While the researchers did not routinely perform a systematic post-cryoablation prostate biopsy as part of the study, follow-up MRI revealed no suspected region for remaining prostate cancer in any of the 11 treated patients [20]. The hope is that their long-term results will be as good, if not better, than the previous cohort of patients treated with cryoablation. In that population, a multicenter registry (the Cryoablation-On-Line-Database registry) has reported pooled 5-year biochemical disease-free rate using the Phoenix definition of nadir plus 2 as: 91 % in the low-risk group at 5 years, 78 % in the intermediate-risk group, and 62 % in the high-risk group [26].

High-Intensity Focal Ultrasound

High-intensity focal ultrasound (HIFU) is a minimally invasive procedure directing increased intensity ultrasound waves compared to those used during imaging exploration. Ultrasound waves are focused on specific pathologic regions from a transducer, generating high local tissue temperatures. Absorbed ultrasound energy is rapidly converted to heat in prostatic tissue, via a thermal effect, yielding cellular disruption and coagulative necrosis. Tissue is heated for approximately 5 seconds, attaining temperatures up to 90 °C (194 °F), and its focal application to targets allows for preservation of the surrounding tissue. In addition to the thermal effect of HIFU, cavitation results from ultrasound waves interacting with intraprostatic, intracellular water to cause microbubbles, which are responsible for dispersion of energy and enhancement of tissue ablation. Use of ultrasound waves to destroy human tissue was first proposed in the 1940s by John G. Lynn before its implementation in soft-tissue tumor ablation in the 1950s, followed by the use of MRI guidance with HIFU in prostate cancer in the 1990s [27–30].

While MRI-guided HIFU is not approved in the USA as of 2015, the therapy is approved for use in 30 countries and clinical trials are underway. The utility of MRI-guided HIFU is in real-time monitoring using quantitative MRI thermometry to report tissue temperature and ensure accurate ablation without compromising other key structures of the pelvis, including the urethra and neurovascular bundles [31]. Additionally, coregistration of ultrasound and mpMRI has been used in identifying treatment margins, up to 5 mm in one study [31], both prior to and during HIFU therapy [32–34], providing a means for serial follow-up imaging to detect recurrence and to assess need for re-treatment.

Prior work applying MRI-guided focused ultrasound that led to its application in prostate cancer was performed in uterine fibroids before extending to other organs, including breast, liver, and bone [35–38]. Preliminary work in canine prostate models again confirmed the feasibility of MRI-guided HIFU with small transition zones between ablated and viable tissue ranging from 0.4 to 2.0 mm [39–41]. Two cohorts of males underwent initial MRI-guided HIFU in 2010 prior to radical prostatectomy; approximately 30 % of the prostate volume was ablated post-prostatectomy with no complications during or after surgery [40, 42]. MRI guidance proved to be advantageous in overcoming rectal damage and urethral damage previously documented in patients undergoing HIFU sans MRI [43]. Despite this, the initial cohorts did reveal technological limitations: average ablation times were extensive, ranging from 2–2.5 hours, with incidental peaks greater than 6 hours [44] and tumor and prostate mobility allowed aberrant movement to create focal spot losses and misalign treatment. A similar study by Napoli et al. found no evidence of disease on follow-up MRI or residual viable tumor in the ablation area on final pathology [31]. However, histologic examination revealed a nonsignificant bilateral residual tumor according to the Epstein criteria outside the treated area in three out of five patients and bilateral Gleason 7 tumor in the other two patients.

HIFU has also been implicated in a promising future clinical application with targeted drug delivery. It has been proposed that systemic therapeutic agents, like chemotherapy, can be delivered to the body in encapsulated form and then stimulated to locally release upon activation by the heat from the mechanical oscillation of the focused ultrasound waves [45].

Laser Interstitial Therapy

Laser interstitial therapy (LIT) is also commonly referred to as focal laser ablation (FLA). This thermoablative technique employs high-energy laser light to generate rapid heat and incite coagulation in target tissue. Previously popularized as a means to destroy hepatic and renal lesions, most recent adaptations of FLA in tumor destruction have arisen in the field of neuro-oncology, with applications in several brain lesions — both primary gliomas and cerebral metastases have been treated with promising outcomes [46]. First attempts at FLA of prostate cancer were documented in the 1980s when neodymium-doped yttrium aluminum garnet (Nd:YAG) lasers were employed, but FLA has since come to use 980 nm diode lasers [47–49]. Energy is delivered to the prostate using transperineally inserted laser fibers that produce and spread laser energy from the fiber tip through the immediate surrounding absorption zone, causing an increase in temperature to exposed tissues. Initial results in canine and cadaveric prostate models demonstrated easy handling and good penetrating laser fiber power [50–52].

The first patients to undergo FLA under MRI-guidance did so in 2010, using a 1.5 T MRI, 980 nm diode lasers, and the assistance of MRI thermometry, similar to cryoablation. Both of these males underwent in-bore treatment, were discharged within 3 hours of undergoing therapy, and suffered no adverse events within 1 month of follow-up [49]. The application of transperineal focal laser treatment in these two patients represented initial feasibility work with regard to this focal therapy technique. Subsequently, in-gantry multiparametric MRI was employed to locate tumors, guide laser placement, and confirm optical laser application. Use of MRI thermometry provided precise assessment of ablated zones. Use of post-treatment multiparametric MRI therefore should be able to confirm overlap of cancerous lesions and necrotic areas [53] (Fig. 13.3).

Since its inception, results of phase I laser interstitial therapy trials have shown potential, as developments of phase II trials are underway. Two phase I trials concluded in 2013, applying laser interstitial therapy to a total of 47 men. In one study, seven of nine showed no signs of cancer at the ablation site after 6 months of follow-up, while the remaining two individuals showed recurrence of Gleason $3+3$ disease [54]. The second study reported nearly identical results, mirroring minimal complications post-treatment; the group published that 26 % of their 38 male cohort showed positive biopsy at the time of their 4-month follow-up appointment, with no incidences of incontinence, rectal wall injury, or other complications [55]. Both study groups on retrospective review cited failure to completely cover the lesions using the ablation zone produced by FLA as likely cause for cancer recurrence.

A concern about the accuracy of ablation zones therefore arises as MRI-identified tumor volumes must correlate with treatment volumes for sufficient treatment application. Preclinical trials were performed in dogs and rats; these studies aimed to assess efficacy of FLA prior to their human counterparts. One study in dogs showed that histological examination of ablation zones consistently showed central areas of unviable tissue surrounded by coagulative necrosis and strong correlations of thermal damage on MRI thermometry and post-treatment MRI volume with histologic volumes ($r^2=0.94$) [51]. A study in rats found that the mean necrosis volume on MRI at 48 hours after FLA strongly correlated with histologic volumes as well, again revealing ellipsoid lesions consistent with coagulative necrosis [56]. In an early case series, ablated volumes measured on MRI correlated strongly with the ablation volume in four patients who underwent FLA 1 week prior to RP [57]. These pathology findings support accurate volume correlations and have since spurred assessment of mpMRI in distinguishing tissue response to treatment. MpMRI modalities, including T2 and ADC, were analyzed for co-occurrence of tissue-specific responses and indicated to have a high sensitivity for identifying change in tissue patterns [58]. This suggests that mpMRI alone may continue to improve in hopes of functioning as a sole quantitative assessment of prostate cancer burden in post-focal therapy patients, in addition to aid in clinical planning and treatment application.

Major criticism of these initial studies has come from inconsistent selection criteria for men treated with FLA. Generally, patients have low to intermediate-risk prostate cancer: PSA <15 ng/mL, Gleason score 6–7, and clinical stage T1c–T2a; disease burden assessed by mpMRI is fundamental to determining eligibility and

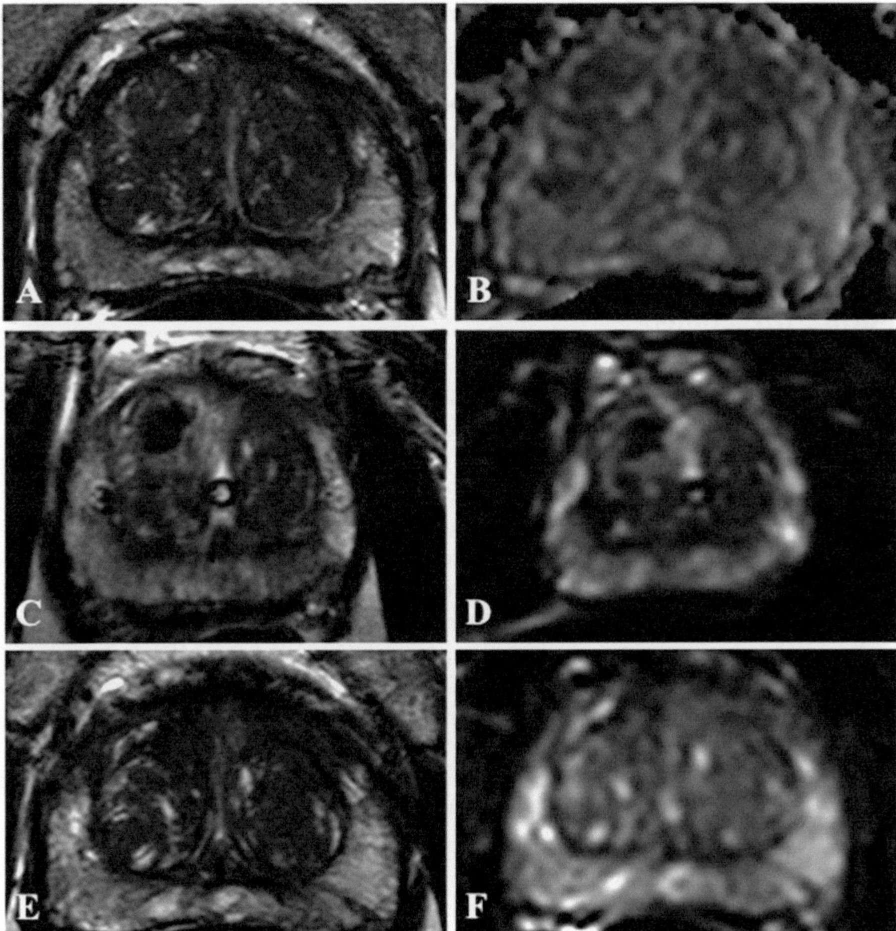

Fig. 13.3 Example of Focal Laser Ablation (FLA). A 58-year-old gentleman presented with multiple prior negative biopsies, an elevated PSA, as high as 12.7 ng/mL, and referred for mulitparametric MRI. On imaging, he was found to have a 1.3 cm lesion in the right apical to mid-central gland lesion; preoperative T2 (**a**) and DWI (**b**) sequences of his multiparametric MRI are shown. On biopsy, he was found to have Gleason 3+3=6 disease. He consented for focal laser ablation. Images 1 day post-treatment (T2 in (**c**), DWI in (**d**)) and at 1 year of follow-up (T2 in (**e**), DWI in (**f**)) are also shown. At 1 year of follow-up, his imaging reported diffuse hypointensity suggestive of tissue necrosis in the ablated area. Subsequent multiparametric MRI/TRUS fusion-guided biopsy of the target did not show disease

planning treatment as FLA maximum ablation zones have been cited to be up to approximately 2 cm^3 [59]. As such, patient selection and treatment planning additionally require specialized prostate MRI radiologists that work in conjunction with urologists, merging anatomical location of lesions on mpMRI with those on prostate biopsy. During the FLA, radiologists aid in MRI thermometry interpretation and further assist with laser repositioning feedback; this highlights the dependence of FLA on MRI in gantry performance of focal therapy (Video 13.1).

Acutely, the side-effect profile of FLA appears to be minimal, but long-term oncological outcomes remain to be seen. The short treatment times, MRI-visualized distinct ablation zones, and promising success rates using real-time MRI remain key features of laser ablation therapy, as future work hopes to elucidate the therapeutic efficacy of laser interstitial therapy. At present, post-treatment quality of life scores do not suggest a significant change from baseline in symptom scores or mean sexual function scores [60]. Phase II trials to investigate oncologic efficacy are in progress.

Future Directions

Other focal therapies are on the verge of development, similarly utilizing multiparametric MRI to benefit patient selection, treatment application, and assess outcomes. One such example is focal photodynamic therapy whereby free radicals and antioxidant enzymes are stimulated from the interaction of light from laser fibers and photosensitive agents administered orally or intravenously [61]. Reactive oxidative species directly induce damage to tumor cells, propagating cell apoptosis and necrosis and producing an acute inflammatory reaction. This cytotoxic method of induced cell destruction requires intraprostatic fibers to target lesions in a darkened room under MRI guidance, allowing for strong correlation between MRI-volumes and lesion targeting [62]. Several agents currently under investigation include temporfin, padoporfin, and padeliporfin. Concerns with these agents include vessel constriction and thrombosis [63].

Similarly, use of localized radiation sources can be placed near or inside the treatment area, as is the case for brachytherapy and brachytherapy seed implantation. MRI guidance of seed implantation aided in MRI-guided microwave and radiofrequency ablation techniques. The first focal therapy modality, microwave ablation, applies an applicator emitting electromagnetic waves that generate heat and cause tissue destruction. These electromagnetic waves, however, can create noise and interfere with the MRI signals themselves. Initial work regarding the signal-to-noise ratio and accuracy of MRI thermometry revealed a negative influence in patient outcomes [64]. Radiofrequency ablation (RFA) utilized a needle electrode inserted into tumor to again use electromagnetic waves producing friction-generated rising of temperature and subsequent cell death. MRI-guided prostate RFA is still very limited, but initial work in liver malignancies showed technical feasibility with no signal-to-noise effects [65].

Conclusion

Use of mpMRI and focal therapy techniques employed in targeting other types of malignancies (i.e., breast, liver cancer) provide promise in developing new alternative therapies applicable to prostate cancer in hope of replacing current standards of care, including surgical intervention and radiation therapy. Focal therapy was once referred to as the "lumpectomy" of prostate cancer [66], as urologists hope to hone multiparametric magnetic resonance imaging, providing better detection of disease, localization and extent of disease involvement, and spatial accuracy to determine optimal candidates for targeted therapy. By melding imaging and intervention in a minimally invasive and centralized manner, these focal therapy techniques and technologies will continue to improve; more results of long-term oncologic outcomes will aid in clinical decision-making for improved patient disease management.

Disclosures This work was supported by the Intramural Research Program of the National Institutes of Health (NIH), National Cancer Institute, Center for Cancer Research, and the Center for Interventional Oncology. NIH and Philips Healthcare have a cooperative research and development agreement. NIH and Philips share intellectual property in the field.

This work was also made possible through the National Institutes of Health Medical Research Scholars Program, a public–private partnership supported jointly by the NIH and generous contributions to the Foundation for the NIH from Pfizer Inc., The Doris Duke Charitable Foundation, The Alexandria Real Estate Equities, Inc. and Mr. and Mrs. Joel S. Marcus, and the Howard Hughes Medical Institute, as well as other private donors. For a complete list, please visit the Foundation website at: http://fnih.org/work/education-training-0/medical-research-scholars-program.

References

1. Klotz L. Active surveillance: patient selection. Curr Opin Urol. 2013;23(3):239–44.
2. Chou R, Croswell JM, Dana T, Bougatsos C, Blazina I, Fu R, et al. Screening for prostate cancer: a review of the evidence for the U.S. Preventive Services Task Force. Ann Intern Med. 2011;155(11):762–71.
3. Schröder FH, Hugosson J, Roobol MJ, Tammela TLJ, Zappa M, Nelen V, et al. Screening and prostate cancer mortality: results of the European Randomised Study of Screening for Prostate Cancer (ERSPC) at 13 years of follow-up. Lancet. 2014;384(9959):2027–35.
4. Wilt TJ, Brawer MK, Jones KM, Barry MJ, Aronson WJ, Fox S, et al. Radical prostatectomy versus observation for localized prostate cancer. N Engl J Med. 2012;367(3):203–13.
5. Stephenson SK, Chang EK, Marks LS. Screening and detection advances in magnetic resonance image-guided prostate biopsy. Urol Clin North Am. 2014;41(2):315–26.
6. Da Rosa MR, Milot L, Sugar L, Vesprini D, Chung H, Loblaw A, et al. A prospective comparison of MRI-US fused targeted biopsy versus systemic ultrasound-guided biopsy for detecting clinically significant prostate cancer in patients on active surveillance. J Magn Reson Imaging. 2014;21:00.
7. Fradet V, Kurhanewicz J, Cowan JE, Karl A, Coakley FV, Shinohara K, et al. Prostate cancer managed with active surveillance: role of anatomic MR imaging and MR spectroscopic imaging. Radiology. 2010;256(1):176–83.
8. Turkbey B, Rastinehad AR, Linehan WM, Wood BJ, Pinto PA. Prostate cancer: can multiparametric MR imaging help identify patients who are candidates for active surveillance? Radiology. 2013;268(1):144–52.
9. Turkbey B, Mani H, Shah V, Rastinehad AR, Bernardo M, Pohida T, et al. Multiparametric 3T prostate magnetic resonance imaging to detect cancer: histopathological correlation using prostatectomy specimens processed in customized magnetic resonance imaging based molds. J Urol. 2011;186(5):1818–24.
10. Yerram NK, Volkin D, Turkbey B, Nix J, Hoang AN, Vourganti S, et al. Low suspicion lesions on multiparametric magnetic resonance imaging predict for the absence of high-risk prostate cancer. BJU Int. 2012;110(11 Pt B):E783–8.

11. Siddiqui MM, Rais-Bahrami S, Turkbey B, George AK, Rothwax J, Shakir N, et al. Comparison of MR/ultrasound fusion–guided biopsy with ultrasound-guided biopsy for the diagnosis of prostate cancer. JAMA. 2015;313(4):390.

12. Baco E, Ukimura O, Rud E, Vlatkovic L, Svindland A, Aron M, et al. Magnetic resonance imaging-transectal ultrasound image-fusion biopsies accurately characterize the index tumor: correlation with step-sectioned radical prostatectomy specimens in 135 patients. Eur Urol. 2014;17.

13. Turkbey B, Mani H, Aras O, Rastinehad AR, Shah V, Bernardo M, et al. Correlation of magnetic resonance imaging tumor volume with histopathology. J Urol. 2012;188(4):1157–63.

14. Cornud F, Khoury G, Bouazza N, Beuvon F, Peyromaure M, Flam T, et al. Tumor target volume for focal therapy of prostate cancer-does multiparametric magnetic resonance imaging allow for a reliable estimation? J Urol. 2014;191(5):1272–9.

15. Cooper SM, Dawber RP. The history of cryosurgery. J R Soc Med. 2001;94(4):196–201.

16. Copper IS. Cryogenic surgery: a new method of destruction or extirpation of benign or malignant tissues. N Engl J Med. 1963;268:743–9.

17. Finley DS, Pouliot F, Miller DC, Belldegrun AS. Primary and salvage cryotherapy for prostate cancer. Urol Clin North Am. 2010;37(1):67–82. Table of Contents.

18. Rees J, Patel B, MacDonagh R, Persad R. Cryosurgery for prostate cancer. BJU Int. 2004;93(6):710–4.

19. Tatli S, Acar M, Tuncali K, Morrison PR, Silverman S. Percutaneous cryoablation techniques and clinical applications. Diagn Interv Radiol. 2010;16(1):90–5.

20. Gangi A, Tsoumakidou G, Abdelli O, Buy X, de Mathelin M, Jacqmin D, et al. Percutaneous MR-guided cryoablation of prostate cancer: initial experience. Eur Radiol. 2012;22(8):1829–35.

21. Abdelaziz S, Esteveny L, Renaud P, Bayle B, Barbé L, De Mathelin M, et al. Design considerations for a novel MRI compatible manipulator for prostate cryoablation. Int J Comput Assist Radiol Surg. 2011;6(6):811–9.

22. Caviezel A, Terraz S, Schmidlin F, Becker C, Iselin CE. Percutaneous cryoablation of small kidney tumours under magnetic resonance imaging guidance: medium-term follow-up. Scand J Urol Nephrol. 2008;42(5):412–6.

23. Josan S, Bouley DM, van den Bosch M, Daniel BL, Butts PK. MRI-guided cryoablation: In vivo assessment of focal canine prostate cryolesions. J Magn Reson Imaging. 2009;30(1):169–76.

24. Van den Bosch MAAJ, Josan S, Bouley DM, Chen J, Gill H, Rieke V, et al. MR imaging-guided percutaneous cryoablation of the prostate in an animal model: in vivo imaging of cryoablation-induced tissue necrosis with immediate histopathologic correlation. J Vasc Interv Radiol. 2009;20(2):252–8.

25. Woodrum DA, Kawashima A, Karnes RJ, Davis BJ, Frank I, Engen DE, et al. Magnetic resonance imaging-guided cryoablation of recurrent prostate cancer after radical prostatectomy: initial single institution experience. Urology. 2013;82(4):870–5.

26. Babaian RJ, Donnelly B, Bahn D, Baust JG, Dineen M, Ellis D, et al. Best practice statement on cryosurgery for the treatment of localized prostate cancer. J Urol. 2008;180:1993–2004.

27. Lynn JG, Zwemer RL, Chick AJ. The biological application of focused ultrasonic waves. Science. 1942;96(2483):119–20.

28. Bradley WG. MR-guided focused ultrasound: a potentially disruptive technology. J Am Coll Radiol. 2009;6(7):510–3.

29. Hynynen K, Damianou C, Darkazanli A, Unger E, Schenck JF. The feasibility of using MRI to monitor and guide noninvasive ultrasound surgery. Ultrasound Med Biol. 1993;19(1):91–2.

30. Cline HE, Hynynen K, Watkins RD, Adams WJ, Schenck JF, Ettinger RH, et al. Focused US system for MR imaging-guided tumor ablation. Radiology. 1995;194(3):731–7.

31. Napoli A, Anzidei M, De Nunzio C, Cartocci G, Panebianco V, De Dominicis C, et al. Real-time magnetic resonance-guided high-intensity focused ultrasound focal therapy for localised prostate cancer: preliminary experience. Eur Urol. 2013;63(2):395–8.

32. Dickinson L, Ahmed HU, Kirkham AP, Allen C, Freeman A, Barber J, et al. A multi-centre prospective development study evaluating focal therapy using high intensity focused ultrasound for localised prostate cancer: the INDEX study. Contemp Clin Trials. 2013;36(1):68–80.

33. Dickinson L, Hu Y, Ahmed HU, Allen C, Kirkham AP, Emberton M, et al. Image-directed, tissue-preserving focal therapy of prostate cancer: a feasibility study of a novel deformable magnetic resonance-ultrasound (MR-US) registration system. BJU Int. 2013;112(5):594–601.

34. Partanen A, Yerram NK, Trivedi H, Dreher MR, Oila J, Hoang AN, et al. Magnetic resonance imaging (MRI)-guided transurethral ultrasound therapy of the prostate: a preclinical study with radiological and pathological correlation using customised MRI-based moulds. BJU Int. 2013;112(4):508–16.

35. Funaki K, Fukunishi H, Sawada K. Clinical outcomes of magnetic resonance-guided focused ultrasound surgery for uterine myomas: 24-month follow-up. Ultrasound Obstet Gynecol. 2009;34(5):584–9.

36. Furusawa H, Namba K, Thomsen S, Akiyama F, Bendet A, Tanaka C, et al. Magnetic resonance-guided focused ultrasound surgery of breast cancer: reliability and effectiveness. J Am Coll Surg. 2006;203(1):54–63.

37. Liberman B, Gianfelice D, Inbar Y, Beck A, Rabin T, Shabshin N, et al. Pain palliation in patients with bone metastases using MR-guided focused ultrasound surgery: a multicenter study. Ann Surg Oncol. 2009;16(1):140–6.

38. Kopelman D, Inbar Y, Hanannel A, Dank G, Freundlich D, Perel A, et al. Magnetic resonance-guided focused ultrasound surgery (MRgFUS). Four ablation treatments of a single canine hepatocellular adenoma. HPB (Oxford). 2006;8(4):292–8.

39. Jolesz FA. MRI-guided focused ultrasound surgery. Annu Rev Med. 2009;60:417–30.

40. Siddiqui K, Chopra R, Vedula S, Sugar L, Haider M, Boyes A, et al. MRI-guided transurethral ultrasound therapy of the prostate gland using real-time thermal mapping: initial studies. Urology. 2010;76(6):1506–11.

41. Chopra R, Burtnyk M, N'djin WA, Bronskill M. MRI-controlled transurethral ultrasound therapy for localised prostate cancer. Int J Hyperthermia. 2010;26(8):804–21.

42. Chopra R, Colquhoun A, Burtnyk M, N'djin WA, Kobelevskiy I, Boyes A, et al. MR imaging-controlled transurethral ultrasound therapy for conformal treatment of prostate tissue: initial feasibility in humans. Radiology. 2012;265(1):303–13.

43. Rouvière O, Souchon R, Salomir R, Gelet A, Chapelon J-Y, Lyonnet D. Transrectal high-intensity focused ultrasound ablation of prostate cancer: effective treatment requiring accurate imaging. Eur J Radiol. 2007;63(3):317–27.

44. Uchida T, Shoji S, Nakano M, Hongo S, Nitta M, Murota A, et al. Transrectal high-intensity focused ultrasound for the treatment of localized prostate cancer: eight-year experience. Int J Urol. 2009;16(11):881–6.

45. Deckers R, Rome C, Moonen CTW. The role of ultrasound and magnetic resonance in local drug delivery. J Magn Reson Imaging. 2008;27(2):400–9.

46. Rahmathulla G, Recinos PF, Kamian K, Mohammadi AM, Ahluwalia MS, Barnett GH. MRI-guided laser interstitial thermal therapy in neuro-oncology: a review of its current clinical applications. Oncology. 2014;87(2):67–82.

47. Sander S, Beisland HO. Laser in the treatment of localized prostatic carcinoma. J Urol. 1984;132(2):280–1.

48. Sander S, Beisland HO, Fossberg E. Neodymion YAG laser in the treatment of prostatic cancer. Urol Res. 1982;10(2):85–6.

49. Raz O, Haider MA, Davidson SRH, Lindner U, Hlasny E, Weersink R, et al. Real-time magnetic resonance imaging-guided focal laser therapy in patients with low-risk prostate cancer. Eur Urol. 2010;58(1):173–7.

50. Woodrum DA, Gorny KR, Mynderse LA, Amrami KK, Felmlee JP, Bjarnason H, et al. Feasibility of 3.0T magnetic resonance imaging-guided laser ablation of a cadaveric prostate. Urology. 2010;75(6):1514.e1–6.

51. Stafford RJ, Shetty A, Elliott AM, Klumpp SA, McNichols RJ, Gowda A, et al. Magnetic resonance guided, focal laser induced interstitial thermal therapy in a canine prostate model. J Urol. 2010;184(4):1514–20.

52. Peters RD, Chan E, Trachtenberg J, Jothy S, Kapusta L, Kucharczyk W, et al. Magnetic resonance thermometry for predicting thermal damage: an application of interstitial laser coagulation in an in vivo canine prostate model. Magn Reson Med. 2000;44(6):873–83.

53. Hoang AN, Volkin D, Yerram NK, Vourganti S, Nix J, Linehan WM, et al. Image guidance in the focal treatment of prostate cancer. Curr Opin Urol. 2012;22(4):328–35.
54. Oto A, Sethi I, Karczmar G, McNichols R, Ivancevic MK, Stadler WM, et al. MR imaging-guided focal laser ablation for prostate cancer: phase I trial. Radiology. 2013;267(3):932–40.
55. Cepek J, Chronik BA, Lindner U, Trachtenberg J, Davidson SRH, Bax J, et al. A system for MRI-guided transperineal delivery of needles to the prostate for focal therapy. Med Phys. 2013;40(1):012304.
56. Colin P, Nevoux P, Marqa M, Auger F, Leroy X, Villers A, et al. Focal laser interstitial thermo-therapy (LITT) at 980 nm for prostate cancer: treatment feasibility in Dunning R3327-AT2 rat prostate tumour. BJU Int. 2012;109(3):452–8.
57. Lindner U, Lawrentschuk N, Weersink RA, Davidson SRH, Raz O, Hlasny E, et al. Focal laser ablation for prostate cancer followed by radical prostatectomy: validation of focal therapy and imaging accuracy. Eur Urol. 2010;57(6):1111–4.
58. Viswanath S, Toth R, Rusu M, Sperling D, Lepor H, Futterer J, et al. Identifying quantitative in vivo multi-parametric MRI features for treatment related changes after laser interstitial thermal therapy of prostate cancer. Neurocomputing. 2014;144:13–23.
59. Wenger H, Yousuf A, Oto A, Eggener S. Laser ablation as focal therapy for prostate cancer. Curr Opin Urol. 2014;24(3):236–40.
60. Lee T, Mendhiratta N, Sperling D, Lepor H. Focal laser ablation for localized prostate cancer: principles, clinical trials, and our initial experience. Rev Urol. 2014;16(2):55–66.
61. Bozzini G, Colin P, Nevoux P, Villers A, Mordon S, Betrouni N. Focal therapy of prostate cancer: energies and procedures. Urol Oncol. 2013;31(2):155–67.
62. Betrouni N, Lopes R, Puech P, Colin P, Mordon S. A model to estimate the outcome of prostate cancer photodynamic therapy with TOOKAD soluble WST11. Phys Med Biol. 2011;56(15): 4771–83.
63. Da Rosa MR, Trachtenberg J, Chopra R, Haider MA. Early experience in MRI-guided therapies of prostate cancer: HIFU, laser and photodynamic treatment. Cancer Imaging. 2011;11 Spec No:S3–8.
64. Chen JC, Moriarty JA, Derbyshire JA, Peters RD, Trachtenberg J, Bell SD, et al. Prostate cancer: MR imaging and thermometry during microwave thermal ablation-initial experience. Radiology. 2000;214(1):290–7.
65. Terraz S, Cernicanu A, Lepetit-Coiffé M, Viallon M, Salomir R, Mentha G, et al. Radiofrequency ablation of small liver malignancies under magnetic resonance guidance: progress in targeting and preliminary observations with temperature monitoring. Eur Radiol. 2010;20(4):886–97.
66. Onik G, Vaughan D, Lotenfoe R, Dineen M, Brady J. The "male lumpectomy": focal therapy for prostate cancer using cryoablation results in 48 patients with at least 2-year follow-up. Urol Oncol. 2008;26(5):500–5.

Conclusions

Prior to the mid-1980s, prostate cancer was most commonly diagnosed when patients presented with systemic symptoms or if found by digital rectal exam with locally extensive disease. Within 10 years of the introduction of PSA testing, prostate cancer death rates had declined and local disease was more often confined to the gland. Today cancer death rates are down 40 % from their high, and most cancers are detected with no palpable disease present. The 5-year survival rate for locally detected disease approaches 100 %.

The dilemma today is who not to treat once prostate cancer is diagnosed. The authors of *The Prostate Cancer Dilemma: Selecting Patients for Active Surveillance, Focal Ablation and Definitive Therapy* have presented a detailed description of the newest technology and thinking regarding this problem. From pathology, new serum and genetic markers, diagnostic modalities such as elastography and mpMRI, to novel biopsy strategies utilizing a mapping and targeted MRI approach and lastly to no longer treating the entire gland but rather providing a focal approach, the authors have covered it all.

This project was conceived after the editors and authors Drs. Stone and Crawford taught a course on this subject matter at the 2014 American Urologic Association meeting. The need for a concise, state-of-the-art book became obvious. We wish to thank all of the coauthors for their valuable contributions. Each of them and their colleagues are the best and brightest in their areas of expertise, and it was no small endeavor for them to take the time out of their busy schedules to write their respective chapters.

We hope you have learned from and enjoyed reading the text. Whether you are a primary care physician, urologist, radiation oncologist, or other health care provider, we believe this book provided helpful and meaningful insight on how to best manage men diagnosed with early prostate cancer.

Sincerely,

The Editors

© Springer International Publishing Switzerland 2016
N.N. Stone, E.D. Crawford (eds.), *The Prostate Cancer Dilemma*,
DOI 10.1007/978-3-319-21485-6